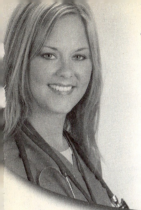

"The review modules are so helpful because they give bulleted highlights  To top it off, you These books a been the greatest review item I have found."

Kimberly Montgomery
Nursing student

Terim Richards *Nursing student*

"I immediately went to my nurse manager after I failed the NCLEX® and she referred me to ATI. I was able to discover the areas I was weak in, and focused on those areas in the review modules and online assessments. I was much more prepared the second time around!"

Molly Obetz *Nursing student*

"The ATI review books were very helpful in preparing me for the NCLEX®. I really utilized the review summaries and the critical thinking exercises at the end of each chapter. It was nice to review the key points in the areas I was weak in and not have to read the entire book."

Lindsey Koeble *Nursing student*

"I attribute my success totally to ATI. That is the one thing I used between my first and second attempt at the NCLEX®....with ATI I passed!"

Danielle Platt *Nurse Manager • Children's Mercy Hospital • Kansas City, MO*

"The year our hospital did not use the ATI program, we experienced a 15% decrease in the NCLEX® pass rates. We reinstated the ATI program the following year and had a 90% success rate."

"As a manager, I have witnessed graduate nurses fail the NCLEX® and the devastating effects it has on their morale. Once the nurses started using ATI, it was amazing to see the confidence they had in themselves and their ability to go forward and take the NCLEX® exam."

Mary Moss *Associate Dean of Nursing and Health Programs • Mid-State Technical College • Wisconsin Rapids, WI*

"I like that ATI lets students know what to expect from the NCLEX®, helps them plan their study time and tells them what to do in the days and weeks before the exam. It is different from most of the NCLEX® review books on the market."

Practical Nurse Nursing Care of Children Review Module Edition 6.1

Contributors

Penny Fauber-Moore, RN, MS
Director, School of Practical Nursing
Stonewall Jackson School of Practical Nursing
Lexington, Virginia

Catherine Miller, RN, BSN
Johnson County Pediatrics, PA
Shawnee Mission, Kansas

Diana Rupert, RN, MSN
Assistant Professor
Conemaugh School of Nursing
Johnstown, Pennsylvania

Teri Scott, RN, MSN
Associate Professor of Nursing
Johnson County Community College
Overland Park, KS
University of Missouri— Kansas City
Kansas City, Missouri

Lucille F. Whaley, RN, MS
Associate Professor of Nursing
San Jose State University
San Jose, California
Textbook Author

Michele Wolff, RN, MSN, CCRN
Associate Professor of Nursing
Saddleback College
Mission Viejo, California

Editor-in-Chief

Leslie Schaaf Treas, RN, PhD(c), MSN, CNNP
Director of Research and Development
Assessment Technologies Institute™, LLC
Overland Park, Kansas

Editor

Jim Hauschildt, RN, EdD, MA
Director of Product Development
Assessment Technologies Institute™, LLC
Overland Park, Kansas

All rights reserved. Printed in the United States of America. No part of this book shall be reproduced, stored in a retrieval system, or transmitted by any means, electronic, mechanical, photocopying, recording, or otherwise, without written permission from the publisher.

Sixth Edition Copyright© 2006 by Assessment Technologies Institute™, LLC. Previous editions copyrighted 1999-2005.

Copyright Notice

All rights reserved. Printed in the United States of America. No part of this book shall be reproduced, stored in a retrieval system, or transmitted by any means, electronic, mechanical, photocopying, recording, or otherwise, without written permission from the publisher. All of the content you see in this publication, including, for example, the cover, all of the page headers, images, illustrations, graphics, and text, are subject to trademark, service mark, trade dress, copyright and/or other intellectual property rights or licenses held by Assessment Technologies Institute™, LLC, one of its affiliates, or by third parties who have licensed their materials to Assessment Technologies Institute™, LLC. The entire content of this publication is copyrighted as a collective work under U.S. copyright laws, and Assessment Technologies Institute™, LLC owns a copyright in the selection, coordination, arrangement and enhancement of the content. Copyright © Assessment Technologies Institute™, LLC, 1999-2006.

Important Notice to the Reader of this Publication

Assessment Technologies Institute™, LLC is the publisher of this publication. The publisher reserves the right to modify, change, or update the content of this publication at any time. The content of this publication, such as text, graphics, images, information obtained from the publisher's licensors, and other material contained in this publication are for informational purposes only. The content is not providing medical advice, and is not intended to be a substitute for professional medical advice, diagnosis, or treatment. Always seek the advice of your primary care provider or other qualified health provider with any questions you may have regarding a medical condition. Never disregard professional medical advice or delay in seeking it because of something you have read in this publication. If you think you may have a medical emergency, call your primary care provider or 911 immediately.

The publisher does not recommend or endorse any specific tests, primary care providers, products, procedures, processes, opinions, or other information that may be mentioned in this publication. Reliance on any information provided by the publisher, the publisher's employees, or others contributing to the content at the invitation of the publisher, is solely at your own risk. Healthcare professionals need to use their own clinical judgment in interpreting the content of this publication, and details such as medications, dosages or laboratory tests and results should always be confirmed with other resources.[†]

This publication may contain health or medical-related materials that are sexually explicit. If you find these materials offensive, you may not want to use this publication.

The publishers, editors, advisors, and reviewers make no representations or warranties of any kind or nature, including, but not limited to, the accuracy, reliability, completeness, currentness, timeliness, or the warranties of fitness for a particular purpose or merchantability, nor are any such representations implied with respect to the content herein (with such content to include text and graphics), and the publishers, editors, advisors, and reviewers take no responsibility with respect to such content. The publishers, editors, advisors, and reviewers shall not be liable for any actual, incidental, special, consequential, punitive or exemplary damages (or any other type of damages) resulting, in whole or in part, from the reader's use of, or reliance upon, such content.

Introduction to Assessment–Driven Review

To prepare candidates for the licensure exam, many different methods have been used. Assessment Technologies Institute™, LLC, (ATI) offers Assessment–Driven Review™ (ADR), a newer approach for customized board review based on candidate performance on a series of content-based assessments.

The ADR method is a four-part process that serves as a type of competency-assessment for preparation for the NCLEX®. The goal is to increase preparedness and subsequent pass rate on the licensure exam. Used as a comprehensive program, the ADR is designed to help learners focus their review and remediation efforts, thereby increasing their confidence and familiarity with the NCLEX® content. This type of program identifies learners at risk for failure in the early stages of nursing education and provides a path for prescriptive learning prior to the licensure examination.

The ADR approach may be preferable to a traditional "crash course" style of review for a variety of reasons. Time restriction is a fundamental barrier to comprehensive review. Because of the difficulty in keeping up with the expansiveness of information available today, a more efficient and directed approach is needed. Individualized review that starts with the areas of deficit helps the learner narrow the focus and begin customized remediation instead of a blanket A-to-Z approach. Additionally, review that occurs sequentially over time may be preferable to after-the-fact efforts after completion of a program when faculty are no longer available to assist with remediation.

Early identification of content weaknesses may prove advantageous to progressive program success. "Smaller bites" for content achievement and a shortened lapse of time between the introduction of course content and remediation efforts is likely to be more effective in catching the struggling learner before it is too late. Regular feedback keeps learners "on track" and reduce attrition rate by identifying the learner who is "slipping." This approach provides the opportunity to tutor or implement intensified instruction before the learner reaches a point of no return and drops out of the program.

Step I: Proctored Assessment

The ADR program is a method using a prescriptive learning strategy that begins with a proctored, diagnostic assessment of the learner's mastery of nursing content. The topics covered within the ADR program are based on the current NCLEX® Test Plan. Proctored assessments are administered in paper-pencil and online formats. Scores are reported instantly with Internet testing or within 24 hours for paper-pencil testing.

Individual performance profiles list areas of deficiencies and guide the learner's review and remediation of the missed topics. This road map serves as a starting point for self-directed study for NCLEX® success. Learners receive a cumulative Report Card showing scores from all assessments taken throughout the program—beginning to end. Like reading a transcript, the learner and educator can monitor the sequential progress, step-by-step, an assessment at a time.

Step II: Modular Reviews

A good test is one that supports teaching and learning. The score report identifies areas of content mastery as well as a means for correction and improvement of weak content areas. Eight review modules contain concise summaries of topics with a clinical overview, therapeutic nursing management, and client teaching. Key concepts are provided to streamline the study process. The ATI modules are not intended to serve as a primary teaching source. Instead, they are designed to summarize the material relevant to the licensure exam and entry-level practice.

Learners are taught to integrate holistic care with a critical thinking approach into the review material to promote clinical application of course content. The learner constructs responses to open-ended questions to stimulate higher-order thinking. The learner may provide rationales for actions in various clinical scenarios and generate explanations of why the solution may be effective in similar clinical situations. These exercises serve as the venue to shift from traditional didactic memorization of facts toward the use of analytical and evaluative reason in a client-related situation. The clinical application scenarios involve the learner actively in the problem-solving process and stimulate an attitude of inquiry.

These exercises are designed to provoke creative problem solving for the individual learner as well as collaborative dialogue for groups of learners in the classroom. Through group discussion, learners discover the technique of elaboration. Learners use group dialogue to increase their understanding of nursing content. In study groups, they may pose questions to their peers or explain various topics in their own words, adding personal experiences with clients and examples from previously acquired knowledge of the topic. Together they learn to reframe problems and assemble evidence to support conclusions. Through the integration of multiple perspectives and the synergy involved in the exchange of ideas, this approach may also facilitate the development of effective working relationships and patterns for lifelong learning. Critical thinking exercises for each topic area situate instruction into a problem-solving environment that can capture learners' attention, increase motivation to learn, and frame the content into an application context. Additionally, the group involvement can model the process for effective team interaction.

Step III: Non-Proctored Assessments

The third step is the use of online assessments that allow users to test from any site with an Internet connection. This online battery identifies specific areas of content weakness for further directed study. The interactive style provides the learner with immediate feedback on all response options. Rationales provide additional information about the correctness of an answer to supplement learners' understanding of the concept. Detailed explanations are provided for each incorrect response to clarify topics that learners often confuse, misunderstand, or fail to remember. Readiness to learn is often peaked when errors are uncovered; thus, immediate feedback is provided when learners are most motivated to find the answer. A Performance Profile summarizes learners' mastery of content. Question descriptors for each missed item are used to stimulate inquiry and further exploration of the topic. The online assessment is intended to extend the learners' preparation for NCLEX® in a way that is personally suited to their deficiencies.

Step IV: ATI-PLAN™ DVD Series

This 12-disk set contains more than 28 hours of nursing review material. The DVD content is designed to complement ATI's Content Mastery Series™ review modules and online assessments. Using the ATI-PLAN™ navigational points, learners can easily find the content areas they want to review.

Recognizing that individuals process information in a variety of ways, ATI developed the ATI-PLAN™ DVD series to offer nursing review in a way that simulates the classroom. However, individuals viewing the ATI-PLAN™ DVDs can navigate through more than 28 hours of material to their topics of choice. Nursing review is available at the convenience of the learner and can be replayed as often as necessary to ensure mastery of content.

The regulation of personal learning goals and the ability to plan and pursue academic intentions are the keys to successful learning. The expert teacher is the one who can determine individual learning needs and appropriate strategies to master learning. The ADR program is an efficient method of helping students prepare for the nursing licensure exam using frequent and systematic content review directed by the identified areas of content weakness. The interactive approach for mastery of nursing content focused in the areas of greatest need is likely to increase student success on the licensure exam.

ATI's ADR method parallels the nursing process in concept and in design. Both provide a framework for solving actual and potential problems purposefully and methodically. Assessment ADR-style is accomplished with ATI's battery of proctored assessments. Diagnosis is facilitated by the individual and group score reports the proctored assessments generate. Planning for improving performance in identified areas of weakness incorporates ATI's modular review system. Implementation begins with modular review and culminates in use of ATI's online assessments to validate improvement. Evaluation is reflected in the score reports, and performance can then be strengthened or further improved with the ATI-PLAN™ DVD series. Just like the nursing process, ATI's ADR prescriptive learning method often leads to specific, measurable results and highly desirable outcomes.

Table of Contents

1 Basic Concepts 1
    Vital Signs 1
    Pain 6
    Hospitalization and Illness 10
    Death and Dying 15
    Nutrition 21
    Medications 28
    Growth and Development 33

2 Respiratory System 50
    Oxygen Therapy 50
    Cystic Fibrosis 55
    Asthma 60
    Tonsillitis and Tonsillectomy 66
    Common Respiratory Illnesses 70

3 Cardiovascular System/Blood Disorders 80
    Congenital Heart Disease 80
    Hodgkin's Disease 87
    Leukemia 92
    Iron Deficiency Anemia 99
    Hemophilia 104
    Sickle Cell Disease 108
    Blood Transfusion 113

4 Neurosensory System 117
    Seizures 117
    Bacterial Meningitis 122
    Reye's Syndrome 126
    Head Injury 130
    Brain Tumor 135
    Cerebral Palsy 140
    Strabismus 146

5 Endocrine System 150
    Type I Insulin-Dependent Diabetes Mellitus 150
    Diabetic Ketoacidosis 159

6 Musculoskeletal System 163
Clubfoot (Talipes Equinovarus) 163
Fractures 167
Traction 173
Scoliosis 177
Juvenile Rheumatoid Arthritis 182
Muscular Dystrophies 187

7 Integumentary System 192
Burns 192
Eczema 198
Impetigo 202
Diaper Rash 205
Head Lice (Pediculosis Capitis) 208
Dermatophytosis (Ringworm) 212

8 Lymphatic/Infectious/Immune System 216
Immunizations 216
Oral Candidiasis (Thrush) 222
Human Immunodeficiency Virus (HIV) and
   Acquired Immunodeficiency Syndrome (AIDS) 225
Otitis Media 231
Varicella-Zoster Infection (Chickenpox and Shingles) 236
Rubeola (Measles) 241
Rubella (German Measles) 245
Epstein-Barr Viral Infection (Mononucleosis) 249
Rheumatic Fever 253

9 Gastrointestinal/Hepatic System 258
Gastroenteritis/Diarrhea 258
Cleft Lip and Palate 263
Pinworm Infection (Enterobiasis) 268

10 Genitourinary/Reproductive System 271
Hypospadias 271
Wilms' Tumor (Nephroblastoma) 274
Nephrotic Syndrome 278
Acute Glomerulonephritis 283
Urinary Tract Infections 289
Sexually Transmitted Disease 293

11 Special Pediatric Emergencies 297
- Sudden Infant Death Syndrome 297
- Abused Child 300
- Lead Poisoning (Plumbism) 306
- Acetaminophen Poisoning 311
- Substance Abuse 314
- Child in a Suicidal Crisis 318

12 Developmental or Psychosocial Disorders 323
- Down Syndrome 323
- Autism 327
- Attention Deficit Hyperactivity Disorder 332
- Failure to Thrive 336
- Anorexia Nervosa 342
- Adolescent Pregnancy 347

Critical Thinking Exercise Answer Keys 352

References 478

Basic Concepts CHAPTER 1

Nursing Management of the Child's Vital Signs

Key Points

- Normal vital signs for children will vary according to age and condition.
- Infants normally have the highest heart and respiratory rates and the lowest blood pressure.
- Tachycardia is a common response to acute illness or stress in infants and children.
- Bradycardia in infants and children is most frequently related to poor airway control.
- Hypotension is a late sign of shock or inadequate circulation in infants and children.
- Goals of collaborative management:
  - Identify normal and abnormal vital signs based the child's age and baseline.
  - Accurately measure, record, and interpret vital signs.
  - Identify cause of changes in baseline vital signs.
  - Respond appropriately to conditions resulting in vital sign changes.
  - Monitor vital signs on a routine basis and as needed according to the child's condition and care needs.
- Important nursing diagnoses (actual and potential) are:
  - Altered body temperature
  - Decreased cardiac output
  - Altered tissue perfusion
  - Activity intolerance
  - Fluid volume, deficit, and excess
  - Risk for injury
  - Knowledge deficit
  - Anxiety and fear
- **Key Terms/Concepts**: Tachycardia, bradycardia, hypertension, hypotension, apnea, hypoventilation, hyperventilation, hyperthermia, hypothermia and neutral thermal environment

Overview

The measurement of vital signs includes: heart rate, respiratory rate, blood pressure, and body temperature. This data provides a baseline regarding the child's clinical condition. Listed below are average ranges for vital sign parameters in children. A variety of factors may influence the accuracy of the measurements and variation from expected normal ranges. The most common factors are age, size, emotional state, physical condition, equipment, movement, and underlying disorders.

Nursing Management of the Child's Vital Signs

Heart Rate

Although the heart rate may be counted at any of the peripheral pulse points, an apical pulse is recommended for infants and small children. A child's heart rate should be counted for one full minute. Irregularities in rhythm and/or rate should be documented. Significant tachycardia is usually an indication of a potentially serious underlying condition.

Heart rates lower than expected require immediate attention and intervention. Significant bradycardia is a medical emergency that may require cardiopulmonary resuscitation (CPR).

Average Resting Heart Rate	
Age	Beats/minute
Birth - 1 month	90-160
1 month - 1 year	80-150
1-3 years	80-130
3-6 years	75-120
6-11 years	70-115
11-13 years	70-110
13-18 years	65-105

Respiration

The respiratory rate should be counted for one full minute while observing the movement of the abdominal wall. Assessment of respiration includes monitoring for signs of respiratory distress such as grunting, nasal flaring, retractions, stridor, tachypnea, or cyanosis. It is important to promptly report any abnormalities in respiratory rate or work of breathing to the health care provider. Significant changes in respiratory rate and/or effort can lead to respiratory failure, a medical emergency.

Average Resting Respiratory Rate	
Age	Breaths/minute
Birth - 1 month	30-60
1 month - 1 year	27-40
1-3 years	25-35
3-6 years	20-30
6-11 years	18-24
11-18 years	16-24

Blood Pressure

The most common sites for blood pressure measurement in children are the upper arm and lower leg. It is important to obtain blood pressure readings using the same extremity as baseline in order to determine the trend. A variety of factors may affect the blood pressure measurement in children: time of the day, age, gender, exercise, pain, medications, emotional state, movement, physical condition, and/or equipment (improper cuff size). The width of the cuff bladder should occupy 3/4 of the upper arm segment or length sufficient to completely encircle arm/leg without overlap. Blood pressure readings outside the normal range need to be promptly reported to the health care provider and addressed as soon as possible. Significant hypotension in infants and children requires immediate intervention to prevent cardiopulmonary collapse.

Average Resting Blood Pressure		
Age	Systolic (mmHg)	Diastolic (mmHg)
Birth - 1 month	50-101	42-64
1 month - 1 year	69-105	39-69
1-3 years	76-107	41-69
3-6 years	78-111	42-70
6-11 years	81-119	44-77
11-18 years	90-136	51-84

Quick Systolic Blood Pressure Calculation *		
Classification	Formula	Example: 2 years old
Low blood pressure threshold	70 + 2x age in years	70 + (2 x 2) = 74 mmHg
Average blood pressure	90 + 2x age in years	90 + (2 x 2) = 94 mmHg

* For children over 1 year

Temperature

Temperature is measured in children to determine the presence of hyper- or hypothermia. Cold stress in newborns can lead to metabolic acidosis or respiratory distress and result in general systems deterioration. Hyperthermia increases a child's metabolic rate and can lead to febrile seizures. The nurse's responsibility is to detect abnormal temperature readings, report the findings to the appropriate care provider, and implement care to normalize the temperature for the child's comfort and well-being.

Oral: Children who are able to hold an oral thermometer in the sublingual cavity (typically: age 4) can have the body temperature measured orally. Mercury thermometers are generally avoided for use in the hospital due to the risk of mercury exposure to the health care worker or the child if the glass thermometer breaks. Oral temperature should never be taken on a child who has had oral surgery or who has seizures.

Axillary: An accurate axillary temperature reading is obtained by placing the thermometer in the axilla with direct skin contact for three minutes. Axillary temperature is the preferred route for newborns.

Rectal: Avoid taking a rectal temperature in newborns. This route is contraindicated for children with cancer and bleeding disorders due to the risk of trauma to the rectal mucosa. To obtain a rectal temperature reading, place the child in a comfortable position, either on the side with knees flexed or on the stomach; insert the lubricated thermometer a maximum of 1/2 inch (for infant) to 1 inch (for older children) into rectum for three minutes.

Tympanic: A tympanic temperature is obtained primarily because of the convenience, ease, and rapid measurement. The accuracy of the tympanic temperature measurement can be affected by the ability to achieve a proper seal and correct placement. The tympanic reading is considered a "core" temperature (similar to the rectal route).

Average Temperature Ranges	
Route	Temperature in degrees Fahrenheit
Axillary	96.6-98.0° Fahrenheit
Oral	97.6-98.6° Fahrenheit
Rectal or tympanic	98.6-100.0° Fahrenheit

Critical Thinking Exercise: Nursing Management of the Child's Vital Signs

Based on the following information received during report, identify which of the vital signs for each child are abnormal (increased, decreased) or normal. This should be based on the normal vital signs for the child's age and the child's illness.

1. 4-year-old with asthma. The vital signs are: HR 128-135, RR 30-35, BP 93/48, and axillary temperature 98° Fahrenheit (F).

2. 7-year-old with gastroesophageal reflux who is bundled with 2 thick blankets. The vital signs are: HR 100-110, RR 20-30, BP 96/54, axillary temperature 99.8° F.

3. 8-month-old with pneumonia. The vital signs are: HR 160-180 dropping to 60's occasionally during the previous shift, RR 76, BP 112/72, axillary temperature 99.5° F.

4. 2-month-old with fever and otitis media. The vital signs are: HR 165-175, RR 32-40, BP 108/64, rectal temperature 102.5° F. (Taken immediately prior to report, no intervention initiated.)

Basic Concepts CHAPTER 2

Nursing Management of the Child with Pain

Key Points

- Identifying and addressing pain in infants and children is an important part of nursing care.
- Pain assessment and management in infants and children should be individualized based on physical assessment, developmental level, behavior, pain scale reporting, and coping style.
- Goals of collaborative management:
  - Prevent pain (round-the-clock medication after major surgery and/or injury).
  - Recognize signs of pain in children of various ages.
  - Provide pharmacologic and nonpharmacologic pain management techniques.
  - Prevent analgesic-related complications (respiratory depression, hypotension).
  - Assist child in dealing with pain.
- Important nursing diagnoses (actual and potential) are:
  - Pain management
  - Ineffective individual coping
  - Powerlessness and hopelessness
  - Sleep pattern disturbance
  - Risk for injury
- **Key Terms/Concepts:** Acute pain, chronic pain, pediatric pain rating scales, PCA, EMLA

Overview

Pain assessment and management in infants and children is an important subject. Some health care providers erroneously believe that due to immaturity of the neurologic system, a young child has diminished pain reception. Additionally, some believe that the lack of memory for early pain experiences negates the importance of the painful stimuli. In recent years, research data has increasingly demonstrated the need for nurses to assess pain responses in children of all ages. Pain assessment in children is based on age-related pain scale ratings, emotional and physical signs, and behavioral cues. Nurses need to use nonpharmacologic pain management techniques and administer the appropriate dosage of analgesia that will promote comfort and rest. The nursing assessment of pain in children should include information regarding past pain experiences and ways of coping with pain.

The type and duration of pain affects the child's ability to cope. The child's ethnicity and family coping style influences the expression of pain. The

> developmental stage of the child greatly impacts the response to painful stimuli. Infants respond to pain by grimacing, tensing the body, and crying. Toddlers and preschoolers will protect their sore area and are usually able to point to where it hurts. School-age and adolescent children may be more stoic about pain due to peer pressure and fear of ridicule.

Pain Assessment

FACES Pain Scale(s): In assessing a child's pain, it is important to use a tool or scale appropriate to the developmental age and cognitive level of the child. Several scales that are drawings (cartoons) or actual photos of children displaying degrees of sadness or distress can be used for the child to relate to and communicate about the amount of pain he/she is experiencing. These scales are referred to as FACES Scale(s) and are most effective with younger children. This scale is also effective when there is a language barrier and with developmentally delayed children of all ages.

In older children the numbered rating scale of pain may be effective. As with adults, the children are asked to rate their pain on a scale (1-10 for instance) with 1 being no pain and 10 being the worst pain the child has ever experienced.

Once a child has expressed his/her pain, interventions must be made to interrupt the pain. The use of both pharmacological and non-pharmacological interventions may be appropriate. The pain rating should be documented, followed by the interventions, and then a reassessment of the pain should be recorded. A reassessment of the pain is essential to evaluate the effectiveness of the interventions.

Therapeutic Nursing Management

Pharmacologic

- Using pharmacologic methods to control pain requires attention to the six "rights": right drug, right dose, right route, right time, right child, and right to refuse.
- Nurses need to have an understanding of the essential principles (action, dosage, administration guidelines, side effects, and interactions) of medication for the child's safety and comfort.
- When administering analgesic agents, an accurate weight in order to determine an appropriate dosage is key to safety. The nurse should assess closely for side effects of the medication, particularly when intravenous narcotics are administered.
- Administer pain medication before the pain becomes intense.
- Non-opioids and nonsteroidal anti-inflammatory drugs are suitable for mild-to-moderate pain; opioids are needed for moderate-to-severe pain. A combination of the two types of analgesia can lessen pain on two levels. The non-opioids reverse pain at the peripheral nervous center; the opioids act on the central nervous system.
- Recent data has supported the use of child-controlled analgesia (PCA) as a safe and effective way to manage pain in older children and adolescents.
- Topical pain blocking medications (EMLA) can be used prior to planned procedures.

Nonpharmacologic

- Include parent involvement.
- Use medical play to help child deal with his or her fears.
- Provide distraction (favorite game or video, drawing pictures, telling stories).
- Help the child learn to use relaxation and guided imagery techniques.
- Apply heat or cold to the site.
- Use positive approach to pain control.
- Straighten sheets and place child in a position of comfort.
- Ask child about what would help make him or her feel better (favorite toy, pillow, TV show).

Most specific nonpharmacologic strategies require a child's understanding and cooperation. A child in severe pain may not be able to concentrate or expend the effort necessary to use a pain reduction technique. Those with very mild symptoms may not be motivated to methods that require the effort. Therefore, the nonpharmacologic techniques may be most effective in the management of moderate pain.

Critical Thinking Exercise: Nursing Management of the Child with Pain

Describe the "Reality" and why the "Myth" is false in each of the following statements:

"Myth"	"Reality"
Infants don't feel pain because they have immature neurologic systems.	
A child who is sleeping or lying quietly is not in pain.	
Nurses and doctors are the best people to judge how much pain a child is feeling.	
Children lack the ability to talk about their pain.	
Infants and young children shouldn't be given narcotics because of the side effects.	
Children who receive narcotics for pain are at risk for addiction.	

Basic Concepts **CHAPTER 3**

Nursing Management of a Child's Hospitalization and Illness

Key Points

- Illness and hospitalization have an effect on the child and every member of the family.
- The experience of illness and hospitalization can have a lasting emotional impact on a child.
- It is important to address the child's individual needs based on his/her previous experiences, knowledge base, and developmental level.
- Explanation of the various aspects of hospitalization in an honest and age-appropriate manner helps allay the child's fear of the unknown.
- Goals of collaborative management:
  - Recognize the child's unique responses to illness and hospitalization based on developmental level, past experiences, and coping style.
  - Assist the child in coping with hospitalization and illness through age-appropriate and child-specific interventions.
  - Provide a family-centered approach to care by promoting family roles, providing information and fostering family support of the child.
- Important nursing diagnoses (actual and potential) are:
  - Altered comfort
  - Sleep pattern disturbance
  - Anxiety and fear
  - Ineffective individual coping
  - Ineffective family coping
  - Altered family processes
  - Altered role performance
  - Knowledge deficit
- **Key Terms/Concepts:** Family-centered care, age-related fears, protest, withdrawal, and despair

Overview

A child's coping with hospitalization depends on a variety of interrelated factors: the illness, child's age, preparation for the experience, previous illnesses, support of the family and health professionals, cultural background, and the child's emotional status. Infants and toddlers often have more difficulty coping with hospitalization due to the developmental task of separation anxiety.

Toddlers commonly fear injury and pain. The inability of children to communicate vague symptoms (such as headache, nausea) can make caring for the hospitalized child of this age more challenging. The preschool-age child often experiences some degree of separation anxiety, impacting the child's ability to cope with hospitalization. Children in this age group fear bodily injury. The cognitive operations for preschoolers are concrete; thereby, explanations for care are most effective when short, simple and clear. Hospitalization for the school-age child and adolescent usually represents separation from peers and some degree of social isolation. The child may feel a loss of control with regard to the illness itself and necessary interventions while hospitalized. To promote feelings of self-determination, allow choices when appropriate.

Risk Factors

- Previous hospitalization and/or illness
- Prolonged hospitalization and/or illness
- Competing demands for family members' time and attention (work, siblings, etc.)
- Situational stressors (lack of transportation, financial challenges, etc.)

Assessment and Intervention Strategies for Hospitalized and Ill Children			
Age	Stressors	Behaviors	Interventions
Infant	• Interrupted routine • Parental separation • Lack of stimulation • Delayed response to cry/needs	• Poor feeding • Irritability • Crying • Altered sleep patterns	• Encourage parents to participate in care of their baby. • Deliver consistent nursing care. • Promote home routines. • Provide stimulation (mobile, music, play, rocking). • Respond promptly to cry and other needs. • Arrange for volunteers to hold, rock, and play with infant. • Encourage family to comfort and soothe child. • Encourage family to stay at bedside when possible. • Promote home routines (favorite toy, blanket, books etc.). • Reassure parents that regression is temporary. • Provide age-appropriate toys and activities.

Assessment and Intervention Strategies for Hospitalized and Ill Children

Age	Stressors	Behaviors	Interventions
Toddler	• Interrupted routine and rituals • Separation from parents • Loss of control • Fear of being hurt	• Protest Stage: crying, fighting, clinging to parent, tantrums • Despair Stage: quiet, passive, inactive • Detachment Stage: indifferent to parent, superficial relationship with others, appears happy • Developmental regression (bottle, incontinence, speech) • Refusal to eat • Sleep pattern disturbance	• Encourage family to comfort and soothe child. • Encourage family to stay at bedside when possible. • Promote home routines (favorite toy, blanket, books etc.). • Reassure parents that regression is temporary. • Provide age-appropriate toys and activities.
Preschool Age Child	• Pain/bodily injury • Separation from parents • Loss of control	• Passiveness, withdrawal • Poor appetite • Sleep disturbances, nightmares • Magical thinking, fantasy • Bed wetting • Aggression	• Encourage expression through play (medical play, coloring, dolls). • Cover catheters and wounds. • Have family bring in photos and objects from home. • Use the treatment room for painful procedures. • Encourage parents to stay with the child. • Explain procedures in concrete terms.
School Age Child	• Guilty feelings • Fear of pain • Loss of control • Body image changes • Missing school and friends • Falling behind in school	• Guilty feelings, self blame • Decreased self-esteem • Anxiety • Fearfulness, stalling, bargaining • Stoicism • Boredom • Withdrawal • Sleep pattern disturbance • Acting out, anger • Crying	• Be honest about what the child should expect. • Encourage expression through play (drawing, clay, and storytelling). • Arrange for making up missed schoolwork. • Encourage cards from classmates. • Provide diversional activities. • Provide choices. • Praise accomplishments. • Give comfort after traumatic procedures. • Give permission to cry and express pain.

Nursing Management of a Child's Hospitalization and Illness

Assessment and Intervention Strategies for Hospitalized and Ill Children			
Age	**Stressors**	**Behaviors**	**Interventions**
Adolescent	<ul><li>Loss of control</li><li>Body image changes</li><li>Self concept disturbances</li><li>Social isolation (separation from peers)</li><li>Personal identity issues (being different than peers)</li><li>Falling behind in school</li></ul>	<ul><li>Anger, aggression, being demanding</li><li>Frustration</li><li>Depression, withdrawal</li><li>Altered/disturbed body image</li><li>Social isolation</li></ul>	<ul><li>Provide consistent nurses who can develop a rapport.</li><li>Promote privacy.</li><li>Encourage creative self-expression (decorate walls with art /cards, wear own clothes, fashionable blanket etc.).</li><li>Provide a phone at bedside.</li><li>Allow friends to visit and bring favorite foods (pizza party, etc.).</li><li>Encourage expression through journaling, talking, etc.</li><li>Arrangements for missed schoolwork</li></ul>

Critical Thinking Exercise: Nursing Management of a Child's Hospitalization and Illness

Identify interventions and rationales for each of the following children.

Child	Interventions	Rationale For Intervention
A 7-month-old female with a congenital heart defect is hospitalized for congestive heart failure. She has been irritable and difficult to console.		
A 14-month-old male who is hospitalized with acute gastroenteritis and dehydration has not slept more than one hour without awakening.		
A 4-year-old hospitalized male with acute appendicitis repeatedly wakes up crying after having nightmares.		
An 8-year-old hospitalized female with asthma has eaten very little from her meal trays in the last few days.		
A 15-year-old female with leukemia expresses a desire to be left alone in a darkened room.		

Nursing Management of Death and Dying Involving a Child

> **Key Points**
>
> - The loss of a child is one of the most difficult things that a family will ever experience.
> - Each child and family will deal with death and dying according to their unique needs.
> - Goals of collaborative management:
>   - Recognize unique responses to death based on developmental level, past experiences and coping style.
>   - Assist the child and family to cope with death and dying issues.
>   - Help families understand the grieving process.
> - Important nursing diagnoses (actual and potential) are:
>   - Grieving, anticipatory grieving
>   - Powerlessness and hopelessness
>   - Anxiety and fear
>   - Ineffective individual coping, ineffective family coping
>   - Altered family processes
>   - Decisional conflict
>   - Altered role performance
>   - Social isolation
>   - Spiritual distress
>   - Knowledge deficit
>   - Fatigue and sleep pattern disturbance
>   - Altered comfort
> - **Key Terms/Concepts:** Grief stages, end-of-life care and decisions, "Do Not Resuscitate" (DNR)

Overview

The death of a child is one of the most painful and unforgettable experiences in a lifetime for a family. When death is anticipated, the family is afforded the opportunity to plan the last days prior to death, the funeral, and the degree of resuscitation efforts to be made. It is the nurse's responsibility to provide care to the dying child and family and provide information to the family that will assist them in making an informed decision regarding future resuscitation efforts. If a decision is made not to resuscitate, it is mandatory to clearly communicate this information to all health care team members.

A primary care provider's order needs to be written in the child's medical record regarding the exact nature of the treatments that are to be withheld. With

> sudden, unexpected death, the child and family do not begin the anticipatory grieving process. Families may spend a lengthy period of time progressing through the stages of acceptance for death due to shock and denial.
>
> The child's concept of death will vary with developmental age, nature of the illness, degree of pain, level of consciousness, and prior experience with the death of others. Fear is a natural response, although children express their fear and cope with it in vastly different ways. Many children assume they will die at night during sleep. Therefore, anxiety is likely to be higher at night. The nurse, while caring for the dying child, has an opportunity to explore the child's feelings and help him/her cope with dying in the best way possible.

Age-Related Perceptions of Death	
Infant-toddler	• No understanding of death • Fear and anxiety over separation
Preschool-age	• Something that happens to others • Not permanent • Curious about death and people, animals and plants that have died • Magical thinking; feel that "bad thoughts" might come true • Death is reversible
Young school-age	• Death is final • Believe they may die but only in distant future • May understand that it is universal and suspect parents will die someday • Fear pain associated with death
Preadolescent/Adolescent	• Able to understand death in logical manner • Understand that death is universal and permanent • Fear of disfigurement and isolation from peers • Healthy adolescents often believe that death "will not happen to me" • Invincibility beliefs are linked with high-risk behaviors (dangerous stunts, reckless driving, etc.)

Kubler-Ross' Stages of Death and Dying

Many authors have described stages of grieving. However, there is no single correct way for a person to progress through the grief process, nor a correct length of time in which to do it. Kubler-Ross (1969) has described the stages of dying, which are similar to the stages of grief:

Denial and isolation: Client refuses to believe that he/she will die, isolates self from reality, and represses what is discussed. The person may think, "They must have mixed my records up with someone else's," and may be artificially cheerful in order to prolong the denial.

Anger: Client or family expresses rage and hostility, sometimes at nurse and staff members, about things that normally would not upset them. The person may think, "Why me? I didn't do anything to deserve this."

Bargaining: Client seeks to bargain for more time: "If I can just live until my daughter's wedding, I'll be satisfied." Client may begin putting affairs in order (e.g., making a will and giving away personal items). Guilt for real or imagined past sins may be expressed. Bargaining helps the client to move into the final stages of dying.

Depression: Client accepts that death is a reality and goes through a period of grief. The client may cry and talk freely about the loss, or may withdraw: "I wanted so badly to see my grandchild, but I won't even be here when he is born."

Acceptance: Client comes to terms with dying. He or she has accepted death and is prepared to die. Client may have decreased interest in surroundings and significant others: "Everything is taken care of and I'm tired of fighting it. I'm ready to go."

Characteristics of Normal Grief Reactions	
Physical symptoms	• Feelings of tightness in the throat • Choking • Empty feeling in abdomen • Lack of muscular strength • Subjective distress such as mental pain or distress
Preoccupation with image of the deceased	• Hears, sees, or imagines the deceased person • Feeling of emotional distance from others • Feeling of loss of emotional control
Feelings of guilt	• Searches for ways death could have been prevented • Accuses self or others of negligence or fault
Loss of usual behavior	• Restlessness, inability to sit still, aimless movement • Lack of capacity to initiate usual interests or activities

Therapeutic Nursing Management

- Focus care on pain relief and comfort measures for the child.
- Balance the need to allow time for uninterrupted rest and privacy with the need to do routine nursing assessments and procedures. Focus on the priority needs of the child and family.
- Provide an environment that is calm with minimal external stressors.
- Sit quietly with child and family (therapeutic silence).
- Avoid insensitive phrases such as "I know how you feel," or "You can have another baby."
- Ask open-ended questions to stimulate discussion.
- Supply relevant information based on the child's and family's questions.
- Present accurate information regarding the child's condition. Do not give false hope.
- Involve the family in planning and delivery of care.
- Encourage the family to use formal and informal sources of support to help them with decision-making and coping with the death.
- Provide as normal environment as possible. Encourage play and other activities as tolerated.
- Talk to the child to provide stimulation and to encourage verbalization of feelings.
- Identify the stages of dying that the child is experiencing and preserve his/her

- defenses.
- Spend more time with the child at night.
- Support child's family in dealing with the daily decisions associated with the physical and emotional care of the child.
- Allow the child to do as much self-care as possible.
- Every nurse should be certified in Basic Life Support (BLS). The American Heart Association (AHA) makes guidelines for CPR and classes are generally offered at all hospitals, through community classes, and directly from AHA. Below are the **very basic steps** in CPR for adults (9 years and older), children (1-8 years), and infant (newborn to 1 year).
    - **Adult (9 years and older)**
        - Determine unresponsiveness by asking, "Are you okay?"
        - Dial 911.
        - Open the airway.
        - Assess for respirations for 5 seconds – look, listen, and feel.
        - Give 2 initial breaths by pinching the nose and making a seal over the mouth.
        - Check the carotid pulse for 10 seconds, as you are doing this you should be continuing to look for respirations.
        - Start CPR if there is no pulse.
        - Compressions are 2-handed with the hand over the lower half of the sternum, 1.5 to 2 inches deep at about 100 a minute.
        - The ratio is 15 compressions to 2 breaths.
        - Reassess the carotid pulse and respirations for 5 seconds after 1 minute of CPR, generally that is 4 cycles.
        - Continue if there is no pulse.
    - **Child (1-8 years)**
        - Determine unresponsiveness by asking, "Are you okay?"
        - Shout for help.
        - Open the airway.
        - Assess respirations for 5 seconds – look, listen, and feel.
        - Give 2 initial breaths by pinching the nose and making a seal over the mouth.
        - Check the carotid pulse for 10 seconds. As you are doing this continue to assess respirations.
        - DO NOT DEFIBRILLATE – Begin CPR.
        - Compressions are with the heel of one hand over the lower half of the sternum, 1 to 1.5 inches deep at 100 plus a minute.
        - The ratio is 5 compressions to 1 breath.
        - Reassess the pulse and respirations for 3 seconds after 1 minute, generally that will be 20 cycles.
        - Dial 911 and continue CPR if there is no pulse.
    - **Infant (Newborn-1 year)**
        - Determine unresponsiveness by asking, "Are you okay?"

- Call for help.
- Open the airway.
- Assess for respirations for 5 seconds – look, listen, and feel.
- Give 2 initial breaths by making a seal over the mouth and nose.
- Check the brachial pulse for 10 seconds; continue to assess respirations during this time.
- DO NOT DEFIBRILLATE.
- Begin CPR.
- Compressions are with 2 fingers over the middle of the chest at the nipple line and are to 1 inch deep at least 100 per minute.
- The ratio is 5 compressions to 1 breath.
- Reassess the pulse and respirations after 1 minute of CPR for 3 seconds, this is generally 20 cycles.
- Dial 911 and continue CPR if there is no pulse.

Critical Thinking Exercise: Nursing Management of Death and Dying Involving a Child

Situation: The parents of a 15-year-old boy who has died suddenly from an injury sustained in a motor vehicle accident asks the nurse how to best explain what happened to his 6-year-old brother. The father told the nurse that his 6-year-old son believes that he caused his brother's death because they had a fight that morning.

1. What is the best way to explain the death to the 6-year-old?

2. What grief reactions should the nurse anticipate when caring for this family? What interventions are most appropriate when caring for a family after the death of their child?

Situation: The parents of a 3-year-old with cancer have just been informed that their child's condition is terminal due to extensive metastasis.

3. The parents ask the nurse what a child of this age understands about death. What is the nurse's best response?

4. What are the appropriate interventions for this child?

Basic Concepts **CHAPTER 5**

Nursing Management of the Child's Nutrition

> **Key Points**
>
> - Adequate nutrition is essential to normal growth and development in children.
> - Nutritional needs and self-feeding ability is based on developmental level.
> - The goals of collaborative management:
>   - Promote optimal nutritional intake.
>   - Maintain consistent weight gain.
>   - Prevent nutritional deficits.
>   - Promote optimal growth and development.
> - Important nursing diagnoses (actual or potential) are:
>   - Altered nutrition: less than body requirements; more than body requirements
>   - Breastfeeding (effective, ineffective, interrupted)
>   - Impaired growth and development
>   - Self care deficit (feeding)
>   - Fluid volume deficit
>   - Risk for injury (electrolyte imbalance, nutritional deficit-related complications)
>   - Altered tissue perfusion (gastrointestinal system)
> - **Key Terms/Concepts:** Recommended Daily Allowance (RDA), nutritional supplements, infant formula types

Overview

The quality of nutrition has one of the greatest impacts on growth in children. Dietary factors regulate growth at all stages of development. In the prenatal period, the placental supply of nutrients impacts the development of the fetus. During infancy, the rate of growth is rapid; caloric and protein needs are high. Nutrient needs vary and reflect the rate of growth, energy expended in activity, basal metabolic needs and the interaction of nutrients consumed. Good nutrition is essential to the child's well being, particularly in the first years of life as bones, muscles, and bodily systems are rapidly developing. Good nutrition also plays a vital role in the prevention of disease.

Breast and Bottle-Feeding

- Human breast milk is nature's perfect food because it is designed to meet the nutritive and metabolic needs for human growth and development.
- The decision to wean a child from breast milk is highly individualized for mother and baby. The reasons for weaning may include time, convenience,

Nursing Management of the Child's Nutrition

breast milk supply, satiety, maternal experience, attitudes about breastfeeding, employment circumstance, support from significant family members and friends, growth of the child, sibling demands, and many other situational influences. The weaning process occurs gradually over a period of days or weeks to prevent breast engorgement thus reducing the risk for mastitis. Weaning from the bottle is done gradually over several days or weeks and should not be attempted when the child is ill. Usually weaning occurs after the child has mastered drinking from a cup. Weaning from the bottle is easier during the day. Most children rely on a bottle before bedtime for comfort. Putting a child to bed with a bottle, however, can result in aspiration and/or tooth decay. After a child has been weaned from the bottle, regression may occur during periods of hospitalization or serious illness.

Solid Foods

- The introduction of solid food generally occurs at four to six months of age (after the protrusion reflex disappears).
- Rice cereal is recommended as the first solid food as it is less likely to cause an allergic reaction and contains a rich source of dietary iron.
- As the child continues to grow and develop, foods should be added one at a time due to the potential for food allergies. The most common causes of food allergies include eggs, cow's milk, wheat, legumes (peanuts), fish, shellfish, strawberries, and some spices. The infant's gastrointestinal system is immature and certain foods may not be easily digested.
- Infants less than 12 months should not be given honey, secondary small risk of botulism.
- The appetite of a toddler is irregular and food "jags" may occur. Children of this age may develop "picky" eating habits and peculiar food preferences. For example, a toddler may insist on eating a particular food for every meal then suddenly refuse to eat this food. The amount of cow's milk needs to be less then 16 ounces per day to prevent iron deficiency anemia. This occurs because overconsumption of milk replaces intake of iron rich foods.
- The appetite of many toddlers and preschoolers is decreased. To optimize the nutritional intake, parents may need information regarding healthy food choices in smaller meal portions and healthy snacks.
- Good sources of calcium are important for healthy teeth and bone structure development.
- School-age children require breakfast to provide energy to optimize performance and concentration at school. The rate of growth during the adolescent period is very rapid and the nutrient requirements are increased.
- Adolescents' food consumption patterns may be affected by peer pressure, body image, and socialization patterns (pizza parties, etc.).

Gastrointestinal Dysfunction that may Interfere with Nutrition

Pica is considered an eating disorder. The child ingests both food and non-food substances excessively and compulsively. Commonly ingested substances include: coffee grounds, uncooked foods, clay, soil, paint, ice, hair, and feces. Pica is more common in children and women (most especially in pregnancy), the mentally retarded, clients with anemia and renal failure.

Gastroesophageal reflux (GER) is the movement of gastric contents up into the esophagus. This is unremarkable in most individuals but for some it is a severe problem with harmful complications. Risk factors that lead to GER include abdominal distention, delayed emptying of the stomach, increased abdominal pressure, hiatal hernia, or gastrostomy. The exact cause is unknown but thought to be related to the central nervous system (CNS). The most common symptom in children is regurgitation. Other symptoms include slow weight gain, anemia, and blood in emesis or stool, heartburn, difficulty during/after feedings, and pneumonia or asthma symptoms. Complications include: esophagitis, bleeding, anemia, pneumonia, and respiratory problems. To decrease the symptoms and increase the probability of the child maintaining his/her dietary intake: small frequent feedings are generally recommended; thickened feedings and upright positioning are still being investigated but are currently accepted practices. The parents should be encouraged to position the child at a 30-degree elevation of the head after feedings and for sleeping.

Inflammatory bowel disease (IBD) includes Crohn's disease and ulcerative colitis. These chronic illnesses are not functional in origin; they are inflammatory. Many cases are diagnosed prior to adulthood. Growth failure is associated with IBD (more with Crohn's disease than ulcerative colitis) in pediatric cases. Symptoms include: intestinal bleeding, diarrhea, weight loss, slowed growth, abdominal pain, and anorexia. These diseases have generalized symptoms and complications. Treatment includes anti-inflammatory agents as well as symptom control.

Irritable bowel syndrome (IBS) is a functional disease of the large and small intestine characterized by abnormal motility. Symptoms include: alternating diarrhea and constipation, abdominal bloating and pain, urgency to defecate, and flatulence. These symptoms lead to embarrassment and anxiety in children. They fear the occurrence of the symptoms in front of peers and may isolate themselves. Treatment may include decreasing stress through age appropriate activities, high fiber diet, antispasmodics and anti-diarrheal medications (may help), eliminating carbonated beverages, and slowed eating (should be encouraged).

Peptic ulcer disease (PUD) is a chronic disease where there is an erosion through the mucosal, submucosal, and possibly into the muscular layer of the GI tract. The cause of the erosion is gastric secretions. Secondary ulcers can occur as a result of disease, or medications (salicylates, NSAID, or iron preparations). The presence of Helicobacter pylori has been identified in up to 100% of the adults with PUD but the exact cause in children is unknown. Symptoms depend on the location of the ulcer in the GI tract. Treatment includes antibiotics, antacids, sucralfate, bismuth, anti-secretory drugs, and in cases with severe complications (hemorrhaging) surgery may be indicated.

Hypertrophic pyloric stenosis (HPS) is a result of thickening of the muscle of the pylorus resulting in constriction. This is generally seen in the first few weeks after birth (but can take months to develop) and a hallmark sign is projectile vomiting leading to dehydration, metabolic alkalosis, and little-to-no growth. During this time, prior to surgical repair, the child should be allowed to rest after feedings, with minimal handling and movement to allow for the feeding to move down the GI tract. This is much more common in first-born children and occurs at a rate of 5-to-1 in males versus females. Treatment is surgery. The child must be re-hydrated and any electrolyte imbalance must be addressed prior to surgery. Postoperatively vomiting is common in the first 24 to 48 hours and the parents should be told that this is not unusual. Prognosis with surgery is very good.

Malabsorption syndromes include celiac disease (an intolerance to gluten found in wheat, barley, rye, and oats), and short bowel syndrome (decrease in the absorption surface of the small bowel).

Gastroenteritis: Literally translated, gastroenteritis is an inflammation of the mucous membrane of the stomach and intestine. There are several causes including viral, parasitic, and bacterial, with rotavirus being the most common in young children in the U.S. that require hospitalization for management of their illness. Other causes include: Salmonella, Shigella, and Campylobacter (the most common bacterial causes); Giardia and Cryptosporidium (the most common parasitic causes); complications of respiratory and urinary tract infections; medications (ampicillin, amoxicillin, cefaclor, and penicillin are the most common examples); some foods which contain sorbitol and fructose, if ingested in large quantities, and food poisoning (staphylococcus, Clostridium perfringens, Clostridium botulinum being the causative agents).

Most cases of gastroenteritis present with nausea, vomiting, diarrhea, cramping and can also include fever and headache. Complications of acute gastroenteritis include dehydration, electrolyte imbalance, and malnutrition. Diagnosis can often be made through the history of the illness. If the illness is protracted or complicated then a stool specimen is recommended for culture.

Because of the high risk of dehydration and electrolyte imbalance, the priority should be given to assessing the fluid and electrolyte status, rehydration and maintenance of fluids, introduction of food as early as possible, and administration of antimicrobial agents (in specific cases--depending upon the causative agent) per the orders. Oral rehydration solutions (ORS) are recommended as the first line of therapy in infants and children with diarrhea and dehydration (vomiting is NOT a contraindication). ORS products include: Pedialyte, Rehydralyte, Infalyte, and WHO. ORS's are nutrient-based products that may shorten the duration of the illness. Once rehydration has been completed, it is suggested that the ORS continue to replace stool losses and that the child then should go to maintenance therapy. Maintenance therapy includes: continuation of established breastfeeding; formulas, if tolerated (lactose free or diluted lactose formulas); or cow's milk for infants.

A regular diet should be introduced as soon as vomiting has stopped and rehydration has been achieved or continued throughout the illness if tolerated. A normal diet may decrease the number of diarrheal stools, decrease the amount of weight loss, and shorten the duration of the illness. Clear fluids are no longer encouraged with diarrhea; these often have high carbohydrate and low electrolyte content with a high osmolality. Other common products in the clear liquid diet contain high sodium or caffeine (a natural diuretic). Both may worsen the water loss and electrolyte imbalance. The BRAT (bananas, rice, apples, and toast or tea) diet is contraindicated in the child with acute diarrhea because of low energy, electrolyte, and protein levels, and high carbohydrate content. Finally, anti-diarrheal agents are contraindicated in infants and young children with infectious acute diarrhea.

Parental teaching should include prevention of the spread of the illness to others (good hand washing; immediate disposal of dirty diapers; isolation of the infected child to certain areas of the house; meticulous cleaning of the areas used in caring for the infected child); signs and symptoms of dehydration; dietary and fluid maintenance; limiting use of juices, broths, Jell-O or the BRAT diet, while providing appropriate fluids and a regular diet.

Nutrition in Childhood	
0-3 months	• Breast milk or infant formula with iron • Strong suck reflex
4-6 months	• Breast milk or formula with iron • Begins to use fingers to feed
6-12 months	• Infant cereal and soft foods • Teething crackers and fruits • Limit formula to 30 oz per day • Holds own bottle • Begins to drink from a cup • Begins to indicate taste preferences by refusing unwanted food
12-24 months	• Table foods chopped into small pieces. Avoid round foods like grapes, hot dogs, etc. • Limit milk to 24 oz per day • Enjoys self-feeding with finger foods • Begins to use a spoon • Drinks well from a cup • Develops food jags
3-5 years	• Table foods in larger pieces • Develops mastery of spoons and forks
6-12 years	• Needs approximately 2000 or more calories/day • Learns to cook (8-10 year-old) • Tendency to eat fast food and "junk food"
13-18 years	• Food preferences may be influenced by peers • Strives for ideal body image (diets, may develop eating disorders) • Increased need for calories with growth spurts and athletic activity • May use food for emotional comfort (leads to obesity)

Critical Thinking Exercise: Nursing Management of the Child's Nutrition

Select the appropriate response for the following case study. Explain the rationale for your response.

1. The mother of a 2-year-old is concerned because her son has not been eating well during mealtimes at home. What is the nurse's best response?
    a. "You need to give him a daily multivitamin to help increase his appetite."
    b. "It is common for toddlers to eat less. Try giving him small meals and snacks."
    c. "It is best for children to eat three meals a day. Limit snacks to increase his appetite."
    d. "If you give him more milk and juice, it will make up for his lack of eating at meals."

    Correct answer: _____

    Rationale:

2. The mother of a 13-month-old asks the nurse what finger foods are best. Which of the following is the best answer?
    a. A celery stick
    b. A hot dog
    c. Grapes
    d. Dry cereal

    Correct answer: _____

    Rationale:

3. Matching: Match the age normally associated with development of each eating behavior listed.

6-year-old	a. Eats larger pieces of table food
3-year-old	b. Uses strong sucking reflex
7-month-old	c. Controls diet to lose weight
5-month-old	d. Enjoys cooking simple recipes
13-month-old	e. Eats chopped table food
6-month-old	f. Begins self-feeding
15-year-old	g. Uses a fork and spoon with ease
4-year-old	h. Begins taste preferences
9-year-old	i. Eats breakfast to help with attention at school
3-week-old	j. Begins eating rice cereal

Basic Concepts CHAPTER 6

Nursing Management of a Child's Medications

> **Key Points**
>
> - Accurate and systematic administration techniques help ensure safe delivery of medications.
> - Pediatric medication administration techniques vary according to the type of medication, route, child's age, and individual preferences.
> - Parental support, education, and practice are crucial to successful home medication administration.
> - Goals of collaborative management:
>   - Identify and administer the appropriate medication, dosage, route, and volume based on the child's individual needs.
>   - Promptly recognize and appropriately respond to medication side effects.
>   - Educate the family regarding home medication administration.
>   - Identify conditions that indicate a change in medication, dosage, route, and/or timing is needed/required.
> - Important nursing diagnoses (actual and potential) are:
>   - Altered comfort related to injections and/or medication side effects
>   - Anxiety or fear related to discomfort associated with medication administration
>   - Injury related to medication errors and/or side effects
>   - Knowledge deficit
>   - Caregiver role strain related to multiple medication needs at home
>   - Altered home maintenance related to medication administration needs
>   - Ineffective management of therapeutic regimen related to noncompliance with medication administration plan
> - **Key Terms/Concepts**: Absorption, distribution, excretion, child identification, dosage calculation, concentration, dilution, infusion, documentation, side effects, contraindication, medication administration route

Overview

Many factors, such as absorption, distribution, and excretion, have an impact on the effectiveness of medications usage in children.

Safe and Accurate Medication Administration "Rights"

- **Right Medication**: Ensure that the medication to be administered is correct.
- **Right Dose**: Verify the dose to be administered is correct. Calculate to ensure dose ordered is within the recommended dosage range for the diagnosis, route, and child's age.

- **Right Route**: Verify that the route of administration is appropriate and according to the order.
- **Right Time**: Check when the previous dose was administered and verify against the schedule.
- **Right Volume Concentration**: Calculate that the amount of medication in the syringe or tablet is based on how it is supplied (e.g., mg or mcg/mL).
- **Verify (Right Child)**: Cross-check child's identification with the medication or record.
- **Right Technique/Approach**: Determine the appropriate administration technique based on the medication order, child's developmental level, route, home routine and child's preferences.
- **Documentation**: Document the medication and response (if indicated) on the medical record after administering.
- **Right to refuse**
- **Right to know potential side effects**
- If administering an IV "piggy back" medication, include the following steps:
  - **Volume dilution**— Identify the amount of extra volume to be added to dilute the medication prior to administration.
  - **Infusion time/rate**— Calculate the infusion rate based on the amount of time needed to infuse the medication.

Oral Medications

The administration of oral medications is the most common route for medication administration in children. Although the ingestion of medication is non-invasive, the use of oral medication may not be beneficial to the child who is vomiting or refuses to take it by mouth. Children younger than 5 years may have difficulty swallowing tablets or capsules or taking them in a sublingual form; thus, many pediatric medications are available in liquid suspension. It is not recommended to refer to the medication as "candy" because the well child, taking that description literally, may inadvertently take medication in error. Never attempt to administer oral medication to a crying child because of the risk of aspiration.

An oral dosage syringe is an excellent device for measuring small quantities of liquid medications to infants and young children. The medication should be slowly squirted to the side of the tongue/cheek towards the back of the mouth. Care should be taken to avoid instilling medication with a syringe directly to the back of the throat as this action may elicit a gag reflex. Oral medication can be given to an infant by squirting the liquid into a nipple and eliciting the sucking reflex. Crushed tablets and strong-tasting medications can be mixed with a small amount (teaspoon) of applesauce, ice cream, or pudding to increase the likelihood of getting the child to take the medication. It is not recommended to mix medication in a large volume of food or liquid due to the difficulty of getting the child to finish the entire amount.

Nose, Ear, and Eye Drops

Nose drops can be administered with the infant or child lying flat with the head over the edge of a pillow, placing the head in the "sniffing position." Maintain the child's position for one minute to allow the drops to penetrate the nasal cavity.

Ear drops are instilled after warming to room temperature. For the child under 3 years of age, the affected ear is drawn down and back to straighten the canal. In the older child, the lobe is pulled up and back to obtain a straight canal.

Eye drops are administered with the child in either supine or sitting position. The head is tilted back and drops instilled in the inner canthus of the eye and allowed to roll to the lateral side. The child is encouraged to blink to enhance the penetration of the medication.

Eye ointments are used in the delivery room and when the child has a localized infection. About 1/2 inch of the ointment is distributed along the lower conjunctival sac. The lids and lashes should be cleaned prior to applying the ointment. After the ointment is applied, the child should close the eye and move it from side to side in order to spread the ointment.

Intramuscular Injections

Intramuscular injections should be avoided in children due to the traumatic nature of this route. The child often fears the needle and perceives the invasive stimulus as painful and threatening.

Needle length - the needle must be long enough to deliver the medication to the muscle. The usual needle gauge for an infant and small children is 22 to 25 gauge and the usual needle length is 0.625 to 1". A 1" needle is usually acceptable for delivering 1 mL to 2 mL of medication. When amounts of less than 1 mL are ordered, a tuberculin syringe should be used, which comes with an attached needle, usually 3/8" 28 gauge needle.

The vastus lateralis site is usually the recommended site for infants and children less than 2 years of age. After age 2 the ventral gluteal site can be used. Both of these sites can accommodate fluid up to 2 mL. The deltoid site has a smaller muscle mass and only can accommodate up to 1.0 mL of fluid.

General Guidelines for IM Injections

- Provide emotional support and comfort before, during, and after injection.
- Use proper hand washing and sterile technique when handling syringes and medications.
- Calculate and prepare medication away from the child.
- Select the needle and syringe size based on the child's size, medication amount, muscle mass, and medication viscosity.
- Provide privacy during administration.
- Prepare the child by honestly explaining what will happen in developmentally appropriate terms.
- Enlist assistance for holding the child during injection, as needed.
- Select best route. Rotate sites if appropriate.
- Avoid injecting excess amounts of medication in one site.
- Use appropriate administration technique.
- Dispose of syringes and needles properly.

- Document drug, dosage, route, site, date, time, the person administering the medication, and the child's response to the medication completely and accurately.

Intramuscular Injection Sites			
Site	Age	Technique	Volumes
Vastus Lateralis	Infant-Adolescent	• Locate site on middle third between trochanter of the femur and knee, anterior to the midline area. • Inject perpendicular to skin or at a 45-degree angle toward knee.	• Infant: 0.5-1 mL • Young child: 1-1.5 mL • Adolescent: 1.5-2 mL
Ventrogluteal	Preschool-Adolescent	• Place palm over greater trochanter with the hand pointing upward. • Inject in the "V" between the fingers and thumb.	• Young child: 1-1.5 mL • Adolescent: 1.5-2 mL
Dorsogluteal	Preschool-Adolescent	• Diagonal line between posterior iliac crest and the greater trochanter of the femur • Have child point the toes inward, a technique to avoid tensing. • Do not use this route until the child has been walking for two years.	• Young child: 1-1.5 mL • Adolescent: 1.5-2 mL
Deltoid	School age-Adolescent	• Need adequate muscle mass for this route • Locate site on upper arm two finger widths below the acromion process. • Limit volume injected.	• Young child: 0.5 mL • Adolescent: 1 mL

Critical Thinking Exercise: Nursing Management of a Child's Medications

Situation: Identify the correct order for each of the steps for administering a PRN dose of oral acetaminophen to a 9-month-old child. Explain the rationale for each step.

Step	Order	Rationale for Step
Invite the father to assist and/or give suggestions for techniques.		
Wash hands.		
Educate the infant's father at the bedside regarding the need for the medication.		
Calculate correct dosage.		
Prepare a bottle of juice.		
Calculate amount to be drawn up from the bottle of acetaminophen.		
Draw up the acetaminophen from the bottle using a syringe.		
Offer the infant a sip of juice from a bottle.		
Verify medication order.		
Document the medication administration and response on the medical record.		
Identify the need for the PRN medication based on the order.		
Squirt the medication into the back of the infant's mouth between the teeth and gums.		

Basic Concepts CHAPTER 7

Nursing Management of a Child's Growth and Development

> **Key Points**
>
> - Growth and development is a continual, ongoing process that requires physical and psychological energy.
> - Patterns of growth and development most frequently occur in "spurts" and "lulls."
> - The progression, sequence, rate of growth and development are unique in each child.
> - Goals of collaborative management:
>   - Promote optimal growth patterns.
>   - Recognize the child's developmental level based on progress towards achieving expected developmental milestones.
>   - Promote an optimal pattern of growth and development based on the individual child's capacity.
>   - Provide family education and support regarding the child's level of development.
> - Important nursing diagnoses (actual and potential) are:
>   - Altered growth
>   - Altered development
>   - Impaired communication
>   - Disorganized infant behavior
>   - Knowledge deficit
> - **Key Terms/Concepts**: Growth, development, developmental task, maturation, neurobehavioral development of the infant, locomotion, prehension, pincer grasp, fine motor, and gross motor

Overview

Growth is defined as an increase in physical size. Development represents an increase in the skills needed to function. Development usually results in achievement of increasingly complex tasks. Maturation reflects an increase in ability, competence, and/or functioning at a higher level.

Growth is the physical change and increase in size; growth is measurable.

Development is the behavioral aspect of growth; the capacity and skill of a person to adapt to the environment; and an increase in the complexity of function and skill progression.

Growth and development are independent yet interrelated processes. Growth generally takes place during the first 20 years of life while development persists throughout life. Factors that influence growth and development are both genetic and environmental.

Nursing Management of a Child's Growth and Development

Genetic factors of growth and development are present at conception and remain unchanged throughout life. Genetic factors determine characteristics like sex, physical stature, and race.

Environmental factors include family, religion, climate, culture, school, community, nutrition, exposures, and economics.

The assessment of the psychosocial development of a child should be included in each clinic visit. The extent of that assessment may depend upon the reason for the visit, how the child presents to the health care provider, or the age of the child.

There are several theories that nurses and other professionals use as a reference to assess the child. These theories are the basis for many developmental assessment tools. Aspects of the developmental theories the nurse should be familiar with include:

Piaget's Theory of Cognitive Development: According to Piaget, cognitive development is a sequential, orderly process where a variety of new experiences must exist before intellectual abilities can develop. Piaget's theory is divided into five major phases: sensorimotor, preconceptual, intuitive, concrete operations, and formal operations. In each phase, the individual must use: assimilation, to encounter and react to the new situation which allows one to acquire new knowledge and skills; accommodation, to cognitively process the new information, allowing problems to be solved that may have been unsolvable before (This is possible primarily because the new information has been assimilated.); and adaptation, a coping behavior enabling the individual to handle the demands made by the environment.

Piaget's Phases of Cognitive Development		
Phases	**Age**	**Defining Characteristics**
Sensorimotor Phase	**Birth-2 years**	
Stage 1: Reflexes	Birth-2 months	• Most action is reflexive.
Stage 2: Primary Circular Reaction	1-4 months	• Perception of events is centered on the body. • Objects are an extension of self.
Stage 3: Secondary Circular Reaction	4-8 months	• Acknowledges the external environment • Actively makes changes in the environment
Stage 4: Coordination of Secondary Schemata	8-12 months	• Can distinguish a goal from a means of attaining it
Stage 5: Tertiary Circular Reaction	12-18 months	• Discovers new goals and tries ways to attain goals • Rituals are important
Stage 6: Inventions of New Means	18-24 months	• Interprets the environment by mental image • Uses make-believe and pretend play

Piaget's Phases of Cognitive Development		
Phases	Age	Defining Characteristics
Preconceptual Phase	2-4 years	• Uses an egocentric approach to accommodate the demands of the environment • Everything is significant and relates to "me" • Explores the environment • Language development is rapid. Associates words with objects.
Intuitive Thought Phase	4-7 years	• Egocentric thinking diminishes. • Thinks of one idea at a time • Includes others in the environment • Words express thoughts
Concrete Operations Phase	7-11 years	• Solves concrete problems • Begins to understand relative concepts, such as size • Begins to categorize, serialize and group items • Understands right and left • Cognizant of viewpoints
Formal Operation Phase	11-15 years	• Uses rational thinking • Reasoning is deductive and futuristic

Maslow's Hierarchy of Needs

Maslow's hierarchy of needs is a commonly accepted needs theory used in promoting health. Maslow found that those who satisfy basic needs appropriately are healthier and happier than those individuals that do not.

Maslow's Needs:
- Self-actualization
- Self-esteem
- Love and belonging
- Safety and security
- Physiologic

Maslow's theory states that people will not progress successfully to the next level of needs without appropriately satisfying the lower level needs first.

Physiologic needs include air, food, water, shelter, rest, sleep, activity, and comfortable temperature. These are considered the lowest level needs, which are crucial for survival.

Safety and security needs are both physical and psychological and are the second level of needs.

Love and belonging needs are the third level, which include giving and receiving affection, and achieving and maintaining the feeling of belonging to a group.

Self-esteem needs include feelings of independence, competence, and self-respect. Esteem includes recognition, respect, and appreciation from others.

Self-actualization is the highest level in Maslow's hierarchy of needs. When the self-esteem need is satisfied, one strives for self-actualization, the innate need to develop one's maximum potential and realize one's abilities and qualities.

Erikson's Five-Stage Model of Psychosocial Development

Erik Erikson developed his theory from Freud's theory of development and includes development across the life span. Erikson describes stages of development as levels of achievement. Each task must be achieved at some level: complete, partial or unsuccessful. Erikson believes the greater the task achievement, the healthier the personality. Failure to achieve the task affects the individual's ability to achieve the next task.

Each stage has its developmental task wherein the individual must find balance. Erikson's stages include:

Erikson's Five-Stage Model of Psychosocial Development			
Stage	**Age**	**Central Task**	**Positive Resolution**
Infancy	Birth-18 months	Trust vs. mistrust	Learning to trust others. Trust is relative to something or someone; therefore, consistency in the caregiver and daily routine can be significant. Mistrust can develop when basic needs are not met.
Early Childhood	18 months-3 years	Autonomy vs. shame and doubt	Self-control without loss of self-esteem. Ability to cooperate and to express oneself. The child moves through this stage successfully by learning to control his/her body. Toilet training is significant to this. Doing things for themselves is important. Learning at this stage is often done through imitation. Shame can develop when the child's attempts are unsuccessful; when he/she is scolded for failed attempts or is forced to be dependent.
Late Childhood	3-5 years	Initiative vs. guilt	Learning the degree to which assertiveness and purpose influence the environment. Begins to have the ability to evaluate one's own behavior. In this stage, the child develops his/her conscience and must do as that conscience guides them. If the child's actions are in conflict with the parents' ideas, guilt may develop.
School Age	6-12 years	Industry vs. inferiority	Beginning to create, develop, and manipulate. Developing a sense of competence and perseverance. The focus of this stage is achievement and accomplishment. As the child develops socially he/she learns to compete, cooperate, and follow rules. Setting goals or standards that are too high may cause the child to develop a sense of inferiority or inadequacy. The parents should support the child's development of independence; generally the child is able to separate from the parent and routine of the home without anxiety.

Nursing Management of a Child's Growth and Development

Erikson's Five-Stage Model of Psychosocial Development				
Stage	Age	Central Task	Positive Resolution
Adolescence	12-20 years	Identity vs. role confusion	Coherent sense of self. Plans to actualize one's abilities. At this stage, when the body changes dramatically and rapidly, the child may be anxious over not "knowing" his/her own body. Adolescents are focused on their appearance and have a preoccupation with peer acceptance. They move on to develop their own values within their culture and society at large. Late in this stage they will likely become focused on their choice of an occupation.

Freud's Psychosexual Stages

Freud used sexuality to identify stages of personality development. He used regions of the body to identify several of the stages relative to the area that he felt were significant, at each age, to pleasure and conflict.

Freud's Psychosexual Stages		
Stage	Age	Significance
Oral sensory	Infancy-1 year	At this age, the mouth is the area of most pleasure. Sucking, eating, and vocalizing are examples of activities which provide oral gratification.
Anal-urethral	1-3 years	Associated with the ability to defecate at will and "hold it" is a focus. Toilet training is significant.
Phallic-locomotion	3-6 years	Recognition of the differences between the sexes is a focus and the genital area is now of interest. It is during this stage that Freud presents discussions of Oedipus and Electra complexes, penis envy, and castration anxiety, all of which he felt strongly influenced personality development. These theories are very controversial.
Latency	6-12 years	Play and acquiring knowledge occupy most of the child's time and energy.
Genital	12-19 years	Final major stage in Freud's theory. Focuses on sexual maturation with energy also spent on friendships and readying for marriage.

Denver Developmental Screening Test (DDST)

The DDST is used to screen children from 1 month to 6 years for gross motor skills, fine motor skills, language development, and personal/social development. This tool is easy to administer and potentially can identify developmental issues soon enough to ensure early intervention. It is felt that early identification leads to more effective therapy of children with developmental disabilities. The DDST is an example of secondary prevention.

In assessing the development of a 6- to 10-year old, the nurse should include questions in the following areas:

Ask the child about:
- **Family** - "Who is in your family?" "What do you do with your family?" "How do you get along with your family?"
- **Friends** - "Who are your friends?" "Do you have a best friend?" "What do you like to do with your friends?"
- **School** - "What grade are you in?" "Who is your teacher?"
- **Activities** - "What do you like to do for fun?" "Do you play any sports or have any hobbies?"

Ask the parent about:
- **Family** - "Have there been any major changes in the family?" "How do the children get along?"
- **Friends** - "Who are your child's friends?"
- **School** - "Do you participate in your child's school activities?"
- **Activities** - "What activities does your child participate in outside of school?"

In the adolescent (11-21 years), developmental assessment should include the following areas:

Ask the child about:
- **Family** - "How do you get along with your family?" "How are you disciplined?"
- **Friends** - "Who are your friends?" "What do you like to do with your friends?"
- **Dating/Drug Use** - Start with a declarative statement like: "Some teenagers your age have begun to be sexually active," or "I know that drugs are common on school campuses."
- **School** - "Do you like school?" "Are you in (or planning to go to) college?"
- **Activities** - "What do you do for fun outside of school?"

(Ask the parents about these same areas for the child in early adolescence [11-14 years].)

Language Development

Stage	Significance
Prelinguistic stage (before talking)	From birth to 10/12 months: first crying, then cooing; then "baby talk;" to the first meaningful words.
Holophrastic stage (one word)	Sometimes associated with thoughts; the child uses one word to ask/state something when older children would use a sentence. This stage generally begins at about 1 year of age.
Telegraphic stage	This is the time when the child uses only significant words (nouns, verbs) without prepositions, articles, etc. This generally begins around 18-24 months.
Preschool period	Sometime between 2-5 years, the child begins to talk in full sentences; the vocabulary grows and becomes more complex.
Middle childhood	At this time the child learns the rules of grammar, writing, and complexities of her/his culture's language.

Generally, females develop their language skills more rapidly than boys, as do first-born children of either gender. Children that result from a multiple birth, or later-born children generally develop language skills at a slower pace. There are other factors that can negatively influence the development of language and language skills, these include: congenital or structural abnormalities of the mouth, hearing problems, emotional factors, mental health issues, neurological problems, illness, or trauma.

Play

Onlooker play: The child(ren) only watch others play with no attempt to join them.

Solitary play: The child(ren) play alone. They may be in a room or area with other children and usually enjoy being near them, but do not make any attempt to play or even speak to the other children.

Parallel play: In this type of play, the children play among other children, often with the same types of toys. The children use their toys to play out what they want and how they want things to be. They play among others in an independent fashion. This is a common type of play among toddlers.

Associative play: The children play together, engaged in similar activities. This is a spontaneous type of play with no real organization or assigned roles.

Cooperative play: This type of play is organized with a similar goal among the children.

Age	Type of play
3-12 months	Exploring and examining, the infant learns to grab and hold articles and begins to be able to explore once he/she can crawl.
1-8 years	Imitation is the common type of play, imitating adults using toy replicas (play computers, cash registers, doctor's equipment, firefighter equipment, etc.). Having imaginary friends is typical.
8-12 years	There is less interest in toys, and the children begin to develop more individual interests like hobbies, sports, or playing organized games.
Older children	Play and imagine themselves as the hero liked by everyone, that everyone thinks they are beautiful or wonderful, or may be acting as though they are victims, feeling sorry for themselves.

Principles of Growth and Development

- Self-fueling, ongoing process that requires physical and psychological energy
- Sequence of growth is characterized by "spurts and lulls"
- Progression is highly individualized for each child.
- Variation at different ages for specific structures

Concepts of Death in the Child

- Infants and toddlers have no concept of death, they have separation anxiety and react to change but have no concept of forever.
- Preschoolers often think of death as a temporary state like sleep. Preschoolers are afraid of separation and may see death as a punishment.

- School-age children begin to understand that death is not reversible and may think of it as violent. They may understand that death is natural and going to happen to everyone, but have difficulty understanding that they (themselves) may die.
- Late school-age children understand that death is final and may want to know the biological details and information about funerals and body preparation.
- Adolescents generally understand death, but continue to deny that they could die any time soon. Therefore, adolescents tend to participate in high-risk behaviors. They often have difficulties when there is a death and may not be able to admit that they need the support of others.

Separation Anxiety begins to develop as the 4- to 8-month-old becomes aware of separateness between themselves and others or objects. By 12 months, most children are cued by parental behaviors when their departure is imminent and begin to protest through crying and clinging behaviors. Parents can help overcome this problematic development by having a variety of people around the child or in the home with the parents so the child becomes comfortable with several potential caregivers. Separation anxiety can continue through the toddler and preschool years, though the degree may vary. Generally the reaction is stronger when fearing loss of the mother rather than that of the father. Separation anxiety is often present when the child begins school. Most children deal with this successfully and transition to the school day well. Some children, with strong dependent relationships with the parent, may have a longer and more difficult transition period. Nurses should be aware of the presence of separation anxiety in the hospitalized child. At this time, the reaction of the child to the parents' absence can be much stronger. There is a fear of the unknown environment, fear of unknown people and the likeliness that they have been or will be hurt by a procedure or are not feeling well; all of these will increase the negative reaction to the separation from parents. This may continue in the hospitalized child to an older age, even into adolescence.

Physical Growth Patterns during Childhood

- Very rapid growth during infancy
- Slow, steady growth during childhood
- Growth spurt during puberty
- Maximum height is attained within two inches shortly after the onset of menses in females.

Height

- An infant's length at birth is an average of 20 inches.
- During the first year of life, the child increases birth length by approximately ten inches.
- During the second year of life the child typically grows five inches.
- Growth of three inches per year occurs during the preschool period.
- In the sixth to tenth year the annual height gain is two inches.
- The maximum growth in height occurs during the pubescent period.
- The peak height increase in boys usually occurs at age 14.

Nursing Management of a Child's Growth and Development

- Peak growth rate in girls occurs at age 13.
- The growth in height typically ceases sometime between ages 18 and 20.

Weight

- The appropriate weight for the gestational age infant at term is 5-9 pounds at birth.
- The weight typically doubles by 4th or 5th month.
- A child's weight triples by his/her first birthday.
- During the preschool years the weight may increase five pounds each year.
- Small increases in weight occur during school-age years.
- Rapid weight gain may accompany the pubescent period.

Bone Formation

- Bone development is progressive; the process is completed in the twenties.
- Bone age can be determined by x-ray.
- Growth of long bones is complete when the epiphyses and diaphysis are fused.
- Bone development of the wrist and hand is complete at age 17 for girls and 19 for boys.

Tooth Formation

- At birth, all of the primary (deciduous) tooth buds are present under the gum, and the permanent teeth are developing below the deciduous teeth.
- The two lower central incisors appear at approximately 6 months of age.
- Although the appearance of teeth varies among children, a typical pattern of eruption occurs: the two upper central incisors appear after the central bottom and top incisors.
- Many children have six teeth at 1 year and all twenty by age 2 years.

Motor Development

- Motor development progresses in a cephalocaudal (head-to-toe) manner as evidenced by the following sequence of motor activities: the infant first tracks with his eyes, then follows objects and turns head side to side. The infant learns to lift the shoulders, then the upper body. Rolling from side to side precedes sitting and later crawling. Then the child cruises and learns to walk.
- Motor development proceeds from the center of body to the extremities (proximo distal).
  - **Prehension** is the ability to oppose the thumb to the fingers in picking up an object, known as the pincer grasp. This generally begins to occur in the eighth month. Reaching, grasping, and raking movements precede this fine motor skill.
  - **Locomotion** is the ability to walk independently without support. Due to the variation in the time when walking occurs (9-17 months); some parents may need support and reassurance that their child is developing

normally. The parents with concerns regarding their infant's rate or pattern of growth and development may obtain developmental screening from the health care provider.

Growth Dimensions

Weight, height/length and head circumference are components of the physical assessment of children. An accurate weight is important for correct medication dosing, determination of intake/output and nutritional assessment for children. Gross assessment of the rate of brain growth can be accomplished by plotting serial head circumference measurements on the child's growth curve.

Physical Development and Milestones in Infancy (1-12 Months)		
Age	Gross Motor	Fine Motor
1 month	• Turns head to sides, lifts head for short periods • Head lag • No head control when held up	• Hands usually closed • Strong grasp reflex • May grasp toy
2 months	• Decreased head lag when pulled up • Beginning to lift head • Head bobs to upright when held sitting	• Hands open more • Decreased grasp reflex
3 months	• Holds head up more but still bobs • Only slight head lag remains • Able to lift head 45 to 90 degrees • Bears weight on forearms	• Holds items but won't reach for them • Grasp reflex gone • Pulls and grasps at blankets
4 months	• Holds head up when in sitting position • Able to sit if propped • Lifts head and chest off surfaces • Rolls from back to side	• Pulls blanket over face in play • Tries to grab objects • Plays with small toys but can't grab them • Gets objects to mouth
5 months	• No head lag • Holds head erect when sitting • Sits for long periods when back supported • Turns from stomach to back • Feet to mouth when lying	• Grasps objects voluntarily • Palmar grasps present • Moves items straight to mouth
6 months	• Lifts chest off bed bearing weight on hands • Lifts head when someone is about to pull them to a sitting position • Sits straight in high chair • Bears weight when held in standing position	• Able to retrieve a dropped item • Grabs and pulls feet to mouth • Holds bottle • Manipulates small items
7 months	• Lifts head spontaneously • Sits leaning on hands • Sits erect for short period without support • Bears full weight on feet • Bounces when held standing	• Transfers objects from hand to hand • Holds two items at once • Bangs items on surface

Nursing Management of a Child's Growth and Development

	Physical Development and Milestones in Infancy (1-12 Months)	
Age	Gross Motor	Fine Motor
8 months	• Sits unsupported • May stand holding on • Moves to reach an object	• Beginning pincer grasp • Drops items at will • Can get an item by pulling on a string
9 months	• Creeps on hands and feet • Sits alone for long periods • Recovers when leans forward but not to sides • Pulls to standing and stands holding on	• Uses thumb and index finger to grasp items • Begins to show dominant hand • Compares items by bringing them together
10 months	• Can go from lying to sitting • Stands holding on and sits by falling • Recovers easily in sitting position • When standing lifts one foot to step	• Releases objects
11 months	• Pivots to reach when sitting • Walks around holding on to furniture	• Good pincer grasp • Puts objects in a container one after another
12 months	• Walks being held with one hand • May stand alone or take first steps • Can sit from standing without assistance	• Trying to build with blocks • Can turn many pages at once

	Growth and Development Patterns	
Infant	**Birth-3 months:** • Head circumference increases 1-2 cm/month • Posterior fontanel closes • Steady gains in weight and height • Head control increases • Follows objects with eyes	**3-6 months:** • Birth weight doubles • Head circumference increases by 1cm/month • Increased gross motor skills • Social smile and verbalization
	6-11 months: • Gains 3-5 ounces/week • Length increases 0.5 inches/month • First primary teeth • More vocalization • Crude pincer grasp	**12 months:** • Triples birth weight • Eruption of 6-8 teeth • Walks alone • Picks up small objects with thumb and forefinger • Few words

Nursing Care of Children

Nursing Management of a Child's Growth and Development

	Growth and Development Patterns	
Toddler	**12-18 months:** • Growth rate slows • Abdomen protrudes • Eruption of 8-12 teeth • Anterior fontanel closes • Walks well, can throw, climb stairs, kick a ball • Uses eating utensils • Vocabulary increasing	**18-24 months:** • Grows 3-5 inches and gains 5 pounds; weighs 25-28 pounds • Eruption of 18 teeth • Opens doors, runs without falling • Copies lines, scribbles • Increasing vocabulary use
	24-30 months: • Has all twenty teeth • Slow, steady growth • Undresses self • Builds eight block tower • Says full name, sings, expresses needs • Thrives with routine • Magical thinking • Begins to have bowel and bladder control	**3 years:** • Relatively slow growth (gains about 5 pounds and 3 inches) • Hops on one foot, rides tricycle, balances on one foot • Strings large beads, copies crosses and circles • Increased vocalization to about 900 words • Imaginary playmate • Begins self-care activities (brushes teeth) • Able to identify five body parts
Preschool-Age	**4 years:** • Height 39-41 inches, weight 35-40 pounds, slow growth rate • Climbs, runs, jumps well • Increasing finger dexterity, buttons and unbuttons clothes • Increased vocalization, asks many questions • Magical thinking, sexual curiosity	**5 years:** • Height 43-45 inches, weight 40-45 pounds • May lose lower central incisors • Good muscle coordination • Enjoys simple board games, names all colors and coins, defines seven words, knows opposites, prints name • Dresses and undresses independently

Nursing Management of a Child's Growth and Development

	Growth and Development Patterns	
School-Age	**6-7 years:** • First permanent teeth, loses upper incisors • Annual growth of 2 inches, height 47-48 inches, weight 50-51 pounds • Good balance, advanced throwing, outdoor sports • Penmanship becomes legible, increased dexterity, reads and writes, counts, may tell time • Able to bathe self, is modest and independent	**8-9 years:** • Gradual increase in height and weight • Movements more graceful, complex fine motor skills • Enjoys jokes and reading • Plays well alone or in groups, prefers own gender • Begin to group, serialize, and categorize objects
	10-12 years: Appearance of secondary sex characteristics • Girls: pubic hair, breasts • Boys: increase in muscle mass, penis and scrotum enlarge • Tasks include: emancipation from parents and development of healthy self-concept, beginning skills for future • Understanding psychosexual differences • May begin to see fat deposits increase in hips and legs (most especially in females)	
Adolescent	**12-15 years:** • Wide individual variations of growth maturation • Girls between age 10 and 14 gain 2-8 inches, and 15-55 pounds • Menarche begins 2 years after growth spurt • Boys' growth spurt occurs at age 12-16, increases 4-12 inches in height and 15-65 pounds, growth of pubic, auxiliary and upper lip hair	**16-20 years:** • Spermatogenesis occurs by age 16; boys' height slowly increases, ceasing at 18-20 years; in girls, growth stops at 16-17 years of age

Sexual Maturation

Puberty is the time of the development of secondary sexual characteristics. This maturation occurs in a fairly predictable sequence, though these changes can be very individualized since they begin at different ages and progress at varying rates. When the child asks questions about these changes the caregiver should refer to the Tanner staging system and take the opportunity to talk about other sensitive issues. During puberty, children should be getting accurate information about sexuality, pregnancy, contraception, sexually transmitted infections, as well as continuing education on wellness issues like nutrition, safety, and exercise. It is important to address these issues in a straightforward manner, at the level of the children participating, and to include them in the educational activity. They can assist in planning the subjects to be covered.

Terms

- **Adrenarche:** The appearance of pubic hair
- **Gynecomastia:** Breast enlargement and tenderness in males, occurs during mid-puberty in about 1/3 of males and is generally temporary.

- **Menarche**: The first menstrual period occurs in late puberty.
- **Pubertal delay**: In females, if there is no breast development by age 13, or if menarche has not occurred within four years of the beginning of breast development; in the male when there is no enlargement in the testes or scrotal changes by age 13-14 or if genital growth isn't complete within four years after the enlargement of the testicles begins
- **Pubertal growth spurt**: Is the general acceleration of growth seen in children, for males it is about 14 years (range can be 10 1/2-16) and for females it is about 12 years of age (range can be 9 1/2-14 1/2)
- **Physiologic leukorrhea**: An increase in normal vaginal discharge; occurs in early puberty
- **Thelarche**: Changes in the nipple and areolas area with development of a breast bud. One of the earliest signs of puberty.
- **Tanner Stages**
  - **Females**:
    - **Stage 1** (pre-pubertal): No signs of breast changes or development or any pubic hair growth
    - **Stage 2** (pubertal): Small breast buds with enlargement of the areola area, and dark, downy hair begins to appear in the genital area.
    - **Stage 3**: Increase of breast and areola areas with no separation of their contour, and development/growth of darker, coarser, and curly pubic hair spread over the female triangle.
    - **Stage 4**: Generally, a secondary mound occurs in the breast at the areola, and pubic hair is adult-like in distribution and appearance but not as thick.
    - **Stage 5**: Breasts are now mature and pubic hair is adult-like in type, amount and distribution.
  - **Males**:
    - **Stage 1** (pre-pubertal): No pubic hair or changes in the genital area
    - **Stage 2** (pubertal): Initial enlargement of the scrotum and testicles, reddening and textural changes in the scrotum with appearance of sparse, downy hair at the base of the penis
    - **Stage 3**: Initial enlargement of the penis (usually) in length with continued changes in the testicles and scrotum, hair darker, coarse, and curly in a larger area
    - **Stage 4**: Penis continues to grow in diameter with development of glans (larger and broader) and darkening of the scrotum; hair is more adult-like in appearance.
    - **Stage 5**: Penis, scrotum, and pubic hair is like that of an adult.

Safety

- More infant and children die of unintentional injuries than any other cause. The Agency for Healthcare Research and Quality has documented the following teaching guidelines for infants and young children:
  - Use a car safety seat at all times until your child weighs at least 40 pounds.

- Car seats must be properly secured in the back seat, preferably in the middle.
- Keep medication, cleaning solutions, and other dangerous substances in childproof containers, locked up and out of the reach of children.
- Use safety gates across stairways (top and bottom) and guards on windows above the first floor.
- Keep hot water heater temperature below 120° F.
- Keep unused electrical outlets covered with plastic guards.
- Provide constant supervision for babies using a baby walker. Block the access to stairways and to objects that can fall or cause burns.
- Keep objects and foods that cause choking away from the child (balloons, small toy parts, coins, hot dogs, peanuts and hard candies).
- Use fences that go all the way around pools and keep gates to pools locked.
- **Safety Guidelines for Parents of Children of All Ages** by the Agency for Healthcare Research and Quality:
    - Use smoke detectors in each home. Change the batteries every year, and once a month check to make sure that they work.
    - If there is a gun in the home, make sure the gun and ammunition are locked up separately and kept out of the reach of children.
    - Never drive after drinking alcohol.
    - Use car safety seat belts at all times.
    - Teach children traffic safety. Children under 9 years need supervision when crossing streets.
    - Teach children when and how to call 911.
    - Learn basic life-saving skills (CPR).
    - Post the phone number of poison control near the phone.

Children of all ages and their parents should be educated in the proper fit and need to wear bicycle helmets.

Critical Thinking Exercise: Nursing Management of a Child's Growth and Development

Situation: A 16-month-old is admitted to a pediatric unit for observation after removal of a small toy that she aspirated earlier that day. Select the appropriate response and explain why this is the best answer.

1. When assessing the child for the first time, what is the best approach to initiate contact?
    a. Call the child by name before picking her up.
    b. Reassure the child that you are not going to hurt her.
    c. Smile and get the child to talk by asking her to tell you her name.
    d. Talk softly to the child at her eye level while she is in her mother's arms.
    Correct answer: _____

    Rationale:

2. Which of the following is a priority teaching need for a family with a 16-month-old child?
    a. Toilet training guidelines
    b. Instructions for preschool readiness
    c. Information on home safety assessment
    d. Guidelines for weaning toddlers from bottles
    Correct answer: _____

    Rationale:

3. Matching: Match the age normally associated with the developmental task listed.

3-year-old	a. Fears body mutilation
4-year-old	b. Develops social smile
11-year-old	c. Anterior fontanel closes
5-month-old	d. Vocabulary of 850 words
9-year-old	e. Reads and writes
13-year-old	f. Begins picking up objects with fingers
8-month-old	g. Menarche begins
7-year-old	h. Begins to excel in sports
20-month-old	i. Pubic hair develops
13-month-old	j. Scribbles drawings

Respiratory System CHAPTER 8

Nursing Management of the Child with Oxygen Therapy

Key Points

- Oxygen is a medication that is used to treat actual or anticipated hypoxia.
- Oxygen therapy should be administered promptly in an emergency situation involving a child with respiratory distress or respiratory failure.
- Goals of collaborative management:
  - Restore and/or maintain adequate oxygen to meet tissue metabolic demands.
  - Prevent complications of oxygen therapy (oxygen toxicity and membrane irritation from drying effect).
- Important nursing diagnoses (actual or potential) are:
  - Risk for injury
  - Impaired gas exchange
  - Altered respiratory function
  - Anxiety and fear
  - Altered tissue perfusion
  - Altered tissue integrity
- **Key Terms/Concepts:** Hypoxia, hypoxemia, oxygen toxicity

Overview

Inhalation therapy refers to the interventions that involve changing the composition, volume, or pressure of inspired gases. These therapies include increasing the oxygen content of inspired gas (room air is FIO_2 21%) and using various methods for controlling the positive pressure for ventilation. Humidification is an important factor in the delivery of supplemental oxygen to prevent drying and subsequent injury to the breathing structures. The goal of inhalation therapy in supplying additional oxygen to the respiratory tract is to improve the availability of inspired oxygen for delivery to body tissues. The nurse assessing the oxygen delivery in children monitors oxygen saturation readings (which should exceed 95% in non-cardiac conditions) and blood gas results. However, the clinical assessment of the child is the most important indication of respiratory sufficiency.

Risk Factors

- Prematurity
- Congestive heart failure
- Cystic fibrosis
- Respiratory distress

- Status asthmaticus
- Trauma
- Pneumonia

Methods of O_2 Enrichment

Oxygen Delivery Device	Description	Flow Rate Considerations	Nursing Considerations
Oxygen Hood	Small plastic hood that fits over an infant's head to deliver oxygen	Minimum flow rate of 4-5 L/min to prevent CO_2 buildup. Delivers a higher level of oxygen than the incubator	Do not allow oxygen to blow directly onto infant's face. Prevent hood from rubbing infant's neck, chin or shoulders
Nasal Cannula	Oxygen is administered through plastic tube placed under nares.	1/16-6 L/min	Monitor nares for dry and irritated skin
Face Mask	Mask covers nose and mouth.	Minimum flow rate of 5-6L/min to prevent CO_2 buildup	Children fear masks. Fear of suffocation. Monitor face for skin breakdown
Oxygen Tent	Large plastic tent that fits over the crib or bed. Provides a humid environment. Can deliver oxygen	Flush tent with oxygen to raise oxygen level, then adjust flow meter to desired flow rate before placing child in tent.	Moisture accumulation on linens and walls of tent. Linens and child's clothing are changed frequently to keep child dry. Monitor temperature of child and inside tent. The cool environment can lead to hypothermia. Some children are frightened by the tent. Tent is a physical barrier between child and family. Tent is opened for the least amount of time and as infrequently as possible to help maintain oxygen level. Do not allow toys that may create a spark in the tent.

Nursing Management of the Child with Oxygen Therapy

Additional Devices For Oxygen Delivery

- **Blow-by oxygen**: Up to 100% delivered from reservoir end of a resuscitation bag
- **Incubator (Isolette)**: Free flow oxygen in the isolette provides low concentration of oxygen.
- **Mist tents**: Mist/oxygen tents are a good way to deliver the oxygen to active toddlers and older infants. Oxygen levels are difficult to maintain above 30% to 50% within the tent. It can get warm within the tent so a cooling method is used. The tent must be checked frequently for leaks/openings, and the care should be planned so the tent is opened for the least amount of time and as infrequently as possible. There is a danger of fire due to the high oxygen levels within the environment and potential sources of sparks should be eliminated. The nurse should check the child and the environment frequently for temperature and moisture levels.
- **Continuous positive airway pressure (CPAP)**: Delivered via nasal prongs, face mask, tracheotomy tube, or tracheal tube.
- **Conventional mechanical ventilation**
- **Nitric oxide (NO) Therapy**
- **High frequency oscillatory ventilation (HFOV)**
- **Extracorporeal membrane oxygenation (ECMO)**

Related Diagnostic Tests and Labs

- Pulse oximeter
- Arterial blood gas
- Exhaled CO_2 detector— end tidal CO_2 monitoring or colorimetric device
- Chest x-ray

Therapeutic Nursing Management

- Assess the need for supplemental oxygen based on the child's oxygen saturation, arterial blood gas (ABG), respiratory assessment (work of breathing, color, level of consciousness), and clinical status.
- Collaborate with the respiratory therapist and health care provider regarding the appropriate oxygen delivery device based on the child's age, condition, and oxygen needs.
- Flush incubators/hoods/tents with O_2.
- Ensure that a proper method of ventilation is provided to prevent the build up of CO_2.
- Monitor oxygen saturations on an ongoing basis. Assess ABGs as needed.
- Secure nasal cannula with a small piece of tape on the cheeks for active infants/children.
- Teach home oxygen use and safety prior to discharge if needed.
  - Teach appropriate use and care of oxygen equipment.
  - Avoid open flames, cigarettes, and matches; suggest the family post signs as needed.

- Have electrical appliances safety checked.

Complications

- Retinopathy of prematurity could result in retinal detachment in premature infants.
- Necrosis of nares and nasal septum if using nasal prongs
- Microbial growth if using a tent with high humidity
- Bronchopulmonary dysplasia
- Oxygen toxicity signs and symptoms: a dry, unproductive cough, substernal chest pain, stuffy nose, headache, sore throat, hypoventilation, nausea and vomiting, and fatigue

Critical Thinking Exercise: Nursing Management of the Child with Oxygen Therapy

Situation: A 13-month-old with bronchiolitis is receiving 1 L of oxygen via a nasal cannula. The nurse responds to an alarm of the pulse oximeter. Upon arrival at the room, the nurse notes that the pulse oximeter is reading 75%. The nurse also notes that the child is crying and kicking his legs. The pulse oximeter probe on the right foot has loosened. The oxygen cannula is lying beside the child in the bed.

1. What should the nurse do first? Why?

2. After the initial interventions, the child has the following signs: cyanosis, oxygen saturation level of 86%, moderate retractions, and cough. What actions should be taken next?

3. If this child does not improve, what alternative oxygen delivery devices may be needed? What are the challenges of using these devices with toddlers?

Respiratory System CHAPTER 9

Nursing Management of the Child with Cystic Fibrosis

Key Points

- Cystic fibrosis (CF) is an inherited disorder leading to multi-system organ involvement.
- Children with CF frequently experience problems with chronic lung infection and malnutrition due to blockages from thick mucous.
- Characteristic signs of CF are: large fatty stools; failure to thrive, with distended abdomen and thin arms and legs; pulmonary complications with cough; thick yellow-gray sputum, and abnormal lung sounds.
- Goals of collaborative management:
    - Maintain optimal pulmonary functioning and prevent complications from infection.
    - Maintain adequate nutritional status and prevent failure to thrive.
    - Monitor for signs of complications associated with CF.
    - Promptly intervene with associated pathophysiology.
    - Support optimal growth, development, and coping with a chronic illness.
    - Prevent secondary complications.
- Important nursing diagnoses (actual or potential) are:
    - Ineffective airway clearance
    - Ineffective breathing pattern
    - Altered nutrition: Less than body requirements
    - Fluid volume deficit
    - Altered growth and development
    - Altered protection
    - Activity intolerance
    - Risk for injury
    - Powerlessness and hopelessness
    - Ineffective family coping
    - Caregiver role strain
    - Impaired home maintenance management
- **Key Terms/Concepts:** Autosomal recessive, bronchiole obstruction, hyperinflation, pulmonary infection, pancreatic enzymes, fat soluble vitamins, failure to thrive, meconium ileus, and steatorrhea.

Nursing Management of the Child with Cystic Fibrosis

Overview

Cystic fibrosis (CF) is an inherited autosomal recessive disorder due to mutation of the CF gene on chromosome 7. This multi-system disease involves increased viscosity of mucous causing obstruction of small passageways. The bronchioles, pancreas, small intestine, and bile ducts are most frequently affected. The mucus accumulation in the lungs leads to hyperinflation and chronic pulmonary infection with eventual lung damage. The disturbed function of the pancreatic enzymes leads to impaired digestion and absorption of nutrients. Biliary obstruction and fibrosis can occur. Skeletal maturation and sexual development are delayed. The incidence is 1 in 3500 live births. Caucasians are most frequently affected. The gene associated with CF, identified in 1989, makes it possible to identify carriers of the disease. Recent advances in diagnosis and treatment have led to improved quality of life and longer survival rates. Currently, most children with CF are expected to live into young-to-middle adulthood. Frequent illness and need for home care affect family roles and functioning.

This is particularly an issue for families with more than one child with cystic fibrosis. Physiological changes and frequent hospitalization can cause disruption of normal growth and development.

Risk Factors

- Family member with CF (autosomal-recessive trait)
- Increased incidence of genetic carriers in Caucasian population

Signs and Symptoms

System	Pathophysiology	Symptoms
Lungs	<ul><li>Bronchial obstruction</li><li>Pneumonia</li><li>Obstructive emphysema</li><li>Atelectasis</li></ul>	<ul><li>Thick mucous</li><li>Chronic cough</li><li>Dyspnea</li><li>Wheezing</li><li>Cyanosis</li><li>Difficulty with expiration</li><li>Irritability and/or fatigue</li><li>Positive sputum cultures</li><li>Fever</li><li>Barrel-shaped chest</li><li>Cor pulmonale</li><li>Clubbing of fingers and toes</li></ul>
Gastrointestinal Tract/Pancreas/Nutrition	<ul><li>Pancreatic duct blockage</li><li>Pancreatic degeneration</li><li>Loss of pancreatic enzyme secretion</li><li>Impaired absorption of fats, proteins, and to a limited degree, carbohydrates</li><li>Failure to thrive</li></ul>	<ul><li>Loose stools (large, fatty, foul-smelling: steatorrhea)</li><li>Impaired digestion</li><li>Failure to gain weight</li><li>Delayed growth patterns</li><li>Distended abdomen</li><li>Thin arms and legs</li><li>Buttocks and thighs atrophy</li></ul>

System	Pathophysiology	Symptoms
Gastrointestinal Tract: Newborn Infant	• Meconium ileus (may be first indication in the newborn)	• Abdominal distention • Failure to pass stool • Vomiting • Rapid deterioration
Integumentary System	• Increased sodium and chloride in sweat glands	• Sweat, tears, and saliva abnormally salty • Parent report of salty taste when kissing their baby • Positive sweat chloride test
Growth and Reproduction	• Growth delay • Infertility due to mucous blockage	• Delayed puberty • Viscous cervical mucous (female) • Decreased or absent sperm count (male)

Diagnostic Tests and Labs

- History and physical
- Abnormally high sweat chloride levels (2 positive tests)
- DNA testing
- Chest x-ray
- Abdominal x-rays
- Pulmonary function tests
- Stool analysis
- Pancreatic function tests
- Sputum cultures and white blood cell count (pneumonia)

Therapeutic Nursing Management

- Provide oral pancreatic enzyme replacement and fat-soluble vitamins (A, D, E, and K).
- Control pulmonary infection.
- Perform routine postural drainage and percussion.
- Administer intermittent aerosol therapy.
- Administer oxygen therapy with humidity as needed.
- Encourage breathing exercises.
- Maintain nutrition: high calorie, high protein, moderate fats, and increased salt.
- Provide nutritional supplements and enteral nutrition via gastrostomy or nasogastric tube as indicated.
- Protect the skin: proper skin care, frequent position changes, good oral hygiene.
- Provide emotional support to child and family.
- Support normal growth and development.

- Provide home care and ongoing support instructions:
  - Teach family to recognize signs of infection, dehydration, and nutritional deficiency.
  - Instruct child and family members to perform postural drainage and percussion, aerosol breathing treatments, medication administration, and nutritional support at home.
  - Instruct family in the proper use of vascular access devices and/or feeding tubes.
  - Provide information regarding support resources for children and families with CF (national and local organizations, case manager, home health agency, etc.).

Pharmacology

- Pancreatic enzymes: Pancrease
- Supplementary vitamins
- Antibiotics
  - Prophylactic and/or to fight infection
  - Oral, inhaled, intravenous
- Bronchodilators
  - Meter-dose inhalers
  - Hand-held nebulizer
- Pulmozyme (recombinant human deoxyribonuclease)
- May receive routine immunizations

Complications

- Rectal prolapse
- Peptic ulcer
- Intestinal obstruction
- Hepatic dysfunction
- Infertility
- Malnutrition
- Retinal hemorrhage
- Pulmonary fibrosis
- Cor pulmonale
- Osteoporosis
- Death

Critical Thinking Exercise: Nursing Management of the Child with Cystic Fibrosis

Situation: A 10-month-old male infant with a neonatal history including meconium plug is admitted with respiratory difficulty, recurrent bronchitis, and poor weight gain. The health care provider suggests a potential diagnosis of cystic fibrosis.

1. What additional history questions should the nurse ask the family?

2. What are the most important interventions for the infant and family at this time?

Respiratory System CHAPTER 10

Nursing Management of the Child with Asthma

Key Points

- Asthma is the most common cause of chronic illness in children.
- "Asthma triggers" such as allergens, airway irritants, stress, or acute illness frequently precipitate exacerbation of asthma.
- Airway obstruction occurs from airway edema, bronchospasm, and mucous thickening.
- Wheezing, air trapping, and lung hyperinflation results from narrowed airways.
- Goals of collaborative management:
  - Maintain long-term control and prevent acute asthmatic exacerbations.
  - Restore and/or maintain adequate gas exchange (O2, CO2) during exacerbation.
  - Prevent secondary complications.
- Important nursing diagnoses (actual or potential) are:
  - Ineffective airway clearance related to tracheobronchial secretions, spasms of the bronchi and bronchioles, and ineffective coughs
  - Gas exchange, impaired, related to decreased functional lung tissue secondary to fibrotic, non-ventilated areas of lung parenchyma
  - Risk for fluid volume deficit related to inadequate fluid intake secondary to difficulty in breathing or increased insensible water losses from rapid respiration
  - Activity intolerance
  - Risk for injury
  - Anxiety related to air hunger
  - Ineffective family coping
  - Knowledge deficit
  - Anxiety related to fear of suffocation, dying, or recurrence
  - Risk of infection related to suboptimal nutrition and or stasis of respiratory secretions
- **Key Terms/Concepts:** Allergy, chemical mediators, respiratory distress, airway clearing, bronchospasm, blood gas exchange, and respiratory failure

Overview

Asthma is a reactive airway disease resulting in obstruction of the large and small airways. Airway hyper-responsiveness and bronchospasm are associated with chemical mediators (acetylcholine, prostaglandins, and histamine) and various triggering agents. These may be related to both allergic and nonallergic etiology.

> Thickening of the tracheobronchial mucosa and alterations of the bronchial epithelial integrity cause airway edema. Accumulation of thick secretions results in mucous plugging. Airway narrowing and obstruction results in alveolar air trapping. Infants and young children have relatively narrow airways with poor elastic recoil of the airways resulting in increased expiratory obstruction.
>
> Increased work of breathing occurs because of the increased effort required to move air through narrowed airways. Respiratory muscle fatigue occurs from increased energy expenditure, poor diaphragm support, and ineffective airway clearing.
>
> Approximately 50% of the new cases of asthma are diagnosed before 1 year of age and 80% before 5 years of age. Generally, the younger the child is at the onset of symptoms and the more severe the symptoms, the greater the chance that asthma will persist. Current data has shown an increasing incidence of acute exacerbation, hospitalizations and asthma-related death in children.

Risk Factors

- Family history
- Chronic illness (prematurity, bronchopulmonary dysplasia, recurrent pneumonia)
- Exacerbation of symptoms increases with exposure to "asthma triggers"
  - Allergens (pollen, foods, dust, mold, animal dander)
  - Airway irritants (cigarette smoke, cold air, humidity, dust, chemicals)
  - Medications
  - Respiratory tract infections
  - Overexertion
  - Stress/emotional distress

Signs and Symptoms

- Abrupt onset after exposure to allergen or over a period of days
- Initially a tight, non-productive cough
- Expiratory wheezing
- Respiratory distress (dyspnea, tachypnea, retractions, accessory muscle use, pallor)
- Tachycardia
- Difficulty talking
- Lethargy progressing to decreased LOC
- Slowed capillary refill

Nursing Management of the Child with Asthma

Asthma Symptoms

	Mild	Moderate	Severe
Respiratory Effort	No accessory muscle use or mild intercostals retractions	Moderate intercostal and supraclavicular retractions, additional accessory muscle use	Severe intercostal, tracheal retractions, nasal flaring, or decreased respiratory effort
Speech Patterns	Speaking in complete sentences	Speaking in short panting phrases	Speaking only single words or no speech
Respiratory Rate	Mild to moderate tachypnea	Moderate tachypnea	Severe tachypnea, apnea
Color	Pink	Pale (may have flushing)	Cyanotic, dusky, mottled, ashen
Breath Sounds	Expiratory wheeze, diffuse coarseness	Increased expiratory wheeze, inspiratory wheeze	Decreased over all lung fields (decreased wheezing with severe distress is an ominous sign)
LOC	Alert, restless	Irritable, agitated, combative, (air hunger)	Lethargic, somnolent, indifferent to painful stimulation
Positioning	Relaxed in a recumbent position	Upright, tripod, refusing to lie down	Passive
Oxygen Saturation	>95% in room air	90%-95% in room air	<90% in room air
PaCO$_2$	<35-40 mmHg (normal to low)	40-65 mmHg	>65 mmHg
PaO$_2$	70-100 (normal)	<70 on room air	<70 on 40% oxygen
pH	Elevated	7.35-7.45 (normal)	Decreased
Blood Gas Analysis	Mild respiratory alkalosis	Physiologic	Respiratory and metabolic acidosis
Peak Flow Expiratory Rate	70%-90% of predicted or personal best	50%-70% of predicted or personal best	<50% of predicted or personal best

Diagnostic Tests and Lab

- Peak flow monitoring (peak flow meter)
- Pulmonary function tests
- Oxygen saturation
- Arterial blood gases
- Allergy skin testing (IgE)
- Radio allegro sorbet test (RAST)
- Chest x-ray
- CBC (White blood cell count)

Therapeutic Nursing Management

- Acute exacerbation:
    - Closely monitor vital signs, breath sounds, and work of breathing, oxygen saturation, and level of consciousness.
    - Position upright (position of comfort).
    - Administer bronchodilators and monitor for effectiveness.
    - Administer oxygen.
    - Administer intravenous steroids.
    - Administer antibiotics as ordered.
    - Maintain hydration with intravenous fluids and/or by encouraging clear, oral fluids (if respiratory distress is not severe).
    - Monitor intake and output, assess for dehydration.
    - Provide emotional support to child and family.
- Long-term control:
    - Teach child and family appropriate use of medications and metered-dose inhaler.
    - Assist child in identifying and avoiding factors that trigger exacerbations.
    - Teach family treatment plan based on peak expiratory flow rates. Plan consists of three color-coded zones. Each zone lists expected peak flow rate, symptoms and medications:
        - Green zone is 80%-100% of expected peak flow rate. This zone is when the child is generally symptom free.
        - Yellow zone is 50%-80% of expected peak flow rate. This zone indicates an asthma attack may be developing.
        - Red zone is below 50% of expected peak flow rate. The child is experiencing an asthma exacerbation. Call the health care practitioner.

Pharmacology

- Bronchodilators
    - Albuterol (Proventil/Ventolin)
    - Isoetharine (Bronkosol); levalbuterol (Xopenex)-neb solution only
    - Metaproterenol (Alupent/Metaprel)
    - Terbutaline (Brethine)
    - Pirbuterol (Maxair)
    - Theophylline (Aminophylline)
    - Mast Cell Stabilizer
    - Cromolyn sodium (Intal)
    - Nedocromil
- Corticosteroids
    - Beclomethasone
    - Prednisone (Solu-Cortef); Ora-pred (Prelone) in liquid form
    - Methylprednisolone (Solu-Medrol)

- Leukotriene modifiers-montelukast sodium (Singulair)
- Anticholinergics
- Epinephrine for acute attacks
- Skin test for allergens

Complications

- Status asthmaticus
- Atelectasis
- Pneumothorax
- Dehydration
- Respiratory failure
- Respiratory arrest
- Cardiopulmonary disease (chronic bronchitis, pneumonia, emphysema, Cor pulmonale)
- Death

Critical Thinking Exercise: Nursing Management of the Child with Asthma

Situation: A 6-year-old boy is admitted into the emergency department because of dyspnea, coughing, and wheezing. The boy states that he feels tightness in his chest. Physical findings include pallor with tachypnea and tachycardia.

1. Which health information is most important for the nurse to collect from the parents?

Situation: The child is given a bronchodilator and a metered dose inhaler.

2. Assuming that this is the child's first episode of asthma, prioritize the discharge instructions. (1 is most important).

Instruction	Priority
Avoid milk/milk products.	
Drink large amounts of water.	
The child should trigger the inhaler as he breathes in.	
Bronchodilators can cause tachycardia and restlessness.	
Asthma decreases the size of the airway causing distress.	
If an attack occurs at home, the child should sit or stand.	
Attacks of asthma can be prevented by avoiding environmental and emotional triggers.	

3. Which of the following needs of the child in the case study should be addressed first? Which need should be addressed next?
    a. Difficulty breathing
    b. Anxiety
    c. Risk for potential adverse reaction to medications

Respiratory System **CHAPTER 11**

Nursing Management of the Child with Tonsillitis and Tonsillectomy

> **Key Points**
>
> - Tonsils are lymphatic tissue that act as a filter to protect from invading organisms.
> - Viral or bacterial organisms can cause tonsillitis.
> - Enlarged or infected tonsils can lead to breathing, eating, sleeping, and hearing difficulties.
> - Tonsillectomy and adenoidectomy may be indicated with recurrent infection and/or sleeping difficulties.
> - Goals of collaborative management:
>   - Provide symptomatic support with tonsillitis.
>   - Prevent complications associated with a tonsillectomy.
> - Important nursing diagnoses (actual or potential) are:
>   - Altered breathing pattern related to anesthesia and accumulation of secretions
>   - Ineffective airway clearance related to edema, collection of blood in oropharynx, vomiting, and sedation
>   - Risk of infection
>   - Fluid volume deficit related to blood loss of the highly vascular site or related to decreased fluid intake resulting from throat pain and blood swallowing
>   - Nutrition: Less than body requirements related to loss of appetite, sore throat, and difficulty swallowing
>   - Anxiety and fear
>   - Pain related to surgery procedure or edema
> - **Key Terms/Concepts:** Nasopharynx, adenoiditis, peritonsillar abscess, obstructive apnea, tonsillitis, adenoidectomy

Overview

The tonsils are masses of lymphatic tissue located in the pharyngeal cavity. Their function is to filter and protect the respiratory and alimentary tracts from the invasion of pathogenic organisms. They may also have a role in the formation of antibodies to protect the upper respiratory system from infection. Tonsillitis is an inflammation or infection of the 2 palatine tonsils. The incidence peaks at 4-7 years (organism exposure with preschool). Peritonsillar abscess occurs in older children and adolescents. Adenoiditis is an inflammation or infection of the adenoids (located above tonsils on posterior wall of nasopharynx).

Tonsillectomy may be indicated with repeated tonsillitis, airway obstruction, sleep apnea, and/or chronic feeding difficulty. Adenoidectomy may be indicated with hypertrophied adenoids and obstructed nasal breathing. Contraindications for a tonsillectomy include: cleft palate, acute infection at the time of surgery, and bleeding disorders.

Risk Factors

- Chronic respiratory tract infections
- Chronic illness
- Large tonsils and/or adenoids

Signs and Symptoms

- Tonsillitis
    - Tonsillar inflammation (redness with edema)
    - Mouth odor
    - Sore throat, difficulty swallowing
    - Mouth breathing
    - Bright red enlarged tonsils, "kissing tonsils," exudates on tonsils
    - Snoring, sleep apnea
    - Fever
    - Nasal qualities in the voice
    - Otitis media, hearing difficulty
- Peritonsillar Abscess
    - Displaced uvula
    - Refusal to talk or drink due to pain
- Adenoiditis
    - Nasal Speech
    - Enlarged glands

Diagnostic Tests and Labs

- History and physical
- CBC
- Throat culture
- Rapid strep screen
- Sleep apnea diagnostic test
- Preoperative lab
- Coagulation studies

Therapeutic Nursing Management

- Tonsillitis (care most frequently provided at home by family)
    - Provide comfort measures for sore throat (gargle warm salt water, throat sprays, hot tea, popsicles, etc.).
    - Administer antipyretics and cooling measures for fever.
    - Administer antibiotics when indicated.

- Encourage fluid intake and monitor hydration status.
- Assess for airway complications related to enlarged tonsils.
- Postoperative care after tonsillectomy
  - Position on side to facilitate drainage.
  - Assess frequently for signs of bleeding, the most common postoperative complication of tonsillectomy (frequent swallowing, throat clearing, restlessness, bright red emesis, tachycardia, and pallor).
  - Assess airway and vital signs frequently.
  - Monitor for breathing difficulty related to oral secretions, edema or bleeding.
  - Provide ice collar.
  - Provide analgesics.
  - Discourage cough, throat clearing and nose blowing (protect surgical site).
  - Encourage clear liquids and fluids after gag reflex returns (avoid red colored liquids and milk based foods initially).
  - Advance diet with soft, bland foods.
  - Provide discharge instructions regarding bleeding precautions, assessment and actions; pain assessment, medication and comfort measures; diet and fluid recommendations, and when to call the health care provider (breathing difficulty, bleeding, lack of oral intake, signs of infection, etc.).

Pharmacology

- Acetaminophen with or without codeine

Complications

- Otitis, difficulty hearing
- Airway obstruction
- Sleep apnea
- Poor concentration and/or school performance (from obstructive apnea and sleep deprivation)
- Postoperative hemorrhage
- Dehydration
- Wound Infection

Critical Thinking Exercise: Nursing Management of the Child with Tonsillitis and Tonsillectomy

1. Which of the following children is most likely to receive a tonsillectomy?
   a. 4-year-old with viral adenoiditis with nasal speech
   b. 2-year-old with bronchopulmonary dysplasia and gastroesophageal reflux
   c. 5-year-old with obstructive sleep apnea and frequent sore throats
   d. 1-year-old with recurrent otitis media and bronchiolitis

   Correct answer:

2. List three indications for tonsillectomy in children.

3. Identify each of the following nursing intervention as Appropriate or Not Appropriate when caring postoperatively for a child who has just tonsillectomy and explain your responses.
   _____ Placing in a side-lying position
   _____ Suctioning of the oropharynx routinely
   _____ Providing bright colored red Jell-O
   _____ Providing warm milk and cookies
   _____ Administer pain medication

4. Identify the earliest sign of hemorrhage in a child who has had a tonsillectomy.
   a. Labored breathing and increased respiratory rate
   b. Decreased heart rate
   c. Frequent throat clearing with restlessness
   d. Dark brown emesis
   e. Pallor

   Correct answer:

   Rationale:

Respiratory System CHAPTER 12

Nursing Management of Common Respiratory Illnesses in Children

> **Key Points**
>
> - Upper respiratory problems include those affecting the respiratory tract from the nose to the larynx (nose, sinuses, pharynx, glottis, epiglottis, and larynx).
> - Lower respiratory problems include those that affect the respiratory tract from the trachea to the alveoli (trachea, main stem bronchi (2), lobar, segmental and sub-segmental bronchi, bronchioles, alveolar ducts, alveoli, and lungs).
> - Respiratory infections are the most common cause of acute illness in children.
> - The incidence of respiratory infections in children remains high up to the age of 5 years.
> - After 5 years of age the frequency of respiratory infections decreases.
>   - Young children are at risk for respiratory infections due to:
>   - Decreased surface area for gas exchange
>   - Alveoli continue to bud until 8 years of age.
>   - Disproportionately small airways compared to adult
>   - Airways are easily obstructed with mucous or edema.
>   - Young infants are obligate nose breathers
>   - Airway cartilage is easily compressible.
>   - Sternal retractions
>   - Reduction in diameter of airway during respiratory distress
>   - Primary muscle of respiration for infants and young children is the diaphragm.
> - Respiratory infections in children are generally more common in the winter and spring; exceptions include mycoplasma infections, which occur at a higher frequency in fall and early winter.
> - Younger children (ages 2 months to 3 years) have a more serious reaction to respiratory illness, often presenting with tachypnea and more generalized symptoms than older children.
> - Goals of collaborative management:
>   - Maintain current level of participation in ADLs.
>   - Conserve energy.
>   - Verbalize the need for rest.
>   - Understand the basic disease process and care.
>   - Maintain urine output, normal vital signs, and skin turgor.
>   - Educate the parent(s)/family on the importance and means to prevent fluid loss.
>   - Prevent dehydration related to hyperthermia.

- Maintain or improve gas exchange, respiratory effort, and lung sounds.
- Teach effective coughing technique.
- Identify ways to maintain respiratory secretion removal.
- Identify and understand the significance of change in sputum.
- Understand activities that inhibit effective airway clearing.
- Maintain adequate caloric intake with normal feeding.
- Remain free of symptoms of superinfection.
- Reduce spread of the infection to other clients, staff, and parent(s)/family.
- Identify signs and symptoms of infection.
- Practice good hand hygiene.
- Important North American Nursing Diagnosis Association (NANDA) nursing diagnosis:
    - Activity intolerance
    - Anxiety
    - Fluid volume deficit
    - Hyperthermia
    - Nutrition imbalance: Less than body requirements
    - Impaired gas exchange, airway clearance, and/or breathing pattern
    - Aspiration risk
    - Infection: Risk for contamination to others
    - Infection: Risk for superinfections
    - Risk for airway obstruction

Upper Airway Illnesses

Common Cold

The common cold is an upper respiratory infection (URI) or acute nasopharyngitis. It is generally a self-limiting viral illness lasting from seven to ten days.

Signs and Symptoms

- **3 months to 3 years**
    - Fever
    - Nasal inflammation
    - Rhinorrhea
    - Decreased appetite
    - Irritability
    - Lethargy
- **Older children**
    - Dry throat
    - Sneezing
    - Cough
    - Nasal inflammation
    - Nasal discharge
    - Nasal qualities to the voice

Treatment
- Home management
- Antipyretics (most commonly acetaminophen)
- Rest
- Decongestants (after 6 months of age)
- Antitussives (dextromethorphan)
- Encourage fluids
- Follow up with primary care provider

Strep Throat

Caused by Group A beta-hemolytic streptococcus (GABHS) and is a common URI in children. The illness in and of itself is self-limiting. As a healthcare provider prevention of the complications of strep, namely rheumatic fever and acute glomerulonephritis are the primary goal of treatment. Education on the necessity of completing the ordered antibiotics is a major role of the nurse.

Signs and Symptoms
- Inflamed throat
- Exudates in the throat (present in up to 80% of the cases)
- Headache
- Fever
- Abdominal pain
- Cervical lymphadenopathy
- Pain in the throat increased with swallowing
- Difficulty swallowing
- Truncal, axillary and perineal rash

Diagnostic Tests
- Rapid strep testing done initially
- Throat culture for GABHS
- Antibody titer (antistreptolysin O)

Treatment
- Amoxicillin
- Omnicef

Complications
- Rheumatic Fever
- Acute Glomerulonephritis

Acute Epiglottitis

Considered a medical emergency due to the speed with which it develops and progresses. The major concern is for a blockage of the airway due to swollen epiglottis. An examination with a tongue blade or a throat culture is contraindicated in this situation unless there are the emergency personnel and equipment available to intubate and/or perform tracheotomy. This illness is generally caused by haemophilus influenzae. The incidence of epiglottitis caused by haemophilus influenzae has substantially declined due to use of the Hib vaccine.

Signs and Symptoms
- The Four D's
    - Dysphonia (muffled voice)
    - Dysphagia (difficulty swallowing)
    - Drooling
    - Distress
- Child sits in the tripod position to ease the work of breathing
    - Chin pointed out
    - Mouth open
- Inspiratory stridor
- Sore throat
- High fever
- Tongue protrusion
- Elevated pulse and respiration
- Restlessness
- Irritability
- Retractions

Diagnostic Tests
- Lateral neck film

Treatment
- Maintain an upright position for the comfort of the client and to ease breathing
- Antibiotics for 7 to 10 days
- Rest
- Encourage fluids if child can safely swallow
- Monitor IV for rate of flow and signs and symptoms of infiltration
- Intubation or tracheostomy may be necessary in very severe cases

Complications
- Respiratory distress
- Airway obstruction

Acute Laryngitis

When acute laryngitis is secondary to viral infection, hoarseness is often the only symptom. Laryngitis may follow a URI or may be accompanied by the symptoms of a URI. This illness is self-limiting.

Acute Laryngotracheobronchitis

Acute Laryngotracheobronchitis (LTB) is the most common croup syndrome that requires hospitalization. It may not be severe enough to require hospitalization but does so more commonly than the other croup syndromes.

Signs and Symptoms
- Low grade fever
- URI symptoms
- Restlessness
- Hoarseness
- Barky cough (sounds like a seal bark) - nonproductive
- Respiratory distress
- Inspiratory stridor
- Retractions

Treatment
- Humidified air
- Encourage fluids (if there is no respiratory distress)
- IV fluids (if the client is unable to tolerate oral fluids)
- Nebulized epinephrine (racemic epinephrine)
- Corticosteroids

Acute Spasmodic Laryngitis

Acute spasmodic laryngitis is characterized by spasmodic episodes of laryngeal tightening. This generally occurs at night and most often in children 1 - 3 years of age. Some children are seemingly predisposed to the illness. Generally, this is a self-limiting illness that is treated at home. Many times the condition will clear when the parents take the child outside in the cool air while transporting them to the care provider.

Signs and Symptoms
- Classic barky cough
- Restlessness
- Recurrences
- Difficulty breathing
- Hoarseness of the voice

Treatment
- Cool mist
- Nebulized epinephrine (racemic epinephrine) in more severe cases
- Corticosteroids

Bacterial Tracheitis

Bacterial tracheitis is an infection of the lining of the trachea. This is most often seen in children from 1 month to 6 years of age. The illness presents with the symptoms of both croup and epiglottis. The hallmark symptom of this disease is thick, purulent drainage from the trachea (into the throat), which can obstruct the airway and cause respiratory distress.

Treatment
- Humidified oxygen
- Antipyretics

- Antibiotics
- Suctioning (the primary treatment to prevent obstruction of the throat with the thick drainage)
- Intubation may be necessary in severe cases

Lower Respiratory Problems

Bronchitis

Bronchitis is generally associated with a URI and results in a persistent cough as a result of the inflammation of the trachea and bronchi. This illness is generally self-limiting, requiring only symptomatic treatment to include: analgesics, antipyretics, humidified air and antitussives.

Bronchiolitis

Caused, in up to 75% of the cases, by respiratory syncytial virus (RSV), and rarely occurs in children over 2 years of age. RSV occurs most often in the winter and spring and can be of a very serious nature. The virus literally causes cells to fuse with the infected cells creating a mass and a loss of the cilia in those cells. There are increased amounts of mucus and exudates that prevent expiration of air. This causes overinflation of the lungs (emphysema). Mucous plugs may obstruct the bronchioles and cause collapse of the lung tissue. Maintaining the airways through suctioning of the copious amounts of mucus and exudates is a priority to prevent overinflation of the lungs. RSV is transmitted by direct contact or inhalation of the large infected droplets expired by a contagious sufferer. The incubation period of RSV is 4 to 8 days from exposure to the first symptoms. The virus may be spread from the infant for about 12 days. RSV occurs most frequently in 2-5 month-old infants but continues to be severe in those up to 2 years of age and occurs more frequently in males. Unfortunately, the younger the child, generally, the more severe the symptoms of this illness are, due to the smaller airways. A large percentage of infants that contract bronchiolitis have reactive airway disease later in their lives.

Signs and Symptoms

- Rhinorrhea (lasting several days)
- Symptoms of URI
- Fever (about 102° F)
- Decreased or lack of appetite
- Respiratory distress
- Cough
- Wheeze (in some)
- Increased respiratory rate
- Nasal flaring
- Retractions
- Cyanosis
- Rhonchi, fine crackles, wheezes

Diagnostic Tests

- CBC with differential
- Arterial blood gases (ABGs)

- Pulse oximetry
- Bacterial cultures (to determine cause)
- Immunofluorescence analysis of nasal swab (for RSV)
- Chest x-ray (for air trapping, overinflation from inflammation or mucous plugs)

Treatment
- Cool, oxygenated mist (for severely ill)
- Nebulizer treatments-albuterol or levalbuterol
- IV hydration
- Tube feeding if the child is unable to eat
- Prop up the head of the child/infant.
- Observe and maintain the airway for patency.
- Rest
- Limit treatment disturbances to ensure rest.
- Comfort measures to decrease crying and restlessness
- Lubricate oral mucosa and lips to decrease irritation from mouth breathing and suctioning (primary care provider's order may be required).
- Private room or room with other RSV-infected children
- Good hand washing by family and staff
- Limit the number of providers to limit the potential for spread of the illness.
- Provide emotional and educational support to the parent(s) and family.
- Use of antiviral drugs in even the very severely ill infant or child is controversial.
- Antipyretics (generally acetaminophen)
- Prevention of RSV bronchiolitis in high-risk children under 24-months-of-age
  - Palivizumab (Synagis) is a monoclonal antibody and is the preferred product
  - RSV-IGIV (RSV immune globulin)

Allergic Rhinitis

Allergic Rhinitis is also known as "hayfever" or as "allergies," and is usually a seasonal reaction to airborne allergens. The seasonal type of allergic rhinitis (most often symptomatic in the fall and/or spring) is usually a reaction to pollens and, in most cases, takes a client a season or two to become sensitized to the allergen. Year-round (also known as perennial or chronic) allergies are caused by household pollutants that are inhaled (feathers, dust, mold, and dander). While young children can have allergic rhinitis, it is most common in the adolescent and post-adolescent period.

Allergen: An antigen that stimulants immunoglobulin E (IgE) release by the beta lymphocytes. IgE-specific antigens bind to the basophiles and mast cells triggering release of histamine, prostaglandins, leukotrienes, and cytokines.

Anaphylaxis is the most severe form of type I hypersensitivity reaction. This is a life-threatening response to the exposure to an allergen. Common allergens include: antibiotics, opiates, blood, local anesthetics, allergen extracts, shellfish, eggs, nuts, berries, preservatives, snake venom, fire ants, bees, wasps and hornets. The initial symptom is the client's sense of anxiety, commonly referred as to a feeling of "impending doom." This is followed by hives and itching, erythema, angioedema (swelling of the eyes, lips, or tongue), and bronchospasm with mucosal edema and increased mucus production leading to respiratory distress. Respiratory failure can quickly follow the respiratory distress; lifesaving interventions must be immediate.

Histamine is a vasoactive amine, which causes vasodilation, mucosal edema (nasal stuffiness), mucus production (rhinorrhea), itching, and erythema.

Signs and Symptoms
- Watery rhinorrhea
- Nasal stuffiness/congestion
- Sneezing
- Itching of the nose, eyes, pharynx
- Itchy watery, eyes
- Nasal quality to the voice
- Headache or pressure over sinuses
- Dry, scratchy throat (from post-nasal drip)
- Presence of the "allergic salute" (rubbing of the nose)
- "Allergic Shiners" dark circles under the eyes
- Snoring while sleeping and mouth open for breathing
- Symptoms associated with poor sleep: decreased performance in school, fatigue, and malaise
- Upper respiratory infection (can also be present)

Diagnostic Tests and Lab
- Nasal smear for eosinophils
- Blood test for total IgE and elevated eosinophils
- Phadiatop (tests for allergies to a group of common allergens through the presence of IgE antibodies in the blood)
- Radioallergosorbent tests (RAST): Used to determine the level of specific IgE antibodies to specific allergens
- Skin testing is the most common type of allergy testing, first by scratch or pinprick. The results are positive if a wheal develops within 20 minutes. Injection of a specific allergen (intradermally - at up to 3 dilutions) is used for a suspected allergy non-reactive to scratch/prick testing. A reaction does not always indicate the presence of an allergy that will be seen clinically. The child's medication history must be taken since antihistamine and corticosteroid protection lasts for 5 days. These medications should be discontinued prior to testing to prevent interference with the results. Nasal anti-inflammatory sprays may be continued.

Treatment
- Immunotherapy (hyposensitization or desensitization to the allergen through injection of diluted extracts of the specific allergen) usually takes 4-8 months with maintenance injections every 3-4 weeks for up to another 5 years.

- Antihistamines (H1 receptor antagonists for children over 12 years of age: Benadryl [diphenhydramine], Chlor-Trimeton [chlorpheniramine], Hismanal [astemizole])
- Antihistamines that are less sedating include; Claritin [loratadine], Zyrtec [cetirizine hydrochloride] and Allegra [fexofenadine hydrochloride])
- Adrenergic and anticholinergic drugs (nasal decongestants: pseudoephedrine, phenylpropanolamine, ephedrine, phenylephrine)
- Mast cell stabilizers (cromolyn sodium [NasalCrom])
- Nasal steroids (to decrease inflammatory and immune response: Beconase (beclomethasone), Flonase [fluticasone]), Nasonex (mometasone), Rhinocort (budesonide)
- Avoidance therapy: If possible, avoid the known allergen. Specific foods or drugs may be easy to avoid. Air conditioning, covering ducts, pillows and mattresses with plastic or mesh, removing carpet, cloth curtains, and upholstered furniture, plus frequent clipping and bathing of pets may eliminate some airborne exposures. May need to wash hair nightly to remove pollen during peak season.
- Skin testing and immunotherapy are generally considered safe but can illicit an anaphylactic reaction. It is recommended that clients remain in the office for 20 minutes after testing or injection.
- Epi Pen should be carried at all times for those with a history of anaphylactic reaction.
- Medical alert bracelet/necklace if a severe allergy.

Critical Thinking Exercise: Nursing Management of Common Respiratory Illnesses in Children

Situation: A pediatric nurse is working at a community walk-in clinic. It is one of the most common months for respiratory infections and the nurse assesses a variety of respiratory conditions.

1. Match the symptoms on the left with the illness on the right.

___ Hoarseness of the voice with no associated symptoms	a. Allergic Rhinitis
___ Exudates in the throat, headache, fever, painful swallowing	b. Epiglottis
___ Body aches and chills, nasal discharge and inflammation, cough	c. Anaphylaxis
___ Tonsillar edema and inflammation, difficulty swallowing	d. Common Cold
___ High fever, protrusive tongue, drooling	e. Tonsillitis
___ Watery eyes and nose, headache, itching of eyes, nose, and pharynx	f. Laryngitis
___ Hives, itching, swelling of eyes, lips and tongue, respiratory distress	g. Strep Throat

2. What is the most common cause of bronchiolitis?

3. Who is at greatest risk of severe illness with respiratory syncytial virus (RSV)?

4. What diagnostic test is definitive for RSV?

Cardiovascular System/Blood Disorders CHAPTER 13

Nursing Management of the Child with Congenital Heart Disease

> **Key Points**
>
> - Congenital heart disease (CHD) is the most common cardiac problem in children.
> - Anatomic defects of the heart prevent the proper flow of blood to the lungs and/or body.
> - Children with symptomatic CHD have chronic problems related to decreased cardiac output, congestive heart failure, hypoxia and cardiac rhythm disturbances.
> - Goals of collaborative management:
>   - Support maximal growth and nutrition.
>   - Reduce the cardiac workload.
>   - Prevent and treat congestive heart failure.
>   - Maintain optimal cardiac output.
>   - Correct the underlying defect.
>   - Maintain fluid and electrolyte balance.
>   - Prevent secondary complications (failure to thrive, cardiogenic shock, thromboembolism, infection, respiratory compromise, cardiac dysrhythmia).
>   - Improve respiratory function.
>   - Maintain adequate nutritional intake to meet metabolic demands.
>   - Prevent infection by observing standard precautions. Assess for early signs of infection and report to primary care provider.
>   - Reduce anxiety by providing emotional support to child and family.
>   - Provide information regarding the plan for care to client and family.
> - Important nursing diagnoses (actual or potential) are:
>   - Decreased cardiac output
>   - Altered tissue perfusion
>   - Altered respiratory function, ineffective breathing pattern, and impaired gas exchange
>   - Activity intolerance, fatigue
>   - Altered growth and development
>   - Fluid volume excess
>   - Risk of infection
>   - Risk of injury (stroke, sudden cardiac arrest)
>   - Anxiety and fear
>   - Self-care deficit
>   - Knowledge deficit
>   - Ineffective family coping

Nursing Management of the Child with Congenital Heart Disease

- **Key Terms/Concepts**: Congestive heart failure, cyanotic lesion, acyanotic lesion, hemodynamic, dysrhythmia, shunt, palliative procedure, corrective procedure

Overview

Any structural lesion in the heart or blood vessels that is directly proximal to the heart is described as a congenital heart defect. Approximately 8-10 per 1000 live-born children have a congenital heart defect. The majority are diagnosed within the first year of life; although with some types of cardiac malformations the child does not exhibit signs of cardiac decompensation until later on in childhood. The nurse's role is to identify children with signs and symptoms of congenital or acquired heart disease and report them to the health care practitioners for immediate medical evaluation. The nurse also provides supportive care of and education to the family caring for the child at home.

There are two major types of congenital heart diseases acyanotic and cyanotic. Hemodynamic classification further categorizes congenital heart anomalies based on movement of blood through the heart. Acyanotic defects characteristically have a left-to- right shunt (oxygenated-to-unoxygenated blood flow); a cyanotic defect involves a right- to-left shunt (unoxygenated-to-oxygenated blood flow).

Types of Congenital Cardiac Defects		
Hemodynamic Classification	**Acyanotic**	**Cyanotic**
Increased pulmonary blood flow **Left-to-right shunts** **Acyanotic anomalies**	• Ventricular septal defect (VSD)-most common CHD • Atrial septal defect (ASD) • Patent ductus arteriosus (PDA)	
Obstructive lesions **Prevent blood flow from moving forward**	• Pulmonary stenosis • Aortic stenosis • Coarctation of the aorta	
Decreased pulmonary blood flow **Right-to-left shunts** **Cyanotic anomalies**		• Tetralogy of Fallot • Tricuspid atresia
Mixed anomalies		• Transposition of the great vessels

Risk Factors

- Maternal
    - Rubella in early pregnancy

Nursing Care of Children

- Alcoholism
- Exposure to coxsackie virus (commonly known as hand, foot and mouth disease)
- Diabetes mellitus
- Ingestion of lithium
- Advanced maternal age
- Genetic factors
  - History of congenital heart disease in other family members
  - Trisomy 21 (Down's syndrome)
  - Multifactorial

Signs and Symptoms

- Tachycardia
- Decreased peripheral perfusion (cool extremities, delayed capillary refill, weak pulses)
- Heart murmurs
- Active precordium
- Cyanosis
- Dysrhythmias
- Pulmonary congestion (crackles, coarseness)
- Increased work of breathing (flaring, retractions, grunting)
- Stridor or choking spells
- Recurrent respiratory infections
- Difficulty feeding
- Failure to gain weight
- Polycythemia
- Cerebral thrombosis
- Anoxic episodes (fainting spells)

Specific Cardiac Defects

- Ventricular Septal Defect (VSD): Hole between the two ventricles; most common of the cardiac defects. Closes naturally or with surgical correction.
  - Loud, harsh murmur that begins at about 4-8 weeks of age
  - Congestive heart failure is common.
  - Failure to thrive
  - Small defects may be asymptomatic.
- Atrial Septal Defect (ASD): Hole between the two atria. Closes naturally, with therapeutic catheterization or surgery.
  - Loud, harsh murmur
  - May develop enlarged right side of the heart
  - Increased oxygen saturation in the right atrium

- May develop mild congestive heart failure
- May be asymptomatic
- If untreated the client is at risk for the following as an adult:
  - Atrial dysrhythmia
  - Pulmonary vascular obstructive disease
- Patent Ductus Arteriosus (PDA): Accessory fetal vessel between the pulmonary artery and the aorta that fails to close. PDA is common in premature infants. Closure occurs naturally, with Indomethacin, therapeutic catheterization, or surgery.
  - Murmur
  - Wide pulse pressure
  - Bounding pulses
  - May be asymptomatic
  - May develop CHF
- Pulmonary Stenosis: Narrowing of the pulmonary valve or pulmonary artery. Opened with balloon procedure or surgery.
  - Right ventricular enlargement
  - Systolic ejection murmur
  - Exercise intolerance
  - CHF
  - Cyanosis with severe narrowing
- Aortic Stenosis: Narrowing of the aortic valve. Opened with balloon procedure or surgery.
  - Left ventricular enlargement
  - Murmur
  - Chest pain
  - Decreased cardiac output
  - Exercise intolerance
  - Faint pulses
  - Hypotension
  - Dizziness
  - Syncope
- Coarctation of the aorta: Narrowing of the aorta usually at or near the ductus arteriosus. Surgical repair and reconstruction are usually needed.
  - Increased blood pressure and oxygen saturation in the upper extremities as compared with the lower extremities
  - Headache
  - Vertigo
  - Nosebleeds
  - Weak or absent femoral pulses
  - Leg pain
  - Decreased cardiac output
  - CHF

- Transposition of the Great Arteries: The aorta arises from the right ventricle instead of the left, and the pulmonary artery arises from the left instead of the right. This condition is incompatible with life if there is no connection between right and left sides. Emergency septostomy is performed to create a connection between the right and left sides. The surgical repair is the atrial switch procedure. Severe cyanosis appears hours-to-days after birth (as PDA closes).
  - Murmur
  - Cardiomegaly
  - CHF
- Tricuspid Atresia: the tricuspid valve is completely closed. Generally requires several complex surgeries. Tricuspid atresia is incompatible with life if there is inadequate pulmonary blood flow. Prostaglandin E infusion is used until an emergency shunt procedure can be performed. A series of palliative and restorative surgeries may be required to repair the anomaly.
  - No blood flow from the right atrium to the right ventricle
  - Severe cyanosis within hours after birth (increased as the PDA closes)
  - CHF
  - Chronic hypoxemia
  - Failure to thrive
- Tetralogy of Fallot: In this syndrome, four anomalies are present: pulmonary stenosis, ventricular septal defect, overriding aorta, and enlargement of the right ventricle. Palliative shunt may be placed until child is able to have the surgical corrective repair.
  - Murmur
  - Cyanosis
  - Polycythemia
  - Clot formation
  - Severe dyspnea
  - Squatting position in an effort to compensate for decreased venous return due to the anomaly
  - Hypercyanotic spells
  - Acidosis
  - Clubbing of the fingers
  - Growth retardation
  - Failure to thrive

Diagnostic Tests and Labs (general)
- History and physical
- Chest x-ray
- Echocardiogram
- EKG
- Labs: ABGs, CBC, electrolyte panel
- Therapeutic and diagnostic cardiac catheterization

Therapeutic Nursing Management

- Avoid situations that increase cardiac demands (fever, pain, agitation, etc.).
- Avoid unnecessarily disturbing the infant.
- Monitor child's weight.
- Provide small frequent feedings. Feed with increased-calorie formula as needed.
- Administer oxygen as needed.
- Administer digoxin and observe for signs of digoxin toxicity: anorexia, nausea, vomiting, and pulse irregularities.
- Administer diuretics as needed. Replace potassium if furosemide (Lasix) is used.
- Maintain accurate input and output record.
- Prepare for cardiac catheterization, surgical palliation, and/or corrective procedures.
- Protect from infection.

Pharmacology

- Digoxin (Lanoxin): Hold dose for low heart rate per health care provider order.
- Diuretics: furosemide (Lasix), chlorothiazide (Diuril), spironolactone (Aldactone)
- Prostaglandin (PGE1) infusion to keep PDA open until surgical palliation can occur
- Indomethacin to promote PDA closure
- Vaccination (to prevent infection)

Complications

- Heart failure
- Cerebral thrombosis
- Failure to thrive
- Death

Critical Thinking Exercise: Nursing Management of the Child with Congenital Heart Disease

1. Fill in the blanks:
   a. Four common signs of digoxin toxicity include: _____, _____, _____, and _____ _____ _____.

   b. Infants with complex congenital heart defects may have difficulty gaining weight because of _____ _____.

   c. _____ are frequently administered to children with complex cardiac defects to prevent fluid retention.

   d. A child who has a high hematocrit related to a congenital heart defect is vulnerable to _____ _____.

   e. Chronic cyanosis leads to _____ of the fingers.

2. Match the heart defect with the symptom or description

Ventricular septal defect	a. Opening between the right and left atrium
Atrial septal defect	b. Increased BP in upper extremities
Patent ductus arteriosus	c. Cyanotic episodes called "Tet spells"
Pulmonary stenosis	d. Aorta and pulmonary artery are reversed
Aortic stenosis	e. Decreased blood flow into the aorta
Coarctation of the aorta	f. Usually closes shortly after birth
Tetralogy of Fallot	g. Decreased blood flow to the lungs
Transposition of the great vessels	h. Opening between the right and left ventricle

Cardiovascular System/Blood Disorders CHAPTER 14

Nursing Management of the Child with Hodgkin's Disease

> **Key Points**
>
> - Hodgkin's disease is a malignancy of the lymphoid system characterized by well-differentiated cells (Reed-Sternberg cells).
> - Approximately 5% of pediatric malignancies in the United States are due to Hodgkin's disease.
> - Hodgkin's disease usually begins as a localized disease at diagnosis that spreads according to predictable patterns.
> - Children with Hodgkin's disease frequently exhibit the following symptoms: firm, painless lymph nodes (cervical, supraclavicular, or mediastinal lymphadenopathy), anorexia, weight loss, malaise, lethargy, night sweats, and fever.
> - Goals of collaborative management:
>   - Control the spread of cancer cells.
>   - Maintain a patent airway and promote adequate oxygenation.
>   - Maintain fluid and electrolyte balance.
>   - Assess and manage pain or promote comfort.
>   - Promote wound healing.
>   - Prevent infection.
>   - Provide child and family education and support.
>   - Promote optimal growth and development.
>   - Prevent complications from radiation and chemotherapy.
> - Important nursing diagnoses (actual and potential) are:
>   - Risk for injury
>   - Impaired tissue integrity
>   - Alteration in fluid and electrolytes
>   - Risk of infection
>   - Impaired gas exchange (lung, mediastinal involvement)
>   - Anxiety and fear
>   - Pain management
>   - Body image disturbance
>   - Altered growth and development
>   - Knowledge deficit
>   - Ineffective family and individual coping
>   - Altered family process
> - **Key Terms/Concepts:** Lymphoma, Reed-Sternberg cells, lymphadenopathy, staging, classification, prognosis, metastasis, chemotherapy, radiation, and bone marrow suppression

Nursing Management of the Child with Hodgkin's Disease

Overview

Hodgkin's disease is a neoplastic disease that originates in the lymphoid system. This type of lymphoma predictably metastasizes to the spleen, liver, bone marrow, mediastinum, and lungs. The cause is unknown. The incidence increases during adolescence and early adulthood and occurs more often in males. There are four subtypes, each with a different age of onset, clinical findings, and prognostic factors. Ann Arbor Staging Classification system is used to determine the extent of involvement. Improved diagnostic techniques, staging, and treatment have resulted in increased survival rates.

Risk Factors

- Close relatives, particularly same gender siblings with the disease
- Immune deficiency
- Most frequently diagnosed in adolescents, rare in children under 5 years of age

Signs and Symptoms

- Painless, firm lymph nodes in the cervical, supraclavicular, axillary, mediastinal or inguinal site(s)
- Movable lymph nodes in the surrounding tissue
- Anorexia
- Weight loss
- Night sweats
- Malaise
- Low-grade fever
- Pruritus

Diagnostic Tests and Lab

- History and physical
- Rule out infectious causes of enlarged lymph glands
- CBC (WBC differential change, anemia)
- Elevated Erythrocyte Sedimentation Rate (ESR)
- Lymph node biopsy shows Reed-Sternberg cells
- Chest x-ray
- CT scan, MRI
- Gallium scan
- Bone marrow aspiration
- Lymphangiography infrequently used

Therapeutic Nursing Management

- Care for the child undergoing surgical procedure for staging.
- Maintain adequate hydration and electrolyte balance.
- Care for the child receiving radiation: sedation as needed.

- Assess and manage radiation-related complications.
- Administer chemotherapy as ordered.
- Assess and manage chemotherapy-related complications as indicated.
- Protect from infection when there is bone marrow suppression (secondary to chemotherapy and radiation).
- Monitor nutritional status and provide nutritional support.
- Protect skin integrity and provide oral care.
- Control vomiting with antiemetics and diet.
- Manage pain with assessment, analgesics, non-pharmacologic and pain management techniques.
- Promote regular elimination by administering fiber, stool softeners, or laxatives as needed.
- Care for the child undergoing a splenectomy.
- Provide support and education to the child and family.
- Provide home care and on-going support instructions:
  - Teach family to recognize signs of infection, skin breakdown, and nutritional deficiency.
  - Teach the family the importance of follow-up care: monitoring for relapse or secondary malignancies and provision for prophylactic.
  - Instruct child and family members to administer medications and nutritional support at home.
  - Instruct family in the proper use of vascular access devices and/or feeding tubes as needed.
  - Provide information regarding support resources for children and families with cancer (national and local organizations, case manager, home health agency, etc.); arrange nutritional and pharmacological care at home.

Pharmacology

- Chemotherapy agents
- Antiemetic medication
- Blood transfusion
- Antibiotics
- Gastrointestinal medications

Teach the importance of follow-up care: monitor for relapse or secondary malignancies, for provision of prophylactic antibiotic therapy, and for pneumococcal and meningococcal immunizations related to the high risk of infection associated with asplenia.

Complications

- Impaired immunity and infection related to decreased WBC from chemotherapy and radiation
- Infertility resulting from radiation therapy
- Hypothyroidism

- Cardiovascular and/or pulmonary dysfunction from treatment or disease process
- Metastasis
- Death

Critical Thinking Exercise: Nursing Management of the Child with Hodgkin's Disease

Situation: A slender 14-year-old female is newly diagnosed with Hodgkin's disease. Her primary care provider first suspected the disease during a routine exam. The girl denied having any symptoms at the time of diagnosis except for feeling tired and not eating much.

1. What is Hodgkin's disease?

2. What symptoms did the primary care provider most likely find during the routine exam that led to the detection of the Hodgkin's disease?

3. What diagnostic tests and assessments should be anticipated to determine if there is spread of the disease to other parts of the body?

Cardiovascular System/Blood Disorders CHAPTER 15

Nursing Management of the Child with Leukemia

> **Key Points**
>
> - Leukemia is a broad term for a group of malignancies that affects the bone marrow and lymphatic system. It is generally divided into 2 groups: acute lymphoid leukemia (ALL) and acute myelogenous or nonlymphoid leukemia (AML/ANLL).
> - Leukemia is the most common form of cancer in children. ALL is the most common form of leukemia.
> - Bone marrow dysfunction caused by leukemia leads to problems associated with anemia, bleeding and decreased immunity.
> - Goals of collaborative management:
>   - Provide early recognition, diagnosis, and treatment.
>   - Promote remission of cancer and prevent metastasis.
>   - Minimize complications from chemotherapy and treatment regime.
>   - Prevent and/or manage bleeding.
>   - Prevent infection.
>   - Assess and manage pain.
>   - Maintain fluid and electrolyte balance.
>   - Promote wound healing.
>   - Provide child and family education and support.
>   - Promote optimal growth and development.
> - Important nursing diagnoses (actual and potential) are:
>   - Risk for injury
>   - Impaired tissue integrity
>   - Alteration in fluid and electrolytes
>   - Risk of infection
>   - Altered nutrition
>   - Body image disturbance
>   - Anxiety and fear
>   - Pain management
>   - Altered growth and development
>   - Knowledge deficit
>   - Ineffective family and individual coping
>   - Altered family processes
>   - Impaired home maintenance management
> - **Key Terms/Concepts:** Acute lymphoid leukemia (ALL) and acute nonlymphoid (myelogenous) leukemia (AML), staging, prognosis, metastasis, chemotherapy, radiation, and bone marrow suppression

Nursing Management of the Child with Leukemia

Overview

Leukemia is a broad term describing a group of malignant diseases of the blood-forming organs of the body, including the bone marrow and lymphatic system. The classification of leukemia is essential since the subtype of leukemia has treatment and prognostic implications. The predominant cell type and level of cell immaturity determine the classification of leukemia.

In children, two forms are generally recognized: acute lymphoid leukemia (ALL) and acute nonlymphoid (myelogenous) leukemia (AML or ANLL).

The pathophysiology involved in leukemia is the unrestricted proliferation of immature white blood cells. Although there is no tumor in this type of cancer, the leukemic cells demonstrate similar neoplastic properties as in other cancers. The three main consequences of leukemia in the child include the risk for: 1) infection due to neutropenia and the of lack white blood cell (WBC) defense; 2) anemia related to decreased red blood cell (RBC) production, and 3) bleeding due to impaired platelet formation. These conditions should be reported to the provider for treatment. The care of the child with leukemia is based on the risk for these complications.

The highest incidence of ALL is in preschool-age children. Approximately 80% of all childhood leukemias are ALL. The goal is to control the disease by using chemotherapeutic agents to induce and maintain remission. A bone marrow transplant may be performed if chemotherapy is not effective. Remission is possible in some types of leukemia. Children who are in remission for five years or more are considered cured.

Risk Factors

- Relationship of leukemia to viral infection is unknown
- Possible genetic correlation
- Risk is higher in children with Down Syndrome
- May be associated with disorders of immune mechanisms

Signs and Symptoms

Early

- Low-grade fever
- Pallor
- Tendency to bruise
- Leg and joint pain
- Listlessness
- Enlarged lymph nodes
- Abdominal pain
- Constipation
- Liver and spleen enlargement
- Petechiae
- Headache

- Vomiting and anorexia
- Unsteady gait
- Adenopathy
- Low platelet and red blood cell count
- WBCs (above 100,000 per mm3)

Late

- Hematuria
- Ulcerations in mouth
- Anemia
- Kidneys enlarge
- Testicles enlarge
- Signs of increased intracranial pressure (headache, stiff neck, irritability, vomiting, lethargy, papilledema, coma)

Diagnostic Tests and Lab

- History and physical
- Bone marrow aspiration (sternum or iliac crest)
- Chest x-ray (mediastinal mass)
- CBC (WBC count and differential, hematocrit, platelet count)
- Absolute neutrophil count (ANC)
- Lumbar puncture to determine CNS involvement
- Kidney and liver function tests to determine baseline function for chemotherapy

Therapeutic Nursing Management

- Administer chemotherapy as ordered.
- Maintain adequate hydration and electrolytes with fluid administration.
- Manage bleeding.
  - Observe for petechiae and ecchymosis.
  - Treat nosebleed with cold and pressure.
  - Observe for burning on urination, may indicate hemorrhagic cystitis.
  - Assess for gastrointestinal bleeding (vomiting or tarry stools).
  - Limit amount of blood sticks and invasive procedures.
- Transfuse platelets, packed RBCs and other blood products as needed. Observe for transfusion reactions and other complications.
- Provide oral care.
  - Inspect mouth for ulceration and hemorrhage from gums.
  - Use a soft toothbrush or soft toothettes for oral care.
  - Rinse and spit chlorhexidine mouthwash, saline or other non alcohol solution.

- Lubricate lips to prevent from cracking.
- Prepare child for hair loss. Suggest use of wig or scarf if the child is self-conscious regarding baldness.
- Provide skin care.
  - Inspect daily.
  - Assess rectal mucosa for fissures.
  - Avoid rectal thermometers.
  - Provide sitz baths as needed.
  - Reposition carefully to promote circulation and prevent pressure ulcers.
  - Use a pressure reduction surface as needed for skin breakdown prevention.
- Control vomiting with antiemetics and diet.
- Manage pain with assessment, analgesics, and non-pharmacologic pain management techniques.
- Promote regular elimination by administering fiber, stool softeners, or laxatives as needed.
- Maintain nutrition.
  - Provide well-balanced diet with preferred foods.
  - Offer small amounts of fluids frequently.
  - Administer enteral nutrition as needed.
- Provide emotional support and teaching for child and family.
- Provide home care and on-going support instructions.
  - Teach family to recognize signs of infection, skin breakdown, and nutritional deficiency.
  - Instruct child and family members to administer medications and nutritional support at home.
  - Instruct family in the proper use of vascular access devices and/or feeding tubes as needed.
  - Instruct the child and family in bleeding precautions: inspect daily for bruising, apply ice for bleeding, avoid aspirin and aspirin-containing products, and avoid contact sports.
  - Instruct child and family to apply pressure at the site of active bleeding and do not dislodge a blood clot. Ice may be applied to site.
  - Provide information regarding support resources for children and families with cancer (national and local organizations, case manager, home health agency, and nutritional and pharmacological care at home).

Pharmacology

- Chemotherapy agents
- Antiemetic medication
- Prednisone and other steroids
- Blood transfusion
- Antibiotics
- Gastrointestinal medications

Complications

- Infection
- Hepatomegaly
- Splenomegaly
- Uncontrolled bleeding
- Metastasis
- Body image changes due to chemotherapy include: hair loss, weight loss, moon face, skin lesions, petechiae and bruising.
- Side effects/complications from chemotherapy:
  - Nausea, vomiting and diarrhea
  - Skin and mucosal breakdown
  - Hemorrhage
  - Infection
  - Altered nutrition
  - Pain
  - Cardiotoxicity
  - CNS complications
  - Cell lysis syndrome
  - Sterility
  - Death

Critical Thinking Exercise: Nursing Management of the Child with Leukemia

1. Which of the following is most frequently associated with the EARLY stages of acute leukemia?
    a. Fever and pallor
    b. Abdominal pain and swelling
    c. Headache with double vision
    d. Painful and frequent urination
    Correct answer: _____

    Rationale:

2. What is the most common cause of death in children with leukemia?
    a. Hemorrhage
    b. Infection
    c. Metastasis
    d. Drug toxicity
    Correct answer: _____

    Rationale:

3. Why are children with leukemia prone to bleeding episodes?

Nursing Management of the Child with Leukemia

4. Which of the following interventions is most appropriate when caring for a child receiving chemotherapy?
   a. Tell the parents that if their child will not have any long-term effects.
   b. Encourage the child to drink orange juice for breakfast.
   c. Monitor rectal temperature every 4 hours.
   d. Administer medication to prevent nausea.

   Correct answer: _____

   Rationale:

5. Which of the following is most appropriate to help 6-year-old girl adjust to her chemotherapy related hair loss?
   a. Wait to discuss the hair loss with the child until it begins to happen
   b. Encourage the girl's parents to help her select a wig or cap to wear
   c. Remove the mirrors from the child's room to prevent her from seeing bald head
   d. Avoid discussing the topic of hair loss because she is too young to understand

   Correct answer: _____

   Rationale:

Cardiovascular System/Blood Disorders **CHAPTER 16**

Nursing Management of the Child with Iron Deficiency Anemia

Key Points

- Iron deficiency anemia is the most common type of anemia in the United States.
- Infants and children with poor nutritional intake, increased iron requirements (bleeding), or impaired absorption (intestinal mucosal impairment) are at greatest risk for this iron deficiency anemia.
- Iron deficiency anemia is easily treated with an iron-rich diet and iron supplementation. If left untreated, it can lead to fatal complications.
- Goals of collaborative management:

  Recognize children at risk for developing the disease.
  - Provide dietary iron and iron supplements at appropriate dosages.
  - Prevent complications.
  - Prevent accidental overdose of iron supplements.
  - Correct the underlying reason for iron deficiency whenever possible.
- Important nursing diagnoses (actual or potential) are:
  - Activity intolerance
  - Altered nutrition
  - Altered growth and development
  - Risk for injury
  - Knowledge deficit
- **Key Terms/Concepts:** Anemia, nutritional deficiency, bleeding, pallor, iron supplement, therapeutic dosage range, developmental delay, accidental overdose

Overview

Iron deficiency anemia is caused by an inadequate supply of dietary iron, impaired iron absorption, or altered synthesis of iron in the body. It is the most common type of anemia in infancy and childhood and the most prevalent nutritional deficiency in the United States. Iron is needed for the manufacture of red blood cells. Premature infants have increased incidence of iron deficiency anemia due to insufficient fetal iron supplies. Adolescents often require additional dietary iron because of their rapid growth coupled with poor nutritional intake. In pregnancy, hemoglobin needs are increased related to the growing fetal demands. Increased incidence and severity of iron deficiency anemia has resulted from the institution of the Women, Infants and Children's Program (WIC), which provides formula to indigent families. The fortification of infant cereals is an excellent source of iron supplementation.

Risk Factors

- Drinking excess amounts of whole cow's milk
- Prematurity
- Bleeding, such as excessive menstrual flow
- Poor dietary intake of iron
- Impaired absorption (severe prolonged diarrhea)
- Infection
- Chronic conditions: folate deficiency, sickle cell anemia, thalassemia major, chronic inflammation

Signs and Symptoms

- Pallor, petechiae, and bruising
- Irritability, short attention span, and restlessness
- Anorexia
- Intolerance to activity
- Poor muscle tone
- Enlarged heart
- Shortness of breath, tachypnea, and dyspnea
- Heart murmur, palpitations, and tachycardia

Diagnostic Tests and Labs

- History and physical
- Hematocrit/hemoglobin
- Dietary history
- Morphological changes in RBC: small (microcytic) and pale (hypochromic) red blood cells

Therapeutic Nursing Management

- Identify children at risk for developing iron deficiency anemia. Work with healthcare team to initiate iron supplements and an iron-rich diet. Important times to check include 9 month and 2 year follow-up.
- Identify dietary habits that may be contributing to the iron deficiency. Provide a dietary plan.
- Administer iron preparation (usually ferrous sulfate administered orally 2-3 times daily between meals).
- Encourage juice or other foods enriched with vitamin C to aid in absorption of iron.
- Give liquid iron preparation via straw to prevent discoloration of teeth.
- Administer intramuscular iron when noncompliance with oral route is a problem.
- Give iron-fortified formula or iron supplements if mother is breastfeeding.

- Provide child/family education:
  - Teach home medication administration techniques.
  - Explain that infants over 6 months should not receive more than 32 oz of formula each day.
  - Teach families to provide cereal for infants and iron-rich foods (muscle meats, eggs, wheat, green-leafy vegetables) for toddlers and older children.
  - Inform families that stools may be tarry, dark-green in color from the iron supplement.
  - Instruct families to avoid giving oral iron with milk, as it interferes with absorption.
  - Return for periodic blood evaluations.
  - Encourage adolescent females to increase iron intake.
  - Stress to family the importance of keeping the iron supplement locked up/secure to prevent accidental poisoning.

Pharmacology

- Iron supplement/replacement therapy
  - Ferrous sulfate
  - Ferrous gluconate
  - Ferrous fumarate
- Vitamin C

Complications

- Related to untreated disease:
  - Poor attention span and learning difficulties
  - Developmental delay
  - Congestive heart failure
- Related to iron supplements:
  - Inadequate dosing
  - Constipation
  - Staining of teeth
  - Accidental overdose

Critical Thinking Exercise: Nursing Management of the Child with Iron Deficiency Anemia

Situation: At a routine clinic visit, the nurse documents the following assessment data for a 22-month-old child: pallor (especially of the mucous membranes), limp muscle tone, restlessness, low energy levels, and a systolic heart murmur. The nurse reviewing the laboratory report notes the hemoglobin is 9.8 g/100 mL and hematocrit is 32%.

1. Place an **X** by the information that should be included in the child's history to support the diagnosis of iron deficiency anemia.

    Amount of milk the child is drinking per day ____

    Child's food preferences ____

    Child's eating patterns ____

    Mother's feelings about the child ____

    Family's socioeconomic status ____

    Family's living arrangements ____

    Number of siblings in the household ____

    Does the child eat dirt or paint? ____

    Percentile ranking of growth and development on a growth chart ____

    Is the child is up to date with immunizations? ____

    Has the child has been taking prednisone or salicylates? ____

After the primary care provider's assessment, the child is started on a daily dosage of ferrous sulfate.

2. Place an **X** by the instructional information that should be given to the child's mother regarding the administration of the medication and treatment of anemia.

    ____ Provide juice enriched with vitamin C, which will aid absorption.

    ____ Give iron supplement via straw to prevent discoloration of teeth.

    ____ Include iron-rich food in diet: including eggs, cheese, green vegetables, dried apricots.

    ____ Children over age 6 months should not receive more than 32 ounces of milk per day.

    ____ Discuss the side effects of the iron supplement: constipation, dark-colored stools, nausea.

    ____ Cost of medication and foods

    ____ Keep iron supplement in a safe place to avoid accidental overdose.

    ____ Provide nutritious snacks and finger foods that reflect the child's developmental stage.

____ Signs and symptoms of anemia
____ Iron stores return to normal after 4-6 weeks of treatment.
____ The importance of returning for follow-up lab work

Cardiovascular System/Blood Disorders **CHAPTER 17**

Nursing Management of the Child with Hemophilia

Key Points

- Hemophilia is an inherited disorder that primarily affects males. It is caused by an X-linked recessive gene from the maternal side.
- A deficiency in clotting factors can lead to uncontrolled bleeding from wounds and into joints, muscles and other body tissues.
- Spontaneous uncontrolled bleeding is associated with severe hemophilia.
- Goals of collaborative management:
    - Provide early recognition, diagnosis, and treatment of the disease.
    - Prevent bleeding.
    - Provide replacement-clotting factors as needed.
    - Treat pain.
    - Prevent complications related to bleeding (blood volume deficit, anemia, pain, joint involvement, intracranial bleeding, etc.).
- Important nursing diagnoses (actual or potential) are:
    - Risk for injury
    - Fluid volume deficit
    - Pain management
    - Impaired physical mobility
    - Activity intolerance
    - Knowledge deficit
    - Ineffective coping
    - Altered family process
    - Impaired home management
- **Key Terms/Concepts**: X-linked recessive genetic inheritance, intrinsic clotting cascade, Factor VIII, Factor IX, anemia, bleeding, pallor, arthropathy, contractures

Overview

Hemophilia refers to a group of bleeding disorders in which there is a deficiency in one of the factors necessary for coagulation. In 80% of the cases of hemophilia, the defect in the clotting mechanism is exhibited in a recessive, X-linked pattern of inheritance. There are many types of hemophilia, each lacking a different clotting factor. The two most common types are hemophilia A or classic type (factor VIII deficiency) and hemophilia B or Christmas disease (factor IX deficiency).

Risk Factors
- Male with a family history of hemophilia or unexplained bleeding
- Mother with recessive gene trait

Diagnostic Tests and Labs
- History and physical
- Complete blood count (CBC)
- Platelet count: normal
- Prothrombin time (PT): normal
- Partial thromboplastin time (PTT): increased
- Bleeding time: normal
- Thrombin clotting time
- Liver biopsy, liver function test to rule out liver disease and other causes of bleeding
- Factor VIII & IX assays

Signs and Symptoms
- Internal bleeding: cerebral hemorrhage indicated by change in mental status
- Hemorrhages in subcutaneous muscle tissue
- Excessive bleeding from trauma: circumcision (if an infant), or any break in skin, nosebleeds, and injections
- Bruises in various stages
- Hematuria
- Hemarthrosis
- Decreased hemoglobin and hematocrit

Therapeutic Nursing Management
- Avoid injections, venipuncture, and invasive procedures as much as possible.
- Apply pressure to insertion sites after needle withdrawal.
- Monitor for bleeding: assess venipuncture sites and joints, urine, stool and nasogastric fluid for occult blood.
- Provide pain relief measures: ice to affected joint, analgesic agents.
- Provide child/family education.
  - Teach family about safety issues: protect toddlers and young children from sharp edges and falls; avoid contact sports and rough physical play, etc.
  - Provide well-balanced meals to avoid excess weight gain. Avoid constipation.
  - Provide good oral hygiene: use a soft toothbrush, avoid high sugar foods, and visit a dentist regularly.
  - Encourage a regular exercise program.
  - Avoid aspirin or aspirin-containing products.

- Do not use rectal thermometers.
- Provide direct pressure over bleeding area.
- Apply ice to affected area.
- Teach caregivers to administer factor replacement at home as needed.
- Provide genetic counseling to parents.

Pharmacology

- Highly purified or recombinant factor VIII concentrate
- Factor IX
- Desmopressin (DDAVP) which increases factor VIII
- Regular immunizations

Complications

- Uncontrolled hemorrhage
- Hemarthrosis (bleeding into the joint which can cause permanent crippling)
- Muscle contractures
- Intracranial bleeding
- Renal impairment
- Death

Critical Thinking Exercise: Nursing Management of the Child with Hemophilia

Situation: A mother brings her 13-month-old son to the emergency department with a small laceration on his forehead from a fall against the edge of a coffee table. The mother sought treatment when she was unable to stop the bleeding. The mother tells the nurse that she noticed that her son seemed to bruise easily and had bleeding with teething. She stated that she didn't think that her son could have hemophilia because no one on his father's side of the family has this disease. She had heard it was a genetic disorder in males.

1. What part of this history is consistent with a diagnosis of hemophilia?

2. What part of the mother's understanding of hemophilia is incorrect?

3. What laboratory studies should the nurse anticipate?

4. Why do children with hemophilia have problems with bleeding?

5. What family teaching should be done with this mother?

Cardiovascular System/Blood Disorders CHAPTER 18

Nursing Management of the Child with Sickle Cell Disease

Key Points

- Sickle cell disease is an inherited disorder that affects the production of hemoglobin.
- African-Americans are primarily affected.
- Complications associated with sickle cell disease are due to red blood cell sickling and obstruction in the vascular beds and subsequent tissue damage.
- The types of sickle cell crises are vaso-occlusive, sequestration and aplastic.
- Goals of collaborative management:
  - Provide early recognition, diagnosis, and treatment of the disease.
  - Prevent sickle cell crisis by avoiding factors associated with sickling (dehydration, stress, acute illness, hypoxia, etc.).
  - Provide pain relief measures.
  - Maintain adequate oxygenation.
  - Provide generous hydration to decrease blood viscosity.
  - Prevent complications related to sickle cell crisis.
- Important nursing diagnoses (actual or potential) are:
  - Risk for injury
  - Altered tissue perfusion
  - Pain management
  - Impaired physical mobility
  - Activity intolerance
  - Knowledge deficit
  - Ineffective coping
  - Altered family process
  - Impaired home management
- **Key Terms/Concepts:** Hemoglobin S, autosomal recessive disease, sickle cell crisis, microvascular obstruction, dactylitis (hand-and-foot syndrome)

Overview

Sickle cell disease is an inherited autosomal recessive disease that affects the hemoglobin in red blood cells. This disease primarily affects individuals of African descent but can occur in individuals of Mediterranean, Indian, or Middle Eastern descent among others. The red blood cells are elongated in a crescent shape and cannot pass readily through the blood vessels. These cells cause an increase in blood viscosity and sluggish blood flow. The tissue becomes ischemic from poor blood supply and results in acute pain, cell destruction, infarcts, and organ damage.

Nursing Management of the Child with Sickle Cell Disease

> Oxygen therapy is a priority for these children to prevent further complications from the disease. Pain management and hydration are also important nursing considerations. Sickle cell crisis may be manifested as vaso-occlusive crisis, acute sequestration crisis, acute chest syndrome, and aplastic crisis. Acute illness, dehydration, respiratory infection, strenuous exercise, hypoxic conditions, or trauma generally precipitates sickle cell crisis. Splenic sequestration caused by pooled blood will lead to splenic enlargement. Large amounts of fetal hemoglobin in the first few months of life obscure the presence of sickle cell hemoglobin, so the symptoms do not usually appear until 4-6 months of life when the fetal hemoglobin is replaced by the adult form.

Risk Factors

- If one parent is a carrier, each offspring has a 25% chance of inheriting the trait.
- If both parents are carriers, each offspring has a 50% chance of inheriting the trait and a 25% chance of inheriting the disease.
- If one parent is a carrier and the other has the disease, each offspring has a 50% chance of inheriting the trait and 50% chance of inheriting the disease.

Signs and Symptoms

- Vaso-occlusive crisis (distal ischemia from vascular occlusion)
  - Pain, particularly in the joints, extremities or back
  - Swollen joints
  - Vomiting
  - Fever
  - Anorexia
  - Dactylitis (hand-and-foot syndrome) in young infants
  - Positive Homans' sign (pain in the calf with dorsiflexion) may indicate a thrombus.
- Acute sequestration crisis (blood pooling causing decreased hemoglobin level)
  - Enlarged liver and spleen
  - Tachycardia
  - Dyspnea
  - Weakness
  - Pallor
  - Shock
- Aplastic crisis (from suppression of RBC production and hemolysis)
  - Weakness, fatigue
  - Pallor
  - Dyspnea
  - Tachycardia
  - Shock
- Acute chest syndrome
  - Chest pain

Nursing Management of the Child with Sickle Cell Disease

- Cough
- Fever
- Abdominal pain

Diagnostic Tests and Labs

- History and physical
- Fetal blood cell testing
- CBC (Hemoglobin, hematocrit, RBC with morphology, WBC count)
- Chest x-ray
- Hemoglobin electrophoresis
- Reticulocyte count
- Sickledex

Therapeutic Nursing Management

- Maintain adequate oxygenation: administer oxygen as needed, monitor pulse oximetry.
- Maintain adequate hydration: administer IV fluids and avoid dehydration.
- Manage pain: provide narcotics analgesia as needed, comfort measures.
- Provide adequate rest.
- Administer blood transfusions as needed.
- Provide oral hygiene.
- Maintain nutrition.
- Prevent infection; administer antibiotics as needed.
- Provide child/family education.
  - Teach child and family to how to avoid factors associated with crisis (cold, dehydration, hypoxia, stress, overexertion, hyperthermia, acute illness).
  - Emphasize the need for adequate hydration.
  - Monitor for signs of infection.
  - Teach importance of routine immunizations.
  - Provide genetic counseling.

Pharmacology

- Antibiotics
- Analgesics (morphine or meperidine)
- Vaccination

Complications

- Secondary infection
- Impaired fertility
- Hypoxia, acidosis
- Cerebral vascular accident

- Hypovolemic shock
- Ocular damage
- Organ damage
- Death

Critical Thinking Exercise: Nursing Management of the Child with Sickle Cell Disease

Situation: A 5-year-old African American female is admitted with complaints of pain in her arms and legs. She has a three-day history of upper respiratory infection with fever, vomiting and decreased oral intake. The nurse caring for the child makes the following assessments: heart rate 136 beats/minute, respiratory rate 30 breaths/minute, blood pressure 90/85 mmHg, temperature 101.3° F, dusky mucous membranes, cough, delayed capillary refill and no tears.

1. What are the most important interventions for this child at this time?

2. What laboratory data is important for this child?

3. What family teaching is appropriate for this child and family?

Cardiovascular System/Blood Disorders   CHAPTER 19

Nursing Management of the Child with a Blood Transfusion

Key Points

- Whole blood or components of whole blood can be administered.
- Incompatibility is a major concern when administering blood or blood products.
- Goals of collaborative management:
  - Administer a compatible blood product.
  - Correct the underlying problem for which the blood is being administered.
  - Prevent reactions to the blood or blood product.
- Important nursing diagnoses (actual or potential) are:
  - Risk for injury (Potential complications of blood transfusion: febrile reaction, hemolytic reaction, hypersensitivity, incompatibility, infection)
  - Fluid volume excess
  - Anxiety and fear
  - Knowledge deficit
- **Key Terms/Concepts**: Incompatibility, febrile reaction, hemolytic reaction, hypersensitivity, thrombocytopenia, ABO typing, Rh typing, autologous transfusion, directed donor transfusion

Overview

The administration of blood components via the intravenous route may be indicated for the child with hypovolemia, anemia, neutropenia, thrombocytopenia, or DIC. Packed red blood cells are the most frequent type of blood transfusion used to provide a concentrated volume of red blood cell without excessive serum load. A blood transfusion may be indicated for an emergency intervention or to provide a therapeutic effect. In spite of technological advances in the screening of blood for infectious disease, some risk remains. Nurses need to be aware of potential complications, promptly identify the onset of a complication (transfusion reaction), and take appropriate interventions in a timely manner.

Indications for Transfusions

- Low red blood cell count
- Hemorrhage
- Hypovolemic shock
- Anemia
- Thalassemia
- Sickle cell anemia

Nursing Management of the Child with a Blood Transfusion

- Low platelets
- Thrombocytopenia
- Platelet dysfunction

Diagnostic Tests and Lab

- History and physical examination
- CBC, hemoglobin, hematocrit
- Arterial blood gases
- ABO and Rh typing and cross match
- Antibody screen for other than anti-A, anti-B

Therapeutic Nursing Management

- Explain procedure to child and family.
- Ensure that the family does not have spiritual or personal reasons to refuse a blood transfusion. Obtain consent as required.
- Obtain a history, including assessment, for previous reactions.
- Place a large bore IV catheter.
- Follow blood identification protocol carefully.
- Use only normal saline to prime IV tubing.
- Use an infusion pump and appropriate blood filter on the tubing.
- Obtain baseline vital signs prior to infusion.
- Premedicate with antihistamines and acetaminophen as needed.
- Administer donated blood or self-donated blood (autologous transfusion) as prescribed.
- Observe child during first 15 minutes of infusion.
- Frequently monitor infusion and vital signs according to hospital protocol.
- Never add medications to blood products.
- Infuse blood within 4 hours.
- A blood warmer may be indicated to decrease potential for hypothermia.
- Monitor closely for signs of a transfusion reaction.

Transfusion Reaction

- Stop transfusion immediately if reaction is suspected.
- Initiate a saline infusion.
- Maintain airway patency.
- Assess and record symptoms of the reaction (most common reaction symptoms are fever and chills, others include itching, weakness, dyspnea, rash, and cough).
- Promptly notify the primary care provider.
- Administer oxygen, antihistamines, and emergency drugs as needed.
- Send blood bag and tubing to blood bank per protocol.

Complications

- Acute hemolytic reaction (the most common symptoms are fever and chills, others include low back pain, tachycardia, flushing, hypotension, tachypnea, cardiovascular collapse, acute renal failure, shock, and death)
- Febrile (non-hemolytic) reaction (most common reaction is rapid-onset fever and chills, other symptoms include fever, flushing, headache, and anxiety)
- Mild-allergic reaction (itching, urticaria, and flushing)
- Anaphylactic reaction (wheezing, dyspnea, chest tightness, cyanosis, hypotension, shock, and death)
- Circulatory overload (dyspnea, chest tightness, tachycardia, tachypnea, headache, hypertension, jugular vein distention, and peripheral edema)
- Sepsis (Fever, nausea, vomiting, abdominal pain, and shock)
- Delayed hemolytic reaction (fever, chills, anemia, jaundice, hemoglobinuria, and back pain)
- Disease transmission (Hepatitis A, B and C, HIV, and CMV)

Critical Thinking Exercise: Nursing Management of the Child with a Blood Transfusion

Situation: A previously healthy 8-year-old lost a large amount of blood after being shot in the upper arm in by his mother's boyfriend during a domestic dispute. The boy's vital signs were stabilized after the bleeding was stopped. A 15-cc/kg blood transfusion was ordered.

1. What are key assessments needed prior to initiating the blood transfusion?

2. The boy tells the nurse that he heard that he could get AIDS or other diseases from a transfusion. How should the nurse respond?

3. Ten minutes into the transfusion the child complains of tightness in his chest and difficulty breathing. The nurse notes that he is wheezing and slightly cyanotic. What interventions are needed at this time?

Neurosensory System **CHAPTER 20**

Nursing Management of the Child with Seizures

> **Key Points**
>
> - Seizures are caused by altered neuronal activity and repetitive electric discharge of brain cells. This activity may be localized (partial seizures) or generalized.
> - Factors commonly associated with seizure activity include: febrile illness, hypoxic brain damage, increased intracranial pressure, trauma, neurological infectious disease, metabolic disorders, toxins, brain tumor, neurodegenerative neurologic disease, genetic factors, and abrupt withdrawal from anticonvulsants.
> - Idiopathic seizures have no identifiable cause.
> - Goals of collaborative management:
>   - Prevent injury during the seizure.
>   - Protect the airway and promote adequate oxygenation.
>   - Prevent recurrent seizures (maintain therapeutic anticonvulsant blood levels).
>   - Provide child and family education (medication administration, therapeutic medication level monitoring and safety measures during a seizure).
>   - Treat causative agent when possible.
>   - Prevent complications related to prolonged seizure activity.
> - Important nursing diagnoses (actual and potential) are:
>   - Risk for injury related to uncontrolled muscle movements during seizure activity
>   - Altered tissue perfusion (cerebral)
>   - Adaptive capacity decreased: intracranial
>   - Altered respiratory function related to weakness and altered level of consciousness
>   - Airway clearance ineffective related to loss of tongue and gag reflexes during seizure activity
>   - Hyperthermia related to seizure activity
>   - Knowledge deficit related to disease process or anticonvulsant medications
>   - Ineffective family and individual coping related to chronic illness
>   - Self-esteem disturbances as related to feelings of being out of control, stigma associated with seizures, perceived as having a weakness
>   - Impaired social interaction related to embarrassment, and fear of having a seizure in public
> - **Key Terms/Concepts**: Partial seizures (simple, complex), generalized seizures (absence, myoclonic, tonic-clonic, atonic), status epilepticus

Nursing Management of the Child with Seizures

Overview

Seizures are brief malfunctions of the brain's electrical system. An excessive and disorganized impulse is discharged from nervous tissue, resulting in involuntary muscular activity or lapses in consciousness. Seizures are not a diagnosis but simply a description of a transient disturbance of the CNS. The site of origin determines the types of seizures that occur. Altered consciousness, involuntary movements, changes in perception and behavior, and loss of voluntary control result from seizures.

The nurse's primary role in the care of the child with seizures is to:
- Provide an environment of safety during the event.
- Implement interventions to minimize the occurrence of seizures.
- Support the child and family and help them cope with the challenges associated with the condition.
- Assist the child and family cope with alterations in self-image.
- Teach the family to identify factors that may trigger the onset of the seizure, administer anticonvulsant therapy as ordered, and protect the child from harm during a seizure.

Risk Factors

- Fever (children from 6-36 months are at greatest risk)
- Increased ICP
- Infection (meningitis, encephalitis, sepsis)
- History of seizures/epilepsy
- Abrupt withdrawal of anticonvulsant therapy with a head injury/trauma
- Anoxic/hypoxic brain damage
- Metabolic disorders
- Fluid/electrolyte imbalance
- Perinatal injury
- Congenital brain deformities
- Toxic agents (medications, chemicals, lead poisoning)
- Kernicterus
- Brain tumors
- Hypoglycemia
- Degenerative neurologic disease
- Genetic factors
- Idiopathic

Signs and Symptoms

- **Partial (focal):** One brain hemisphere is affected; categorized as simple partial or partial complex
    - **Simple partial:** No LOC; alterations in motor function (muscle contractions of the hand, face, one side of the body); autonomic signs (sweating, vomiting, flushing, pupillary changes); sensory symptoms (feeling of

Nursing Management of the Child with Seizures

falling, paresthesia, hearing changes, visual changes, anxiety, fear)
- **Partial complex:** Consciousness is impaired; staring; lip smacking; chewing; unusual hand movements; amnesia
- **Generalized:** Entire brain is involved; categorized as absence or tonic-clonic (consciousness is affected)
  - **Absence (petit mal):** Lack of awareness; unresponsive; lasts less than 15 seconds; eye fluttering; lip smacking; blank stare; abrupt onset and cessation; usually affects children aged 4-14; may be misinterpreted as "day dreaming"
  - **Myoclonic:** No or brief LOC change; sudden onset; synchronous jerking of neck; shoulders; arms and legs; lasts less than 5 seconds
  - **Tonic-clonic (grand mal):** Aura precedes seizure; seizure followed by a postictal period of relaxation; lethargy; confusion and unresponsiveness; amnesia
    - **Tonic phase:** Sudden loss of consciousness; crying out; rigidity of muscles; clenched jaw; apnea with cyanosis; bowel and bladder incontinence; fixed and dilated pupils
    - **Clonic phase:** Alternate periods of contraction and relaxation of the extremities; hyperventilation; eyes roll back; drooling
    - **Atonic:** Sudden loss of tone causing facial/head changes (eyelid drooping; head nod) or fall to ground
- **Status epilepticus:** Prolonged seizures (usually generalized) lasting more than 15-20 min or recurrent seizures without return to baseline. Medical emergency that requires prompt treatment and airway management. Can lead to respiratory failure, hypotension, hypoxic brain damage, hypoglycemia, and other serious complications.
- **Febrile seizures:** Seizures that occur in association with a fever, unrelated to any chronic neurologic condition or epilepsy (in 98% of the cases). Febrile seizures occur between 6 months and 3 years of age and are rare in children over 5 years of age. They occur within families and occur twice as often in males than in females. Generally, the temperature is greater than 38.8o C or 101.8o F. Parental teaching includes: reassurance of the benign nature of febrile seizures, seizure precautions, and, in the event of a reoccurrence, if the seizure lasts more than 5 minutes, the child should be carefully transported to the emergency room.

Diagnostic Tests and Labs

- History and physical
- Neurological exam
- EEG (to define the type, focus and duration of the seizure)
- Brain imaging studies: CT, MRI, PET scan, skull x-ray
- Evoked potentials (auditory, visual)
- Serum labs: CBC, electrolyte panel, glucose level, anticonvulsant levels, toxicology screening
- Urine labs: Urinalysis, toxicology screening
- Lumbar puncture: Culture (bacterial, viral, fungal) and CSF analysis (glucose, protein and cell count with differential)

Nursing Management of the Child with Seizures

Therapeutic Nursing Management

- Protect from injury.
  - Before the seizure:
    - Pad bed or crib rails.
    - Remove any sharp or potentially harmful objects.
  - During a seizure:
    - Turn child to the side (to protect airway in case of vomiting and prevent airway occlusion by the tongue falling backwards).
    - Provide supplemental oxygen (if available).
    - Do not restrain.
    - Loosen any constricting clothing.
    - Do not place anything in the child's mouth.
    - Obtain assistance as needed.
- Observe, record, and report seizure activity.
- Child and family education:
  - Disease process education
  - Home medication administration
  - Appropriate actions to take if child has a seizure (safety, emergency care, etc.)
  - Factors that may trigger the onset of a seizure (fever, stopping medications, etc.)
  - Coping with disease (support groups, Internet resources, etc.)
  - Lifestyle changes: wearing medical alert bracelet, swimming safety, machinery/driving restrictions, avoiding unprotected heights
  - Need for close dental monitoring if on anticonvulsants.

Pharmacology

- Anticonvulsants: Phenobarbital and phenytoin (Dilantin) are most commonly used to treat and prevent recurrent seizures. Carbamazepine (Tegretol), valproic acid (Depakene), primidone (Mysoline), Ethosuximide (Zarontin), and clonazepam (Klonopin) are also used for various types of seizure disorders. Diazepam (Valium) and lorazepam (Ativan) are rapid-acting benzodiazepines used to stop seizure activity during status epilepticus.

Complications

- Status epilepticus
- Hypoglycemia
- Bodily injury
- Brain damage
- Death

Critical Thinking Exercise: Nursing Management of the Child with Seizures

Situation: A 2-year-old male is admitted after a seizure at home. The nurse obtains the following information from the child's mother: the child had generalized jerking of his arms and legs lasting one to two minutes with vomiting and cyanosis. He had been on Phenobarbital since nine months of age when he was diagnosed with a febrile seizure disorder. He has had two prior incidents of seizures since diagnosis.

1. What additional questions should the nurse ask the mother?

2. What child assessment should be made at this time?

3. Shortly after admission, the mother calls the nurse to the room because her child is having another seizure. What interventions are needed for this child during and immediately after the seizure? List in order of priority.

4. The child's mother admits that she had not been giving her son his phenobarbital at home because he hates the taste of the syrup. How should the nurse respond?

Neurosensory System CHAPTER 21

Nursing Management of the Child with Bacterial Meningitis

Key Points

- Bacterial meningitis is a central nervous system (CNS) infection usually caused by *H. influenzae type B*, *Streptococcus pneumoniae*, or *Neisseria meningitidis* in children over 2 months old.
- The *H. influenzae type B* vaccination helps prevent bacterial meningitis in children.
- Prognosis depends on the supportive care given to the child.
- Goals of collaborative management:
  - Provide early and accurate diagnosis (LP, cultures).
  - Provide prompt treatment directed at causative agent (antibiotics).
  - Treat acute symptoms (fever, dehydration, pain).
  - Prevent complications (ICP, sepsis, seizures, neurologic damage, and hearing loss).
  - Prevent fluid and electrolyte imbalance.
- Important nursing diagnoses (actual and potential) are:
  - Risk of infection
  - Altered protection
  - Altered tissue perfusion (cerebral)
  - Adaptive capacity decreased: intracranial
  - Altered respiratory function
  - Risk for injury (complications of meningitis: neurologic damage, sepsis, seizures)
  - Fluid volume deficit
  - Hyperthermia
  - Impaired physical mobility
  - Pain management
  - Knowledge deficit
  - Altered role performance (r/t hospitalization)
- **Key Terms/Concepts**: Photophobia, nuchal rigidity, Brudzinski's sign, Kernig's sign

Overview

Bacterial meningitis is an acute inflammation of the meninges and spinal cord caused by a bacterial infection. Different organisms cause bacterial meningitis and symptoms vary based on the causative organism and the age of the child. The incidence of bacterial meningitis has decreased as a result of the haemophilus influenzae type B vaccine, now a routine immunization schedule for children. Organisms may enter bloodstream from infections in teeth, sinuses, tonsils, and

> lungs or directly through the ear or skull fracture. It is most common in children age 1-5 years during the winter months.

Risk Factors

- Exposure to *H. influenzae* Type B, *Neisseria meningitidis, Diplococcus pneumoniae*, group B *Streptococcus*
- Immunosuppression

Signs and Symptoms

Symptoms may be insidious or acute onset

- History of upper respiratory infection or ear infection
- Irritability
- Restlessness and/or lethargy
- Photophobia
- Severe headache
- Delirium
- Fever
- Vomiting
- Stiff neck and spine
- Characteristic high-pitched cry in infants
- Seizures
- Coma
- Involuntary arching of back in severe cases (opisthotonos)
- Petechiae (suggests meningococcal infection)
- Some children may develop SIADH (syndrome of inappropriate antidiuretic hormone)

Diagnostics Tests and Labs

- History and physical
- CSF (lumbar puncture): cloudy, increased WBC, increased protein, decreased glucose culture and gram stain for causative organism.
- Electrolytes and serum and urine osmolarities to detect for SIADH

Therapeutic Nursing Management

- Administer antibiotics.
- Provide respiratory isolation until 24 hours after antibiotic therapy is started.
- Obtain baseline vital signs and neurologic checks and monitor as indicated.
- Administer intravenous fluids.
- Maintain NPO initially then increase diet as tolerated.
- Measure accurate intake and output.

Nursing Management of the Child with Bacterial Meningitis

- Comfort measures (quiet and darkened room, uninterrupted rest periods, pain medication as ordered for headache)
- Seizure precautions (pad side rails, anticonvulsants as ordered)
- Provide frequent position changes to prevent skin breakdown and maximize lung expansion.
- Monitor temperature.
- Provide oxygen therapy as needed.
- Restrict fluids (if SIADH)
- Report occurrence to local health department.

Pharmacology

- Antipyretics as needed
- Fourth generation cephalosporins
- Ampicillin and gentamicin
- Anticonvulsants for seizures
- Phenobarbital as sedative
- Corticosteroids

Complications

- Epilepsy
- Neurologic damage (cerebral palsy, learning disorders)
- Sensory loss (hearing and vision)
- Hydrocephalus

Critical Thinking Exercise: Nursing Management of the Child with Bacterial Meningitis

Instructions: Place each of the following signs and complications of bacterial meningitis in the correct box(s). Items may be placed in more than one location.

- Apnea
- Behavioral changes Blindness
- Brudzinski sign
- Bulging fontanel
- Cardiovascular collapse
- Cold extremities
- Cranial nerve damage
- Cyanosis Chills
- Diarrhea
- Extreme irritability
- Facial muscle paralysis
- Fever
- Fever or hypothermia
- Full or tense fontanel
- Hallucinations
- Headache
- Hearing loss
- High-pitched cry
- Hydrocephalus
- Irregular breathing pattern
- Irritability
- Kernig sign
- Nuchal rigidity
- Opisthotonos
- Photophobia
- Poor feeding
- Poor muscle tone
- Septic shock
- Seizures
- Sensitivity to noise
- Stupor or coma
- Vomiting
- Weak cry
- Weak suck
- Weight loss

	Early	Late/Complications
Neonate		
Infant/Young Child		
Older Child/Adolescent		

Neurosensory System CHAPTER 22

Nursing Management of the Child with Reye's Syndrome

> **Key Points**
>
> - Children with Reye's syndrome (RS) rapidly become critically ill with encephalopathy, hepatic dysfunction, increased intracranial pressure, and multisystem organ dysfunction.
> - Some attribute the decrease in the incidence of RS with the decreased use of salicylates for children with viral illness.
> - Goals of collaborative management:
>   - Educate caregivers regarding the use of aspirin and the risk of RS.
>   - Implement early recognition and intensive care management.
>   - Provide airway support and promote adequate oxygenation.
>   - Provide circulatory support for shock.
>   - Prevent uncontrolled increased intracranial pressure.
>   - Maintain fluid and electrolyte balance.
>   - Treat hypoglycemia.
>   - Treat coagulopathies.
>   - Prevent complications (hypoxia, sepsis, seizures, neurologic damage, organ damage, and death).
>   - Prevent fluid and electrolyte imbalance.
>   - Provide child/family support and teaching.
> - Important nursing diagnoses (actual or potential) are:
>   - Adaptive capacity decreased: intracranial
>   - Altered tissue perfusion (cerebral, cardiopulmonary, renal, and gastrointestinal)
>   - Risk for injury
>   - Fluid volume deficit
>   - Hyperthermia
>   - Altered respiratory function
>   - Altered protection
>   - Impaired tissue integrity
>   - Risk of infection
>   - Pain management
>   - Knowledge deficit
>   - Anxiety and powerlessness
>   - Altered family processes

- **Key Terms/Concepts:** Influenza, varicella, liver dysfunction, coagulation disorders, metabolic dysfunction, hypoglycemia, shock, cerebral edema, increased intracranial pressure, cerebral herniation, ALT, AST, ammonia levels, hyper-reflexia, obtunded, decorticate, decerebrate, oculocephalic reflexes

Overview

Reye's syndrome (RS) is a disorder defined as a toxic, nonspecific encephalopathy with other organ involvement. Fever, impaired liver function, and a sudden, profound change in the level of consciousness characterize RS. Even with aggressive treatment, RS can rapidly progress to critical illness and death. RS can lead to liver dysfunction, coagulation disorders, metabolic dysfunction, hypoglycemia, shock, myocardial dysfunction, renal damage, pancreatitis, sepsis, gastrointestinal ulceration, cerebral edema, increased intracranial pressure, cerebral herniation, and death.

The cause is unknown but is presumed to be triggered by a viral infection, particularly influenza or varicella and the use of aspirin. The peak incidence occurs between 4 and 14 years of age. RS generally occurs within 5-7 days after a viral illness.

Risk Factors

- Use of salicylates (aspirin) - also found in a form in Pepto-Bismol
- Children <18 years old, most between 4 years and 14 years of age
- Winter months

Signs and Symptoms

Five Clinical Stages	
I.	Quiet, lethargic, vomiting, anorexia, slurred speech, lab evidence of liver dysfunction (elevated ALT-AST; elevated ammonia levels)
II.	Lethargy, confusion, delirium, combativeness, hyperventilation, hyper-reflexia
III.	Obtunded, light coma, seizures, decorticate rigidity, intact pupillary light reaction
IV.	Seizures, deepening coma, decerebrate rigidity, loss of oculocephalic reflexes, fixed pupils
V.	Coma, loss of deep tendon reflexes, respiratory arrest, fixed dilated pupils, flaccidly

Diagnostic Tests and Labs

- History and physical
- Liver function tests including bilirubin
- Serum ammonia levels
- Blood glucose
- Coagulation studies
- Liver biopsy
- CT scan
- EEG

Nursing Management of the Child with Reye's Syndrome

Therapeutic Nursing Management

- Continually assess respiratory status, circulation, and neurological functioning.
- Monitor vital signs, central venous pressure, and arterial pressure.
- Provide oxygen and airway support (intubation may be needed).
- Correct fluid and electrolyte imbalance and treat shock (fluids, electrolyte replacement, and vasopressors).
- Implement measures to treat increased intracranial pressure (positioning, airway support, and mannitol administration).
- Administer glucose for hypoglycemia.
- Observe for bleeding.
- Treat hyperthermia with cooling and medications.
- Insert NG tube.
- Prevent skin breakdown with skin care and pressure relief mattress (if needed).
- Provide enteral nutrition when stabilized.
- Prevent secondary infection.
- Provide supportive care and ongoing information to the child and family.

Pharmacology

- Osmotic diuretics
- Sedatives
- Vitamin K: for coagulopathies
- Analgesics: for pain

Complications

- Speech and hearing impairments
- Developmental delay
- Brain damage
- Renal damage
- Peptic ulcer
- Hemorrhage
- Pancreatitis
- Seizures
- Cerebral edema
- Cerebral herniation
- Death

Critical Thinking Exercise: Nursing Management of the Child with Reye's Syndrome

1. What combination of factors is commonly believed to trigger Reye's syndrome?

    a.

    b.

    c.

2. The parent of a school-age child asks the nurse how she would know if her child had Reye's syndrome. How should the nurse respond?

3. What can happen if Reye's syndrome is not identified and treated promptly and/or if the child does not respond to treatment?

Neurosensory System CHAPTER 23

Nursing Management of the Child with a Head Injury

> **Key Points**
>
> - A mechanical force that leads to pathology of the brain, skull, or scalp causes head injury.
> - Outcomes from head injury are dependent upon the extent and location of the injury and the child's response to treatment.
> - Children with severe head injury may require neurosurgical intervention to decompress and clean the affected areas of the brain. They frequently need aggressive ICP management and extensive rehabilitation following their injuries.
> - Goals of collaborative management:
>   - Provide prompt treatment for severe injury and/or neurological deterioration.
>   - Stabilize neck and spine.
>   - Maintain stable airway and adequate oxygenation.
>   - Control increased intracranial pressure.
>   - Provide neurosurgical intervention as needed.
>   - Prevent infection.
>   - Manage pain and nausea.
>   - Maintain fluid, electrolyte, and nutritional status.
>   - Minimize complications from neurological injuries.
>   - Promote wound healing.
>   - Provide child and family education and support.
>   - Provide rehabilitation to promote optimal growth, development, and functioning.
> - Important nursing diagnoses (actual and potential) are:
>   - Adaptive capacity decreased: intracranial
>   - Altered tissue perfusion (cerebral)
>   - Impaired tissue integrity
>   - Altered fluid and electrolyte balance
>   - Altered protection
>   - Altered respiratory function
>   - Altered nutrition
>   - Pain management
>   - Body image disturbance
>   - Altered growth and development
>   - Self-care deficit

Nursing Management of the Child with a Head Injury

- Knowledge deficit
- Altered family processes
- **Key Terms/Concepts**: Open head injury, closed head injury, skull fracture, concussion, contusion, laceration, intracranial hematoma, epidural hematoma, subdural hematoma, subarachnoid hemorrhage, cerebral hypoxia, cerebral edema.

Overview

Head injuries are the pathologic processes involving damage to the scalp, skull, meninges, or brain as a result of trauma to the head. These are generally caused by blunt trauma, penetrating injuries or shearing forces. Damage from these injuries ranges from minor and temporary to severe, causing permanent changes in the child's level of functioning. The major causes of brain injury in children are related to falls, motor vehicle accidents, bicycle injuries, sports injuries, and gunshot wounds. Multiple traumas are the leading cause of death in children over one year of age. Approximately 75% of childhood deaths caused by mechanical trauma are the result of brain injury.

Terms

Cerebral Edema: Cerebral edema is expected after head trauma and generally peaks 24-72 hours after the injury. Edema of the brain causes venous stasis and tissue anoxia resulting in a change in tissue permeability; further loss of fluid into the brain tissue with further swelling.

Cerebral Hypoxia: Decreased flow of oxygen to the brain

Decerebrate Posturing: Occurs with injury to the midbrain; produces rigid extension and pronation of extremities. The likely cause of unilateral decerebrate posturing is tentorial herniation.

Decorticate Posturing: Results from dysfunction of the cerebral cortex; adduction of the arms, arms flexed on the chest with wrists flexed and hands fisted; legs extended and adducted.

Skull Fracture: Seen in about 25% of children with head injuries; may occur with or without brain damage

Types of Injuries	
Open head injury	Penetrating force which breaks integrity of skull and meninges (increased risk of infection)
Closed head injury	Nonpenetrating force in which skull integrity is not broken; usually caused by blunt force or shearing injury (whiplash, shaken baby syndrome)
Concussion	Temporary period of confusion or unconsciousness that follows a trauma. The most common type of head injury; it is transient and reversible.
Contusion	Bruising of brain
Laceration	Tearing of cerebral tissue
Intracranial hematoma	A hematoma within the head which causes signs of increased intracranial pressure.
Epidural hematoma	Hemorrhage outside the dura, usually a result of the rupture of the middle meningeal artery from skull fractures. Blood accumulates between the dura and the skull to form a hematoma. Associated with skull fractures 75% of time

Nursing Care of Children

Types of Injuries	
Subdural hematoma	Bleeding between the dura and the cerebrum generally from rupture of the cortical veins; these are 10 times more common than epidural hematomas, peaking in incidence at 6 months of age.
Skull fracture	Seen in about 25% of children with head injuries; may occur with or without brain damage.

Risk Factors

- Riding in car without seat belts
- Participating in sports without a helmet: baseball, football, bicycling, skateboarding
- Poor safety practices and lack of supervision in young children

Signs and Symptoms

- Brief loss of consciousness (LOC) change immediately after injury
- Bleeding from the nose or ear and watery nasal drainage from the nose that contains glucose (suggests leaking of cerebral spinal fluid from a skull fracture)
- Headache (fussiness in toddlers)
- Dizziness
- Ataxia
- Blurred/double vision
- Vomiting
- Respiratory pattern changes
- Behavioral changes: irritability, restlessness, agitation
- Vital sign changes
- Seizures
- Lethargy, stupor, coma
- Change in pupillary size and reaction to light and equality

Diagnostic Tests and Labs

- History and physical
- Neuro checks
- X-ray
- Computerized tomography (CT)
- Magnetic resonance imaging (MRI)
- Glasgow coma scale (GCS), modified GCS for children

Therapeutic Nursing Management

- Stabilize neck and spine until cervical trauma/spinal cord injuries are ruled out.
- Support airway management needs (bag-mask ventilation, intubation, and tracheostomy as needed).

- Frequently reassess vital signs, neurological status, LOC, GCS, pupillary responses, eye movement, and motor activity.
- Assess and manage increased ICP as indicated. If injuries are minor, send home instruction sheet regarding signs and symptoms of ICP. (Change in level of consciousness, increasing agitation, confusion and disorientation, drowsiness, headache, change in respirations, elevated temperature, slowed heart rate, vomiting, blurred vision, behavioral changes, pupil changes, progressing weakness, seizure).
- Monitor fluids and control cerebral edema.
- Care for the child requiring surgical intervention (if necessary).
- Examine, clean and dress external wounds as needed.
- Provide nutrition (PO, NG, NJ, GT as appropriate) once stabilized.
- Collaborate with multidisciplinary team in the ongoing care and rehabilitation of the child with a severe neurologic injury.
- Provide education and support to child and family on an ongoing basis.
- Coordinate discharge planning to address the ongoing care and rehabilitation needs (financial assistance, home health, case management, support groups, etc.).

Pharmacology

- Diuretics to control cerebral edema (mannitol)
- Glucocorticoids to control cerebral edema
    - Dexamethasone: Decadron
    - Methylprednisolone sodium succinate: Solu-Medrol
- Anticonvulsants to prevent or treat seizures
- Sedatives and analgesics may be needed during hospitalization: Use with caution in children with decreased LOC and/or increased ICP.

Complications

- Hemorrhage
- Infection
- Respiratory compromise
- Cerebral edema, compression of brain stem, herniation
- Seizures
- Neurological damage
- Failure to thrive
- Developmental delay
- Learning disabilities
- Memory deficits
- Personality changes: Irritability, aggressiveness, poor school performance
- Death

Critical Thinking Exercise: Nursing Management of the Child with a Head Injury

Situation: A 14-year-old male is admitted to a pediatric medical/surgical unit after falling off his skateboard three hours prior to admission. Witnesses at the scene reported a brief loss of consciousness. The child does not recall the events. Initial assessment reveals a healthy appearing adolescent who is alert and oriented. He reports having a headache and vomiting once since the fall.

1. What additional assessments are important for this child?

2. What diagnostics tests should the nurse anticipate for this child?

3. Shortly after admission, the child has a generalized seizure lasting 1-minute followed by a decreased level of consciousness. What are the priority interventions for this child?

Neurosensory System CHAPTER 24

Nursing Management of the Child with a Brain Tumor

> **Key Points**
>
> - Brain tumors are the most common solid tumors in children.
> - The most common pediatric brain tumors are astrocytoma, medulloblastoma, glioma, and ependymoma.
> - Care of children with brain tumors may involve neurosurgical intervention and management of increased intracranial pressure, neurological system dysfunction, and effects of chemotherapy and/or radiation therapy.
> - Goals of collaborative management:
>   - Provide early recognition, diagnosis, and treatment.
>   - Control increased intracranial pressure.
>   - Remove the tumor and/or decrease tumor size through neurosurgical intervention, chemotherapy, and/or radiation.
>   - Prevent metastasis of cancer cells to secondary site.
>   - Minimize complications from tumor damage, surgery, chemotherapy, and/or radiation.
>   - Prevent infection.
>   - Manage pain and nausea.
>   - Maintain fluid, electrolyte, and nutritional status.
>   - Promote wound healing.
>   - Provide child and family education and support.
>   - Promote optimal growth and development.
> - Important nursing diagnoses (actual and potential) are:
>   - Adaptive capacity decreased: intracranial
>   - Altered tissue perfusion (cerebral)
>   - Impaired tissue integrity
>   - Alteration in fluid and electrolyte balance
>   - Altered nutrition, less than body requirements
>   - Altered protection
>   - Anxiety, powerlessness
>   - Pain management
>   - Body image disturbance
>   - Altered growth and development
>   - Knowledge deficit
>   - Ineffective family and individual coping

Nursing Management of the Child with a Brain Tumor

- Altered family processes
- **Key Terms/Concepts:** Cerebral hemisphere, cerebellum, brain stem, astrocytoma, medulloblastoma, glioma, ependymoma, prognosis, metastasis, increased intracranial pressure, projectile vomiting, chemotherapy, radiation

Overview

Brain tumors are second to leukemia as the most common type of cancer in children. Brain tumors may be malignant or benign. Approximately 60% of brain tumors occur in the cerebellum or brainstem. Astrocytoma, the most common type of brain tumor (approximately 50%), invades the cerebral hemispheres and cerebellum.

Medulloblastoma, the second most common brain tumor (approximately 25%), invades the cerebellum. Glioma, the third most common brain tumor (approximately 11%), most frequently invades the brain stem, optic nerve, and the cerebellum. The prognosis depends on the type of tumor, the size, the extent of the disease, and age of the child. Treatment may include surgery, radiation, and chemotherapy.

Risk Factors

- Heredity
- Environmental (toxins, radiation, electromagnetic fields)
- Congenital tumors
- Neurofibromatosis
- Immunosuppression

Signs and Symptoms

- Signs and symptoms will vary according to size and location of tumor.
- Headache
- Vomiting (projectile, especially in the a.m. upon arising)
- Gait changes, loss of balance
- Neuromuscular changes: weakness, hyperreflexia, spasticity, paralysis, clumsiness
- Behavioral changes: irritability, decreased appetite, failure to thrive, fatigue, lethargy
- Visual changes
- Papilledema
- Changes in vital signs: bradycardia, respiratory pattern changes, temperature instability (late signs)
- Seizures
- Tense, bulging fontanel (infants)
- Split cranial sutures (infants)

Diagnostic Tests and Lab

- MRI

- CT scan
- EEG
- Lumbar puncture
- Positive Emission Tomography (PET)
- Single Photon Emission Computed Tomography (SPECT)

Therapeutic Nursing Management

- Care for child undergoing surgical procedure (preoperative teaching and preparation).
- Minimize stimulation and provide a quiet, dimly lit room.
- Position to decrease intracranial pressure - consult with the primary provider to determine correct positioning.
- Provide wound care to surgical incision; assess for edema, bleeding, infection, or other complications.
- Care for the child receiving radiation; provide sedation as needed. Assess and manage radiation-related complications as indicated.
- Administer chemotherapy as ordered. Assess and manage chemotherapy-related complications as indicated.
- Protect from infection with bone marrow suppression (secondary to chemotherapy and radiation).
- Provide nutritional support as needed.
- Protect skin integrity.
- Provide support and education to the child and family. Discuss physical and body image changes: hair loss/shaving, incision, facial edema (postoperative), etc.
- Collaborate with multidisciplinary team in addressing child's medical, nutritional, pharmacological, and rehabilitation needs.
- Provide home care and on-going support instructions:
  - Teach family to recognize signs of infection, skin breakdown, and nutritional deficiency.
  - Instruct child and family members to administer medications and nutritional support at home.
  - Instruct family in the proper use of vascular access devices and/or feeding tubes as needed.
  - Provide information regarding support resources for children and families with cancer (national and local organizations, case manager, home health agency, etc.) support, nutritional and pharmacological care at home.

Pharmacology

- Stool softeners
- Antiemetics
- Pain medications
- Chemotherapy drugs

Complications

- Neurological damage
- Developmental delay
- Behavioral changes
- Increased intracranial pressure
- Seizures
- Coma
- Death
- Pharmacological side effects (organ damage, altered nutrition, infection)

Critical Thinking Exercise: Nursing Management of the Child with a Brain Tumor

Situation: A 7-year-old male is admitted after a large brain tumor was discovered during an MRI scan. The boy has a history of recurrent headaches, vomiting, and blurred vision. Upon admission, the child is awake, alert, and oriented with vital signs within the normal range for his age.

1. What changes in vital signs should the nurse anticipate if the brain tumor were large enough to cause increased intracranial pressure (ICP)?

2. What should the nurse ask the child and parent about the vomiting?

3. What assessments would indicate that the child's neurological functioning and/or level of consciousness are deteriorating?

4. What nursing interventions are indicated for this child and family?

Neurosensory System CHAPTER 25

Nursing Management of the Child with Cerebral Palsy

Key Points

- Cerebral palsy (CP) is a nonprogressive neuromuscular disorder causing impaired posture and movement.
- CP is caused by anoxia, toxins, infection, and unknown reasons in the prenatal, perinatal, and postnatal period.
- Goals of collaborative management:
    - Provide early recognition and diagnosis.
    - Maximize developmental potential by supporting nutritional needs, locomotion and mobility, cognitive capabilities, communication skills, self-care abilities, self-concept and relationships.
    - Prevent complications (seizures, malnutrition, obesity, aspiration, skin breakdown, infection, gastrointestinal alteration, decreased mobility).
    - Maintain effective airway, breathing, and circulation.
    - Maintain functional ability using braces, casts, medications, surgery, adaptive devices, and therapy.
    - Coordinate multidisciplinary care needs (PT, OT, speech therapy, recreation therapy, primary care provider, home health, school nurse and psychologist as needed).
    - Achieve self-care and communication.
- Important nursing diagnoses (actual and potential) are:
    - Impaired physical mobility
    - Risk for injury
    - Self-care deficit
    - Altered nutrition
    - Sensory-perceptual alteration
    - Ineffective family coping
    - Ineffective individual coping
- **Key Terms/Concepts**: Dyskinesis, athetoid, ataxic, hemiparesis, diplegia, dysphagia, dysarthria

Overview

Cerebral palsy (CP) is a nonspecific term that describes disorders characterized by impaired movement and posture. This non-progressive condition affects the motor centers in the brain resulting in abnormal muscle tone and coordination. Perceptual problems, language deficits, and intellectual impairment can accompany the muscular disturbances. A variety of prenatal, perinatal, and postnatal factors can contribute to the etiology of cerebral palsy.

Cerebral palsy may be related to birth asphyxia (lack of oxygen getting to the fetal brain) or perinatal exposure to infection. Congenital problems involving the CNS (hydrocephalus, myelomeningocele) may also be a cause. However, approximately one-quarter of all cases of CP have no determined cause.

Hydrocephalus is a syndrome where cerebral spinal fluid (CSF) accumulates within the intracranial space. In infants, prior to closing of the fontanels, the enlarged head is the hallmark sign. In older infants and in children neurological signs are produced from the increase in intracranial pressure. Treatment goals include removal of the excess CSF, treatment and management of complications of the ICP (serial lumbar punctures, or medications to reduce ICP). Surgical intervention is the most common treatment.

Surgery may include direct treatment of the problem (removal of a blockage) but most frequently is implantation of a shunt to move the CSF from the ventricles of the brain extracranially (usually to the peritoneum). The major concern for a client with a shunt is infection, followed by malfunction of the shunt. Nursing management should include attention to the family needs and concerns with referrals to agencies that can assist them in home care.

Myelomeningocele is a failure of the neural tube to close and fuse. This develops in the first 4 weeks of gestation. Hydrocephalus occurs in up to 95% of these cases and should be monitored for from birth. The amount of neurological involvement is dependent upon the level of the anomaly in the spinal column. The primary nursing goal, prior to surgical repair, is prevention of infection (the repair should take place within 18 hours of the birth). Postoperatively the concerns are for promotion of maximal levels of functioning, management of genitourinary system, and bowel training. Nursing management must include referrals and education to the families to assist them in understanding the anomaly, the prognosis, and in providing home care.

Terms

- **Ataxia (ataxic)**: An inability to coordinate muscle activity in voluntary movement, in coordination, may involve extremities, head, or trunk.
- **Athetosis (athetoid)**: Slow, writhing, involuntary movements; flexion, pronation, extension, and supranational of the fingers and hands and may include the feet and toes. This type of CP involves bilateral involuntary movements, with generalized hypotonia and delayed motor development.
- **Diplegia**: A type of CP with bilateral spasticity; in which the lower extremities are more severely affected
- **Dysarthria**: Disturbance of speech and language
- **Dyskinesis**: Problems with moving voluntarily; difficulty making voluntary movements
- **Dysphagia**: Problems with swallowing
- **Hemiparesis**: Weakness on one side of the body

Risk Factors

- Prenatal teratogens
- Chromosomal abnormalities
- Multiple births
- Complicated labor and delivery, traumatic birth
- Apgar score of 5 or less at birth
- Seizures within 48 hours after delivery
- Prematurity
- Low birth weight under 2500 grams at birth
- Head injuries
- Sepsis
- Meningitis
- Encephalitis
- Toxins

Signs and Symptoms

- Poor head control
- Irritability and persistent crying
- Floppy or limp baby
- Arching or pushing away
- Hypertonicity and/or spasticity
- Feeding difficulties (choking on food, tongue thrust, uncoordinated swallowing)
- Persistent infantile reflexes (Moro, plantar, palmar grasp, tonic neck)
- Drooling
- Speech difficulty
- Delayed gross motor development (missed developmental milestones)
- Early preference for hand dominance
- Involuntary, purposeless movements
- Lack of muscle coordination
- Uses only one side of the body
- Gait changes (toe-walking, wide gait, jerky movements)
- Scissoring or extension of legs
- Seizures
- Mental retardation may or may not be present with CP

Diagnostic Tests and Labs

- EEG
- CT scan
- Screening for metabolic disorders

Nursing Management of the Child with Cerebral Palsy

Therapeutic Nursing Management

- Assist the family in setting realistic long and short-term goals.
- Refer parents to agencies that provide respite care.
- Assist parents with physical, occupational, speech and recreation therapies.
- Assess skin integrity under the braces.
- Assess muscle tone and attempt to prevent contractures.
- Administer medications for muscle relaxation, seizures, and GE reflux as needed.
- Change child's position frequently.
- Ensure appropriate posture using braces and wheelchair.
- Provide adequate nutrition using special feeding equipment and supplements as needed.
- Provide activities that require ROM and use of muscular movements.
- Assist the child with communication skills.
- Assist family in meeting education and schooling needs.
- Collaborate with multidisciplinary team in addressing child's medical, nutritional, pharmacological, and rehabilitation needs.
- Provide home care and on-going support instructions.
  - Teach family to recognize signs of infection, skin breakdown, and nutritional deficiency.
  - Instruct family members to administer medications and nutritional support at home.
  - Instruct family in the proper use of feeding tubes, braces, locomotion devices, and other equipment as needed.
- Range of motion exercises with spastic cerebral palsy clients should stretch and elongate the muscles. This will slow the development of contractures and help to prevent tightening and spasticity.

Complications

- Contractures
- Increased susceptibility to infections
- Skin breakdown
- Compromised self-image
- Caregiver role strain

Critical Thinking Exercise: Nursing Management of the Child with Cerebral Palsy

Situation: A 2-year-old born at 26 weeks gestational age was recently diagnosed with cerebral palsy (CP). The child's parents have many questions about their daughter's diagnosis.

1. Which of the following statements would most help the parents to have an accurate perception of CP?
    a. The child will probably be very intelligent because most children with CP compensate for their disorder by developing significantly superior cognitive abilities.
    b. The child will eventually outgrow the disorder if she has consistent physical and occupational therapy when she is young.
    c. CP is a progressive condition characterized by increasing neuro-muscular deterioration.
    d. CP was most likely caused by hypoxic damage when she was a critically-ill premature infant.

    Correct answer: _____

    Rationale:

2. Which of the following assessments is most characteristic of CP?
    a. Unusual hand and foot creases
    b. Vomiting, diarrhea and high fever
    c. Hypertonicity and developmental delay
    d. Periorbital edema and pulmonary congestion

    Correct answer: _____

    Rationale:

Nursing Management of the Child with Cerebral Palsy

3. What medication should the nurse expect to administer to help decrease muscle tone?
   a. Metoclopramide
   b. Methotrexate
   c. Beclomethasone
   d. Baclofen

   Correct answer: _____

   Rationale:

4. Which of the following are most important to families with children who have cerebral palsy?
   a. Reversing the degenerative processes that have occurred.
   b. Identifying the underlying defect that is causing the disorder.
   c. Promoting optimal cognitive and physical functioning.
   d. Assisting the family in finding counseling resources.

   Correct answer: _____

   Rationale:

Neurosensory System **CHAPTER 26**

Nursing Management of the Child with Strabismus

> **Key Points**
>
> - Strabismus is a misalignment of the eyes causing visual disturbances.
> - Strabismus is a normal finding in the first four months of life due to developing eye muscles.
> - Identification and treatment of strabismus beyond the first few months of life is needed to prevent permanent visual loss.
> - Treatment may be noninvasive (occlusion therapy) or invasive (surgery or intraocular injections).
> - Goals of collaborative management:
>   - Provide early recognition, diagnosis, and treatment.
>   - Identify the associated neurological conditions (if present).
>   - Strengthen eye muscles.
>   - Prevent vision damage.
>   - Provide surgical correction or treatment with intraocular botulinum toxin (if needed).
>   - Provide child and family education and support.
>   - Promote optimal growth, development, and self-image.
> - Important nursing diagnoses (actual and potential) are:
>   - Altered sensory perception
>   - Risk for injury (related to visual impairment)
>   - Body image disturbance
>   - Altered growth and development
>   - Knowledge deficit
>   - Ineffective family and individual coping
>   - Altered family processes
> - **Key Terms/Concepts**: "Lazy eye," "cross-eyed," "squint," strabismus amblyopic, tropia, occlusion therapy, photophobia, and binocular vision

Overview

Strabismus, also called esotropia when it is an inward deviation and exotropia when it is an outward deviation, is an abnormality of the eyes often described as "cross-eye," or "squint." The child with strabismus is not able to focus both eyes toward the same object. It is caused by an imbalance or weakness in the muscles in one or both eyes. Strabismus is a common and benign condition in infants until four months of age due to the initial weakness of the supporting muscles of the eye until normal use serves to strengthen eye muscle. Strabismus causes incomplete fusion of the visual image from two images to one.

This can lead to amblyopia, a loss of vision due to strabismus. Treatment depends on the cause of the strabismus. The condition must be treated early to prevent vision loss. Strabismus is seen in approximately 4% of children under the age of six.

Signs and Symptoms

- One eye deviates from the point of fixation.
- Inaccurate judgment when picking up objects
- Photophobia
- Dizziness
- Headache
- Difficulty focusing from one distance to another
- Squint eyelids together
- Closes one eye to see

Diagnostic Tests

- Corneal light reflex test
- Cover/uncover test (for Amblyopic)

Therapeutic Nursing Management

- Assess for associated neurological conditions.
- Stress the importance of continued eye care may be needed.
- Inform parents that children need books with large letters that are widely spaced.
- Provide bright lighting.
- Instruct parents to monitor for eyestrain.
- Instruct parents that occlusion therapy (patching stronger eye) may be needed.
- Work with parents and child to develop creative ways to ensure compliance with therapy.
- Prepare the child for surgery to shorten the eye muscles (if needed). This allows the eye to realign and develop binocular vision (fusion of the visual fields into one image).
- Provide care to the child receiving botulinum toxin injections in the unaffected eye. This causes temporary weakness in both eyes, causing misalignment.

Complications

- Poor school performance
- Blindness
- Low self-esteem

Critical Thinking Exercise: Nursing Management of the Child with Strabismus

Identify each of the following statements about strabismus as **TRUE** or **FALSE**.

1. The terms "lazy eye," "cross-eyed," or "squint" are commonly used to describe three different conditions of the eye.

2. Strabismus is caused by deformation of the ocular socket and unequal shape of the eyeballs.

3. Assessment of strabismus is done by watching for eye deviation when the child is focusing on an object.

4. Strabismus should be treated as soon as possible during the first 3 months of life.

5. Visual loss is a common result of untreated strabismus.

6. A child with strabismus would be expected to have difficulty building with blocks and assembling puzzles.

7. A child with strabismus who has photophobia, dizziness, and headache probably has meningitis.

8. Treatment involves covering the affected eye to rest the weak muscles.

9. Both young children and older children are at risk for noncompliance with treatment because they don't like wearing an eye patch.

10. Surgical removal of the eye may be needed if noninvasive treatment is ineffective.

Endocrine System **CHAPTER 27**

Nursing Management of the Child with Type I Insulin-Dependent Diabetes Mellitus

> **Key Points**
>
> - Type I diabetes mellitus (Type I DM) causes insulin deficiency and hyperglycemia.
> - Type I DM is believed to be due to a genetic predisposition triggered by an autoimmune response.
> - Type I DM most often presents with polyuria, polydipsia, polyphagia, weight loss, and fatigue.
> - The primary goal of treatment is to maintain stable blood glucose levels and promote optimal growth and development.
> - Goals of collaborative management:
>   - Provide early recognition, diagnosis, and treatment.
>   - Maintain normal blood glucose levels through diet, insulin administration, and related management on an ongoing basis.
>   - Prevent complications – (hyperglycemia, hypoglycemia, infection, renal failure, neuropathies, and retinopathy.
>   - Provide child and family education and support.
>   - Promote child and family competence and motivation to comply with treatment plan.
>   - Promote optimal growth and nutrition.
> - Important nursing diagnoses (actual or potential) are:
>   - Altered pattern of urinary elimination related to polyuria
>   - Fluid volume deficit related to polyuria and dehydration
>   - Risk of injury related to hyperglycemia, hypoglycemia, and disease processes
>   - Knowledge deficit related to new onset, complex disease
>   - Altered nutrition related to dietary changes and metabolic effects of disease
>   - Fatigue related to disease, hypoglycemia
>   - Risk for infection related to delayed healing
>   - Acute pain related to pain in extremities secondary to neuropathy
>   - Altered growth and development related to endocrine involvement
>   - Ineffective individual coping related to lifestyle changes and new diagnosis
>   - Anxiety, fear, powerlessness related to diagnosis of a serious chronic illness
>   - Altered family processes related to family lifestyle changes
>   - Grieving related to loss of "normal" life
>   - Self-concept disturbance related to being "different" from peers
>   - Alteration in coping related to having a chronic illness
>   - Management of therapeutic regimen: effective or ineffective

Nursing Management of the Child with Type I Insulin-Dependent Diabetes Mellitus

- **Key Terms/Concepts**: Hyperglycemia, hypoglycemia, cellular dehydration, lipolysis, ketonemia, ketoacidosis, ketonuria, counter regulatory hormones, polydipsia, polyphagia, neuropathy, and Kussmaul respirations

Overview

Type I diabetes mellitus (Type I DM), also known as insulin-dependent diabetes mellitus and juvenile diabetes, is a chronic, metabolic condition in which the body is unable to metabolize and use carbohydrates, fats and proteins properly due to a deficiency of insulin. Type I DM is believed to occur because of a genetic predisposition for the disease and triggered by an immunologic response to some factor, such as a viral infection.

This response causes damage to the beta cells in the pancreas, which leads to insulin deficiency. This deficiency leads to hyperglycemia, lipolysis, ketonemia, ketoacidosis, ketonuria, polyuria, and cellular dehydration. It also leads to a heightened effect of counter regulatory hormones (epinephrine, glucagon, cortisol and growth hormone) causing glucose production and glucose uptake impedance. Prior to treatment, the blood glucose levels usually exceed 200 mg/dL.

There is currently no prevention or cure. Type I DM, the most common endocrine disorder of childhood, occurs in 1.7 of 1000 people, most of these are children. The highest rate of occurrence is among school-age children. Initial diagnosis occurs most often in the winter. There is an increased incidence of the disease if a family member has the disease, particularly if an identical twin has the disease. The goal for the family of a diabetic child and for the affected child is to receive adequate information through education to allow that child to participate in activities appropriate for his/her age. Adequate education will allow the child to modify behaviors in order to participate in almost all activities. It is important that the child and family know how to control blood glucose levels with appropriate dosing of medications and adjustment of dietary intake.

Risk Factors

- Genetic predisposition: family member with Type I DM, particularly if identical twin
- Autoimmune response trigger: stress, infectious disease, winter months

Signs and Symptoms

- Polyuria may start as bed-wetting
- Glucosuria
- Polydipsia
- Polyphagia
- Weight loss
- Fatigue
- Anorexia
- Nausea
- Lethargy

- Weakness
- Dry skin
- Irritability
- Dehydration (tachycardia, lethargy, decreased perfusion, hypotension)
- Ketones in blood and urine (when the blood glucose reaches 250 mg/dL or higher ketones spill into the urine)
- Frequent infections, delayed healing
- Vaginal yeast infections in girls
- Growth delays

Diagnostic Tests and Labs

- History and physical
- Urinalysis, urine dipstick: glucose, ketones, pH
- Blood glucose levels
- Glycosylated hemoglobin
- Glucose tolerance tests
- Electrolyte profile
- CBC, WBC

Therapeutic Nursing Management

- Monitor glucose and ketone levels.
- Hb A1C levels monitor long-term adequacy of control
- Administer insulin, as needed, based on levels.
- Correct fluid and electrolyte imbalance.
- Provide child and family education regarding:
  - Disease process
  - Recognition of signs of hyperglycemia, hypoglycemia (drink a high sugar/fructose product like fruit juice), and dehydration
  - Monitoring serum glucose
  - Monitoring urine glucose and ketones
  - Diabetic diet customized for child's age and food preferences
  - Insulin administration
  - Activity level and exercise (When adding new activity, the blood sugar should be checked prior to the activity. If the blood sugar is lower than 100, the child should eat a snack. The child should remain alert to signs and symptoms of hypoglycemia during exercise until sugar is available.)
  - Maintaining adequate hydration
  - Prevention of infection
  - Follow-up and care needed during illness or uncontrolled levels
  - Encouraging increased intake of dietary fiber, which slows the rate of absorption of sugar helping to stabilize blood glucose

Nursing Management of the Child with Type I Insulin-Dependent Diabetes Mellitus

Pharmacology

- Insulin (SQ, IV, insulin pump)
  - Rapid-acting
  - Intermediate-acting
  - Long-acting
- Glucose

Complications

- With a deficiency of insulin in the body, glucose is unable to enter the cell thus raising the concentration of blood glucose in the blood stream.
- With an increase in the concentration of blood glucose (hyperglycemia) an osmotic gradient occurs causing a shift in body fluids potentially leading to dehydration and a decreased renal perfusion.
- Long term complications of diabetes involve both the microvasculature and the macrovasculature.
- Sticky glucose compounds enable proteins to stick to vessel walls interfering with blood circulation in the micro/macrovasculature circulatory system.
- The principle microvascular complications of Type 1 diabetes mellitus include nephropathy, retinopathy and neuropathy.
- Hyperglycemia interferes with the normal function of white blood cells which are important in defending the body against bacteria and in cleaning up dead tissue and cells. As a result wounds take much longer to heal and become infected more easily.
- The focus of Type 1 diabetes mellitus management is insulin replacement, diet, and exercise.
- Other Complications:
  - Hypoglycemia
  - Ketoacidosis, DKA
  - Seizures
  - Coma
  - Death
  - Altered growth and development
  - Vascular diseases
  - Depression
  - Body image changes

Hyperglycemia

- Elevated blood glucose.
- Type 1 diabetes mellitus is characterized by destruction of the pancreatic beta cells, which produce insulin, leading to an insulin deficiency.
- Insulin is needed to support the metabolism of carbohydrates, fats, and proteins by facilitation of the entry of these substances in the cell.
- Insulin is needed for the entry of glucose into the muscle and fat cells and

Nursing Management of the Child with Type I Insulin-Dependent Diabetes Mellitus

- storage of glucose and glycogen in the cells of the liver and muscle.
- With the deficiency of insulin, glucose is unable to enter the cell, and the systemic glucose concentration increases.

Signs and Symptoms

- Polyuria
- Glucosuria
- Polydipsia
- Polyphagia
- Fatigue
- Weakness
- Ketoacidosis
- Ketones in the urine

Treatment

- Regular insulin administration (subcutaneous injection or insulin drip depending on glucose level)
- Hydration
- Potassium replacement based on lab values
- Monitoring blood glucose levels closely until stabilize

Hypoglycemia

- Low amount of blood glucose in the blood.
- Fluctuating blood glucose levels are a complication of diabetes mellitus
- Until blood glucose is managed consistently, periods of hyperglycemia and hypoglycemia are common.
- Hypoglycemia can occur by skipping a meal, participating in exercise without having a snack before or by having an interaction with other medication.
- Education on the signs and symptoms and the treatment of hypoglycemia are the role of the nurse.

Signs and Symptoms

- Shakiness
- Headache
- Dizziness
- confusion
- Fatigue
- Restlessness
- Malaise
- Irritability
- Weakness

- Delirium

Diagnostic Tests

- Glucometer
- Venipuncture for blood glucose
- Glycosylated hemoglobin

Treatment

- Give glucose tab or sugar in the form of juice or a candy bar
- Subcutaneous or Intramuscular glucagons
- IV Dextrose

Diabetic retinopathy

- A disorder of retinal blood vessels characterized by capillary microaneurysms, hemorrhage, exudates, and the formation of new vessels and connective tissue.
- Repeated retinal hemorrhage may result in permanent opacity of the vitreous humor, and blindness may eventually occur.

Signs and Symptoms

- Vision difficulties such as cloudiness, floaters, vision threatening lesions

Diagnostic Tests

- Dilated eye examination

Treatment

- Consultation of an ophthalmologist
- Photocoagulation of damaged retinal blood vessels by a laser beam may be performed to prevent hemorrhage from the vessels.
- Rarely, cloudy vitreous humor is surgically removed by a vitrectomy.

Diabetic nephropathy

- A disease which includes inflammatory, degenerative and sclerotic lesions of the kidney.
- As a result of the microvasculature changes decreasing renal perfusion, diabetic renal failure may occur.

Signs and Symptoms

- Decreased urine output
- Edema
- Fluid and electrolyte imbalance
- Hypertension
- Proteinuria

Nursing Management of the Child with Type I Insulin-Dependent Diabetes Mellitus

- Pain in flank

Diagnostic Tests

- Lab work indicating renal function: BUN, Creatinine, Uric Acid, General Chemistry
- 24 hour urine/Urinalysis
- Arterial blood gases
- Ultrasound
- Intravenous pyelography

Treatment

- Restoration of blood flow to the kidney
- Balance intake and output, electrolyte balance
- Dialysis may be indicated

Diabetic neuropathy

- A type of neuropathy in which metabolic and vascular changes caused by long term diabetes mellitus result in damage to peripheral and autonomic nerves.
- Poor sensation leads to undetected injuries.
- Due to the damage to the nerves from diabetes, leg and foot wounds or ulcers heal poorly, become gangrenous and frequently lead to amputation.

Signs and Symptoms

- Sensory loss in the extremities
- Pain in the extremities
- Paresthesia
- Wounds/injuries (poorly healing)

Diagnostic Tests

- Nerve conduction test
- Sensory perception test

Treatment

- Pain medication
- Inspection of extremities (daily)

Critical Thinking Exercise: Nursing Management of the Child with Type I Insulin-Dependent Diabetes Mellitus

1. What factors most commonly lead to hyperglycemia in a client with Type I diabetes mellitus?

2. What factors most commonly lead to hyperglycemia in a client who is taking insulin?

3. What are the most common early signs of Type I diabetes mellitus?

4. Identify the key signs and symptoms for hypoglycemia and hyperglycemia:

	Hypoglycemia	Hyperglycemia
Onset		
Blood Glucose		
Urine Dipstick		

Nursing Management of the Child with Type I Insulin-Dependent Diabetes Mellitus

	Hypoglycemia	Hyperglycemia
Respiratory System		
Cardiovascular System		
Neurological System		
Skin		
Gastrointestinal System		
Fluid status (hydration)		

Endocrine System CHAPTER 28

Nursing Management of the Child with Diabetic Ketoacidosis

Key Points

- Diabetic ketoacidosis is a life-threatening complication of diabetes mellitus that requires immediate intervention due to cerebral edema and complications from electrolyte imbalances (hyperkalemia, hypokalemia, hypocalcemia, and hyponatremia).
- Treatment is directed at gradually restoring serum glucose levels, fluid and electrolyte balance and acid-base balance.
- Goals of collaborative management:
  - Provide early detection and treatment.
  - Correct hyperglycemia.
  - Restore fluid volume, electrolyte and acid base balance.
  - Prevent complications (coma, cerebral anoxia, death).
- Important nursing diagnoses (actual or potential) are:
  - Fluid volume deficit
  - Alteration in acid-base balance related to ketoacidosis
  - Potential for injury related to cerebral edema, electrolyte imbalance, and acid-base imbalance
  - Intracranial adaptive capacity decreased
  - Altered nutrition related to inappropriate intake and/or altered metabolism.
  - Anxiety/fear related to acute, critical illness
  - Knowledge deficit related to status and prevention of DKA
  - Impaired adjustment related to inability to change lifestyle needed for optimal health status
  - Ineffective management of therapeutic regimen
  - Self-concept disturbance
  - Alteration in coping
- **Key Terms/Concepts:** Hyperglycemia, ketoacidosis, Kussmaul's respirations, noncompliance, acid-base balance, hyperkalemia, hypokalemia, hypocalcemia, and hyponatremia.

Overview

Diabetic ketoacidosis (DKA) is caused by an insulin deficiency, hyperglycemia (300 mg/dL or higher), an accumulation of ketones in the blood, and metabolic acidosis. DKA is a medical emergency and can rapidly lead to coma or death. It is most commonly triggered in children and adolescents by infection, missed insulin doses, stress, alcohol intoxication, and/or noncompliance with treatment.

Nursing Management of the Child with Diabetic Ketoacidosis

During this time, the body chooses alternate forms of energy, principally fat and muscle tissue. Fat is broken down by the body into ketones. Excess ketones are eliminated by the kidneys through the urine (ketonuria) or the lungs (acetone breath).

Risk Factors

- Triggered by conditions that increase insulin demand (fever, stress, infection, pregnancy)
- Omission of one or more doses of insulin
- Noncompliance with DM treatment regimen

Signs and Symptoms

- Dry skin, flushed face
- Excessive thirst
- LOC changes: Restlessness progressing to increasing lethargy and coma
- Abdominal pain
- Fruity odor to breath
- Blood pressure and pulse increase
- Kussmaul's breathing: Increase in the rate and depth of respirations in an attempt to blow off more carbon dioxide
- Dehydration (sunken eyeballs, dry lips and membranes, weight loss, decreasing urine output)
- Hyperglycemia (blood glucose > 300 mg/dL)
- Ketones in blood and urine

Diagnostic Tests and Labs

- History and physical
- Blood glucose
- Urine glucose and ketones
- Electrolytes and BUN
- Blood gas analysis

Therapeutic Nursing Management

- Frequently monitor vital signs and perform assessments (including neurological status).
- Frequently monitor serum glucose levels.
- Administer IV fluids.
- Administer insulin (IV or SQ).
- Frequently monitor serum electrolytes.
- Monitor hydration status-assess intake and output.
- Treat any infection.

- Monitor for signs of hyperglycemia, hypoglycemia, and hyperkalemia.
- Provide child and family education and support.
- Reinforce home maintenance routine when stabilized.

Pharmacology

- Regular insulin IV bolus and/or continuous infusion
- Glucose administration (given with insulin to prevent rapid decrease in serum levels)

Complications

- Electrolyte imbalance (hyperkalemia, hypokalemia, hypocalcemia, hyponatremia)
- Acidosis
- Cerebral edema
- Coma

Critical Thinking Exercise: Nursing Management of the Child with Diabetic Ketoacidosis

Situation: A 17-year-old with a seven-year history of Type I diabetes mellitus is admitted after "passing out" at his senior prom. He is currently conscious with slurred speech. He admits to having "a few beers with his friends" earlier that night. His initial serum glucose is 500 mg/dL.

1. List seven additional history questions that would be helpful for this child.

2. List at least five assessments that are most important for this child during initial stabilization.

3. Identify at least ten interventions appropriate for this child (list in order of priority).

Musculoskeletal System **CHAPTER 29**

Nursing Management of the Child with a Clubfoot (Talipes Equinovarus)

Key Points

- Clubfoot is a congenital malformation of the bones, muscles, tendons of foot, ankle, and lower leg leading to plantar flexion, inverted heel, and an adducted forefoot.
- Management of clubfoot may involve stretching, serial casting, and surgery.
- Goals of collaborative management:
  - Provide early recognition, diagnosis, and treatment.
  - Identify the associated conditions (if present).
  - Correct the deformity.
  - Strengthen leg muscles and promote ambulation.
  - Prevent skin breakdown.
  - Provide child and family education and support.
  - Promote optimal growth, development, and self-image.
- Important nursing diagnoses (actual and potential) are:
  - Impaired physical mobility
  - Peripheral neurovascular dysfunction
  - Altered tissue perfusion (related to casts and/or braces)
  - Altered tissue integrity (related to casts, braces, and/or surgical incision)
  - Self-concept disturbance
  - Knowledge deficit
  - Altered family processes
- **Key Terms/Concepts:** Adduction, plantar flexion, metatarsus adductus, serial casting

Overview

Clubfoot (talipes equinovarus) is a deformity of the bone with malposition and resulting contracture of the soft tissue of the ankle and foot (forefoot adduction, mid-foot supination, hind foot varus, and ankle equines). This deformity represents about 95% of clubfoot anomalies and is bilateral in up to 50% of the cases. Early recognition and treatment are imperative. Initial treatment includes manipulation and serial casting until the deformity correction has been achieved. This treatment gradually stretches the contractures on the medial side of the foot. This is done weekly for the first 6 to 12 weeks of life and is successful in up to 50% of the cases. If these interventions are not successful, surgery is recommended.

- **Congenital clubfoot:** Also known as idiopathic or true clubfoot; it occurs in a generally otherwise normal child.

Nursing Management of the Child with a Clubfoot (Talipes Equinovarus)

> - **Positional clubfoot**: Also known as transitional, mild, or postural clubfoot; it is thought to be caused by intrauterine crowding and is successfully treated with mild stretching and casting.
> - **Syndromic clubfoot**: Also known as tetralogic clubfoot; it is associated with other congenital anomalies.
> - **Talipes calcaneus**: Dorsiflexion, toes are higher than the heel
> - **Talipes equines**: Plantar flexion, the toes are lower than the heel
> - **Talipes valgus**: Eversion or bending outward
> - **Talipes varus**: Inversion or bending inward

Risk Factors

- Genetics
- Improper foot position in uterus
- Congenital syndrome associated with clubfoot

Signs and Symptoms

- Anterior half of foot is adducted and inverted.
- Medial border of foot is concave.
- Lateral border of foot is convex.
- Heel is drawn up.
- Underdeveloped calf muscle
- Small foot
- Atrophy of the joint capsule

Diagnostics Tests and Labs

- History and physical exam
- X-ray

Therapeutic Nursing Management

- Provide stretching exercises and manipulation.
- Care for infant with serial casting (cast replaced every week for the first month and then every two weeks until corrected or until surgical intervention is determined).
- Teach family cast care (keep dry, neurovascular checks, skin assessment, and skin care).
- Prepare child and family for surgical correction (cutting tight tendons and placing pins to maintain alignment) if manipulation is not successful.
- Collaborate with physical therapy for muscle strengthening and ambulation.
- Provide education and support to parents.

Complications

- Skin breakdown (from casts)

- Neurovascular compromise
- Difficulty with ambulation
- Delayed motor development
- Multiple surgeries
- Body image disturbance
- Altered parent/infant attachment

Critical Thinking Exercise: Nursing Management of the Child with a Clubfoot (Talipes Equinovarus)

Identify each of the following statements about clubfoot as TRUE or FALSE.

1. Clubfoot is a positional deformity that can be manipulated to a normal position.

2. An infant with clubfoot will need to have foot casts that are replaced every six weeks.

3. A child with clubfoot may need surgery if the casts do not sufficiently correct his feet.

4. Most individuals with clubfoot will be severely deformed for the remainder of their life.

5. Children with clubfoot often do not need treatment because their feet strengthen and straighten as they grow.

6. Surgery should be considered if deformity persists despite casting and manipulation.

7. Most children who have had their clubfoot corrected successfully will have no signs of the defect.

Musculoskeletal System **CHAPTER 30**

Nursing Management of the Child with Fractures

> **Key Points**
>
> - Fractures occur when bone is subjected to greater stress than it can endure.
> - Fractures in children are most frequently caused by trauma.
> - Abuse and/or an underlying condition (osteogenesis imperfecta) should be considered with fractures in children, particularly in infancy.
> - Fractures extending into the growth plate can lead to permanent deformity caused by altered bone growth.
> - The goals of collaborative management:
>   - Prevent hemorrhage.
>   - Relieve pain.
>   - Immobilize and stabilize fractured bone.
>   - Prevent complications (infection, fat embolism, neurovascular compromise, skin breakdown, and immobility related complications).
>   - Prevent deformity and/or alteration in function.
>   - Promote healing and rehabilitation.
> - Important nursing diagnoses (actual or potential) are:
>   - Pain management
>   - Neurovascular compromise
>   - Impaired skin integrity
>   - Activity intolerance
>   - Sleep pattern disturbance
>   - Risk for injury
>   - Impaired physical mobility
>   - Impaired home maintenance management
>   - Self-care deficit
>   - Altered growth and development
>   - Knowledge deficit
> - **Key Terms/Concepts:** Greenstick, simple fracture, complete fracture, incomplete fracture, compression, comminuted, displaced, compound, crepitus; ecchymosis, compartment syndrome, growth plate, spica cast

Overview

A bone fractures when the force exerted on the bone exceeds the strength of the surface to resist the stress. The types of fractures are listed below. Fractures of the long bones occur most frequently in children because of the characteristics of the child's skeletal system, incomplete motor development in children, the activity

Nursing Management of the Child with Fractures

> level of many children, and the nature of traumatic injuries. Child abuse should be considered in children with multiple fractures at various stages of healing and spiral fractures or femur fractures in children less than 1 year of age. Greenstick fractures are most frequently seen in children less than 3 years of age.

Risk Factors

- Child abuse
- Osteogenesis imperfecta
- Ewing's sarcoma, metastatic
- Accidents: MVA, team sports, bicycling, climbing
- High-risk activities and lifestyle
- Nutritional deficiencies (calcium, vitamin D)

Type of fracture	Description
Incomplete	Partial fracture through the width of the bone
Complete	Full separation into two or more parts
Simple (closed)	Bone is fractured with intact skin
Compound (open)	Broken skin (with or without bone protrusion)
Comminuted	Bone splintered or broken into several fragments. Uncommon in children
Compression	Spinal cord injury frequently associated with a fall or sport activity.
Spiral	Twisted or circular break. May be associated with child maltreatment in non ambulating child.
Greenstick	Incomplete fracture on one side with a bend deformity on the other side
Bend	Bone bends but does not break. A child's bone may bend up to 45°.
Buckle	Compression of unossified bone, usually near the metaphysis.

Signs and Symptoms

- Symptoms differ depending on type of fracture
- Protruding bone from the skin
- Generalized swelling or deformity at fracture site
- Pain or tenderness at site
- Diminished function or abnormal mobility
- Crepitus
- Ecchymosis
- Muscular rigidity, spasm
- Linear bruising at the site

Diagnostic Tests and Labs

- History and physical
- X-ray
- Bone scans
- MRI
- CT

Traction

Types

- **Upper extremity**
    - Overhead suspension: Arm is bent and the traction holds the limb vertically by skin or skeletal devices.
    - Dunlop traction: Uses skin or skeletal devices to hold the arm horizontally
- **Lower extremity**
    - Buck extension traction: Skin traction, legs straight, used for short-term, preoperative care in children with hip dislocation or other skeletal muscle deformities.
    - Russell traction: Skin traction to the lower leg with a sling at the knee. Used with femur fractures. Due to the physics of this type of traction, the pull is equal to twice the amount of weight added to the traction.
    - "90-90" traction: Pin in the distal femur with the hip and knee at 90-degree angles, a boot is applied to the lower leg.
    - Balanced skin or skeletal traction: With or without skin or skeletal devices, the limb is balanced and often uses a Thomas splint and a Pearson attachment. This is a balanced traction, so when the client is lifted off the bed surface for care, the traction is maintained.
- **Cervical traction**
    - Intermittent cervical skin traction: Uses a halter to the head and weights to reduce muscle spasm.
    - Crutchfield tong traction: Used in a fracture or displacement of a cervical vertebra, the goal is immobilization until the fracture is healed. The device is a skeletal traction with the weights suspended from the ropes attached to the device.
    - Halo cast: Is a circular device applied to the skull with pins and uses an attachment, which rests on the shoulders to apply traction. This allows ambulation of the client with non-neurological, non-displaced cervical fractures.
- **Pelvic traction**
    - Pelvic belt: Strap at the hips is attached to weight at the foot of the bed, used in low back muscle pain, spasms, strain or sprain.
    - Pelvic sling: A strap at the hips is attached to a bar overhead to maintain space between the hips and the bed, used in pelvic fractures or injuries.

- Assessment
  - Make neurovascular checks frequently to the affected area and any areas with prolonged pressure from immobilization.
  - Maintain traction and alignment at all times unless "rest" periods are ordered.
  - Be certain weights are correct, hanging freely (neither the ropes nor the weights should be touching anything).
  - If there is any break in the skin (from the fracture, surgery, pins, or immobilization) frequent checks for infection or bleeding.
  - Keep the bed surface under the client clean of small objects or food.
  - Assessment and treatment for post-traction muscle spasm and related pain.

Therapeutic Nursing Management

- Provide first-aid stabilization with immobilization/splinting.
- Control bleeding if indicated.
- Prepare child for open or closed reduction.
- Teach parents and child about cast care.
- Assess for pain: administer analgesic agents as needed.
- Keep extremity elevated on pillows while cast is drying and as needed for comfort.
- Monitor for swelling and neurovascular compromise at least every 4 hours and PRN.
- Maintain traction if necessary.
- Encourage a diet high in protein and vitamins to promote healing, high in fiber to prevent constipation.
- Collaborate with physical therapy and occupational therapy for rehabilitation.
- Position the client so that warm, dry, air circulates around and under the cast (support the casted area without pressure under or directly on the cast) for faster drying and to prevent pressure from changing the shape of the cast. If the cast must be handled before it is dry the palms of the hands should be used in a flat position to try to prevent changing the shape of the cast.
- Child and family education:
  - Managing pain (prescription for oral analgesics; ice, rest, elevation)
  - Assessing for complications (skin breakdown, neurovascular compromise, complications associated with immobility)
  - Providing skin/cast care: keep dry (especially pedal edges), cover with plastic for showering/bathing, and teach child not to put anything inside the cast
  - Follow-up appointments and outpatient rehabilitation
  - Report occurrence to SRS/child welfare if abuse suspected (nurses are mandatory reporters)

Pharmacology

- Analgesics

- Antibiotics (compound fractures, surgical reduction)
- Stool softeners or laxatives (with altered mobility)

Complications

- Skin breakdown
- Neurovascular compromise
- Complications associated with immobility
- Embolism (fat, pulmonary)
- Compartment syndrome (swelling causes pressure within the closed space)
- Gangrene
- Contracture
- Refracture
- Limb deformity, leg length discrepancy
- Alteration in movement and/or sensation
- Damage to the joint
- Altered growth (if growth plate is affected)
- Infection (the most likely complication to occur with a compound fracture)

Critical Thinking Exercise: Nursing Management of the Child with Fractures

Situation: A 10-year-old female is admitted to the pediatric unit after an open reduction for a fractured femur. While crossing the street, she was struck by a car and injured. She sustained no other injuries except superficial lacerations. Upon arrival the nurse notes that the child is alert and oriented with an intact spica cast.

1. What nursing assessments are important for this child?

2. What physical and emotional complications is this child at risk for developing within in the next 3-7 days?

3. Identify complications related to skeletal fractures.

Musculoskeletal System **CHAPTER 31**

Nursing Management of the Child with Traction

> **Key Points**
>
> - Traction is used to stabilize injuries, maintain alignment during healing, promote rest, and decrease spasm of affected muscles.
> - Various forms of skin and skeletal traction are used in children based on the child's age and type of injury.
> - Children in traction pose unique challenges due to their age and developmental needs.
> - The goals of collaborative management:
>   - Promote healing through immobilization and stabilization.
>   - Manage pain.
>   - Provide diversional activities.
>   - Promote adequate nutrition.
>   - Prevent complications (infection, fat embolism, neurovascular compromise, skin breakdown, and immobility related complications).
>   - Prevent deformity and/or alteration in function.
>   - Promote healing and rehabilitation.
> - Important nursing diagnoses (actual or potential) are:
>   - Impaired physical mobility
>   - Pain management
>   - Neurovascular compromise
>   - Impaired skin integrity
>   - Activity intolerance
>   - Sleep pattern disturbance
>   - Risk for injury (thrombophlebitis, tissue necrosis, nerve damage, infection)
>   - Self care deficit
>   - Impaired home maintenance management
>   - Knowledge deficit
> - **Key Terms/Concepts:** Counterbalance, skin traction, skeletal traction, pin, Bryant traction, Buck's extension traction, Russell traction, cervical traction, Dunlop traction, 90-degree femur traction

Overview

Bony fragments that cannot be realigned by simple stabilization with casting may require the extended pulling force supplied with traction. Traction is performed with the elevation of the part of bed closest to weights, use of restraints and application of counterweight.

Nursing Management of the Child with Traction

> A forward pulling force is used to reduce dislocation and realign fracture sites. A counter-force (backward pulling) is provided with the child's own body weight. The contact with the bed creates a frictional force to aid in the positioning of the bone into proper alignment.
>
> The three primary purposes of traction for reduction of fractures are:
> - To avoid fatigue of the involved muscle and prevent muscle spasm that would hinder bone alignment.
> - To promote bone healing by interfacing the bone surfaces.
> - To immobilize the site for healing until the injury can be cast or splinted.

Skin traction is applied when there is minimal displacement and little muscle spasticity. It works by indirectly positioning the bone pulling the skin and muscle. A limited amount of weight may be added without causing skin breakdown.

Skeletal traction is used when a significant degree of pulling is needed to properly align and immobilize the fracture or dislocation site. Inserting a mechanical device or pin directly into, or through, the bone and attaching the prescribed weight performs this type of traction.

Traction Types

Name	Type	Description/Use
Bryant traction	Skin traction	Used for fractured femur in child <30 pounds. No longer recommended due to risk for hypotension in lower extremities.
Buck extension	Skin traction	Short-term, used for preoperative care in children with hip dislocation or other skeletal muscle deformities and some fractures.
Russell traction	Skin traction	Skin traction to the lower leg with a sling at the knee. Used with femur fractures. Due to the physics of this type of traction, the pull is equal to twice the amount of weight added to the traction. May incorporate skeletal traction for hip contractures or immobility for fractured femur.
Halo brace	Cervical traction	A circular device applied to the skull with pins and uses an attachment, which rests on the shoulders to apply traction. This allows ambulation of the client with non-neurological, non-displaced cervical fractures.
90-90° Femoral traction	Skeletal traction	The most common type of traction used for fractured femur in the preschool- and school-age child. Pin in the distal femur with the hip and knee at 90° angles, a boot is applied to the lower leg.
Dunlop traction	Skeletal/skin traction	Treatment of fractures of the humerus.

Therapeutic Nursing Management

- Assess frequently for circulatory or neurologic impairment. The five P's of vascular impairment that indicate a neurovascular problem are:
    - Pain
    - Pallor
    - Pulselessness
    - Paresthesia
    - Paralysis
- Avoid moving the weights or interfering with traction, and maintain proper angle.
- Provide skin care and pressure relief to head, back, and buttocks.
- Provide pain relief.
- Provide pin care for skeletal traction.
- Provide diversion and acceptable play activities (these children do not feel sick).
- Report any "burning" sensation to the primary care provider. This symptom is associated with tissue ischemia and can be an indicator of serious neurovascular compromise.
- Encourage a diet high in protein and vitamins (to promote healing) and high in fiber (to prevent constipation).
- Child and family education:
    - Keep child/family informed as to progress of healing.
    - Manage pain (prescription for oral analgesics).
    - Teach setup and care of home traction.
    - Teach family signs of complications (skin breakdown, infection, neurovascular compromise, complications associated with immobility).
    - Provide instructions regarding mobility limitations, skin care, and pin care.
    - Provide information regarding home health care, follow up appointments, and outpatient rehabilitation.

Pharmacology

- Analgesics
- Antibiotics (compound fractures, surgical reduction)
- Stool softeners or laxatives (with altered mobility)

Complications

- Noncompliance with treatment
- Infection
- Skin breakdown
- Hypertension
- Emotional distress, boredom
- Neurovascular compromise
- Constipation

Critical Thinking Exercise: Nursing Management of the Child with Traction

Identify the correct response for each of the following items. Explain the rationale for each response selected.

1. The nurse caring for a child in skeletal traction should question which of the following orders?
    a. Administer acetaminophen (Tylenol®) every four hours PRN pain.
    b. Release traction for 30 minutes every shift.
    c. Elevate the foot of the bed.
    d. Perform neurovascular checks every eight hours.

    Correct answer: _____
    Rationale:

2. Which of the following is most appropriate for assessing circulation and sensation?
    a. Color, temperature, movement, sensation, and capillary refill of the extremity
    b. Degree of motion and ability to position the extremity
    c. Length, diameter, and shape of the extremity
    d. Amount of swelling, intensity of pain, and presence of drainage on the dressing

    Correct answer: _____
    Rationale:

3. A 5-year-old Chinese-American client is hospitalized with skeletal traction for a fractured femur. The nursing assistant tells the nurse that the child has shown little interest in eating the food on his meal trays. Which of the following assumptions is most likely to be accurate?
    a. The child is spoiled and angry that he is in the hospital.
    b. The child needs less food since he is on bed rest and not playing as usual.
    c. The child is probably eating between meals and is spoiling his appetite.
    d. The child may have culturally-related food preferences.

    Correct answer: _____
    Rationale:

Musculoskeletal System CHAPTER 32

Nursing Management of the Child with Scoliosis

Key Points

- Scoliosis is a lateral curvature of the spine that occurs most frequently in adolescent girls.
- Not all spinal curvatures are scoliosis. A curve of less than 10% is considered postural variation.
- Scoliosis can lead to deformity, chronic pain and alteration in mobility, respiratory compromise and altered body image.
- Management of scoliosis for curves greater than 20% or progressive changes involves the use of exercises, shoe lifts, braces, and/or surgical placement of rods for spinal stabilization.
- Goals of collaborative management:
  - Provide early recognition, diagnosis, and treatment.
  - Use noninvasive and invasive methods to stabilize the spine.
  - Manage pain.
  - Prevent complications associated with surgical rod placement (hemorrhage, hypovolemia, pain, skin breakdown, infection, and respiratory compromise).
  - Provide child and family with education and support.
  - Promote optimal growth, development, and self-image.
  - Promote rehabilitation and mobility.
- Important nursing diagnoses (actual and potential) are:
  - Pain management
  - Impaired physical mobility
  - Respiratory compromise
  - Fluid volume deficit (related to surgery)
  - Altered tissue integrity (related to braces and/or surgical incision)
  - Risk for injury
  - Self-concept disturbance
  - Knowledge deficit
  - Altered family processes
  - Ineffective management of therapeutic regimen
- **Key Terms/Concepts:** Scoliosis screening tools, asymmetry, malalignment, Boston brace, TLSO brace, Milwaukee brace, spinal fusion, Harrington rod, and Luque rod, Dwyer cable

Nursing Management of the Child with Scoliosis

Overview

Scoliosis is the most common spinal deformity in children. The condition may be functional or structural and can occur as an isolated deformity or as a component of other diseases. It is characterized by an S-shaped, lateral curvature of the spine of 10 degrees or more. Scoliosis can be congenital, develop during childhood, or occur during the adolescent growth spurt. Eighty percent of the cases in adolescents are idiopathic. New evidence suggests that there is a genetic transmission linked to an autosomal dominant trait. Children with neuromuscular disease and/or cerebral palsy have a tendency to develop scoliosis due to muscular weakness. The condition can lead to physiologic and cosmetic alterations of the spine, pelvis, and chest. Severe scoliosis can lead to interference with normal respiration due to distortion and deformity of the rib cage. Early recognition and treatment are important because the flexible curvature becomes rigid and permanent as the child ages. Current management involves preventing further curvature by use of a brace or straightening by use of surgical fixation techniques.

The two most common types of braces are: the Boston brace, or underarm orthotic device, which is a customized brace from prefabricated shells that provides corrective forces; and the TLSO brace, a customized molded brace. Another type of brace, the Milwaukee brace, an adapted plastic and metal brace with a neck ring is rarely used with scoliosis. The underarm brace is usually more acceptable to the child because loose fitting clothing easily hides it. The Milwaukee brace is necessary for curves higher than T8. Mild-to-moderate scoliosis can be treated with electrical stimulation transmitted to the convex side of the curvature; however use of a brace to prevent further curvature is more effective.

Risk Factors

- Familial inheritance pattern
- Structural caused by congenital abnormalities
- Muscular dystrophy
- Cerebral palsy
- Spinal bifida
- Neuromuscular disease or cerebral palsy
- Poor posture
- Marfan's syndrome

Causes/Types of Scoliosis

- **Congenital** scoliosis may be associated with other congenital anomalies
- **Idiopathic** scoliosis is generally not visible prior to age 10, and is responsible for up to 60% of the cases. This occurs in females 7:1 versus males.
- Other causes of scoliosis include neuromuscular problems, trauma, and formation secondary to tumor, poor nutrition, or metabolic problems

Nursing Management of the Child with Scoliosis

Treatment of Scoliosis	
Degree of curvature	**Treatment**
Up to 20° angle	Does not require treatment but is carefully followed up every 4-6 months
Progressive curvature between 20-40°	Requires bracing until skeletal system is mature. Bracing is required for 23 hours each day.
Angle greater than 40°	Surgical intervention with spinal fusion and internal stabilization (Harrington rods, Luque rod, Dwyer cable)

Signs and Symptoms

- Uneven hemline or difficulty fitting clothes
- Uneven shoulder blades
- Protruding scapula with one side of back higher than the other
- Unequal arm-to-body spaces
- Protruding hip
- Hip and/or buttock asymmetry
- Unequal leg lengths
- Malaligned trunk or pelvis

Diagnostic Tests and Labs

- History and physical
- Spinal radiographs show severity and location of curve

Therapeutic Nursing Management

- Provide routine screening during adolescence.
- Instruct child and caregivers about the application and care of therapeutic braces. Bracing may slow the progression of the deformity until the spine has reached skeletal maturity.
- Encourage an active exercise program to prevent atrophy of the spine and abdominal muscles with bracing. Exercise alone is of little value for correction of curvature.
- Provide ongoing education and support to child and family regarding the brace-wearing schedule, padding and care of the brace and movement exercises.
- Instruct child and caregiver to return for re-evaluation.
- If surgery is indicated, postoperative care includes:
    - Providing IV fluids
    - Monitoring for bleeding, neurovascular compromise
    - Monitoring for edema
    - Log rolling
    - Pain assessment and management (PCA analgesia)
    - Gastric decompression with NG tube

- Urinary catheterization for bladder emptying
- Physical therapy, active and passive range of motion

Pharmacology

- Analgesics
- Antibiotic (if surgical intervention is indicated)

Complications

- Altered growth and development
- Back pain
- Urinary problems (related to surgery)
- Fatigue
- Disability, altered mobility
- Cardiac and pulmonary complications
- Skin breakdown under the brace
- Infection
- Body image changes, depression

Critical Thinking Exercise: Nursing Management of the Child with Scoliosis

Identify five nursing interventions for each of the following problems of a 16-year-old female who has had surgical placement of rods for scoliosis.

Fluid loss
1.
2.
3.
4.
5.

Pain
1.
2.
3.
4.
5.

Difficulty sleeping
1.
2.
3.
4.
5.

Lack of self esteem due to body image changes
1.
2.
3.
4.
5.

Musculoskeletal System CHAPTER 33

Nursing Management of the Child with Juvenile Rheumatoid Arthritis

> **Key Points**
>
> - Juvenile rheumatoid arthritis (JRA) is a disease that causes inflammation resulting in a decreased range of motion and pain in one or more joints.
> - The incidence of JRA occurs in children ages 1-16 years. It is rare in infants under six months old.
> - Each type of JRA has unique incidence, diagnostic indicators, symptoms, and prognosis.
> - Goals of collaborative management:
>   - Provide early recognition, diagnosis, and treatment.
>   - Reduce pain to an acceptable level.
>   - Promote rest and comfort.
>   - Maximize joint function to allow the child to perform normal activities of daily living is the primary goal of therapy.
>   - Promote normal nutrition, growth, and development.
>   - Support the child and family in coping with a chronic, debilitating condition.
>   - Prevent complications.
> - Important nursing diagnoses (actual or potential) are:
>   - Pain management
>   - Hyperthermia
>   - Self-care deficit
>   - Impaired physical mobility
>   - Self-concept disturbance
>   - Risk for injury
>   - Altered nutrition: Less than body requirements
>   - Altered growth and development
>   - Knowledge deficit
>   - Potential complications of drug therapy (infection, gastritis)
>   - Ineffective individual coping
> - **Key Terms/Concepts:** Inflammatory, systemic, polyarticular, pauciarticular, contractures, resistive exercises, range of motion, muscle wasting, uveitis, iridocyclitis, human leukocyte antigens, rheumatoid factor

Overview

Juvenile arthritis (JRA), formerly called juvenile rheumatoid arthritis, is an autoimmune and inflammatory disease of undetermined etiology involving the joints in children. It is commonly believed to be a disorder of the connective tissue. The four major types include: (1) systemic; (2) polyarticular (five or more joints) rheumatoid factor positive; (3) polyarticular rheumatoid factor negative; and (4) pauciarticular onset (four or fewer joints). JA occurs most often in females. Early onset most frequently affects children 1-5 years of age. Late onset JA occurs most frequently in males 8-15 years of age. Growth may be retarded during periods of active disease, usually, with growth spurts during remission where cases that are treated with steroids may experience more significant growth impairment.

Risk Factors

- Autoimmunity
- Infection
- Genetic predisposition (human leukocyte antigens—HLA)
- Stress
- Trauma

Signs and Symptoms

- Systemic
  - High fever spikes several times daily
  - Pale red macular rash on trunk and extremities
  - Hepatosplenomegaly
  - Enlarged lymph nodes
  - Pericarditis
  - Pleuritis
  - Anemia
  - Leukocytosis
  - Arthralgia
- Polyarticular: Rheumatoid factor positive
  - Occurs most frequently in young girls
  - Five or more joints affected, symmetric pattern
  - Involves large and small joints
  - Low-grade fever intermittent
  - Palpable rheumatoid nodules
  - Anemia
  - Fatigue and malaise
  - Morning stiffness, joint pain
- Polyarticular: Rheumatoid factor negative
  - Occurs most frequently in older girls
  - Five or more joints affected, asymmetric pattern
  - Frequently involves knees, wrist, elbows and ankles
  - Low-grade fever intermittent
  - Anemia

- Fatigue and malaise
- Morning stiffness, joint pain
- Pauciarticular onset
  - Occurs during first six months of the disease
  - Four or fewer joints affected
  - Frequently involves knees, ankles and elbows
  - Painless joint swelling
  - Low-grade fever
  - Malaise
  - Anemia
  - Enlarged lymph nodes
  - Uveitis, iridocyclitis
  - Hepatosplenomegaly
  - Ankylosing spondylitis

Diagnostic Tests and Labs

- History and physical
- Complete blood count (CBC)
- Erythrocyte sedimentation rate (ESR)
- C reactive protein (CRP)
- Rheumatoid factor assay
- Antinuclear antibody assay (ANA)
- Human leukocyte antigens (HLA)
- Synovial fluid analysis

Therapeutic Nursing Management

- Assess and manage pain.
- Promote joint mobility and muscular strength.
- Provide care for child with splints.
- Control fevers as needed.
- Apply heat or warm bath for comfort.
- Provide a well-balanced diet.
- Assess body alignment during splinting.
- Collaborate with physical and occupational therapy (exercise, muscle strengthening, and use of adaptive devices as needed).
- Promote normal functioning, growth and development.
- Provide child and family education and support. Provide information regarding community agencies for financial support, home health needs and emotional support.

Pharmacology

- Anti-inflammatory drugs:
    - NSAIDs (ibuprofen, naproxen, tolmetin)
    - Aspirin is no longer the drug of choice due to its association with Reye's syndrome.
- Slow-acting antirheumatic drugs (SAARD) or disease modifying antirheumatic drugs (DMARD)
    - Gold salts
    - Hydroxychloroquine
    - Sulfasalazine
    - D-penicillamine
    - Methotrexate
- Glucocorticoids (for life threatening complications)
- Immunosuppressive agents for unresponsive JRA (azathioprine, chlorambucil, cyclophosphamide, cyclosporine)

Complications

- Uveitis, iridocyclitis (cataracts, glaucoma, vision loss, blindness)
- Anemia
- Malnutrition
- Contractures (may require orthopedic surgery)
- Decreased range of motion
- Muscular weakness
- Joint deformity
- Depression
- Body-image changes
- Social isolation
- Side effects from medications
- Growth impairment

Critical Thinking Exercise: Nursing Management of the Child with Juvenile Rheumatoid Arthritis

Situation: A 10-year-old female is admitted with a diagnosis of juvenile arthritis (JA).

1. What assessments are important for this child?

2. List interventions might be helpful in decreasing the pain associated with JA.

3. List interventions that assist with self-care and mobility in children with JA.

4. Matching: Match the symptoms with the type of JA:

_____ High fever spikes	
_____ Occurs during first 6 months of the disease	a. Pauciarticular
_____ Five or more joints affected	b. Systemic
_____ Red rash on trunk and extremities	c. Polyarticular
_____ Four or fewer joints affected	

Musculoskeletal System **CHAPTER 34**

Nursing Management of the Child with Muscular Dystrophies

> **Key Points**
>
> - Muscular dystrophies (MD) are a group of incurable progressive degenerative disease of the voluntary muscles.
> - Individuals with MD have progressive muscle weakening that frequently leads to loss of ambulation, self-care difficulty, ineffective breathing pattern, poor airway control and a shortened life span.
> - Duchenne (pseudohypertrophic), the most common type, is carried by females and occurs in males. It leads to a delay in motor development, muscular weakness, and gait abnormalities.
> - The multidisciplinary approach to treatment of children is focused on maintaining function, quality of life and preventing complications for as long as possible.
> - Goals of collaborative management:
>   - Provide early recognition, diagnosis, and intervention.
>   - Maximize the child's function by supporting nutritional needs, locomotion and mobility, cognitive capabilities, communication skills, self-care abilities, self-concept and relationships for as long as possible.
>   - Support an effective airway and breathing pattern.
>   - Prevent complications (pneumonia, pulmonary aspiration, obesity, skin breakdown, contractures, scoliosis, and cardiac decompensation).
>   - Maintain functional ability for as long as possible by using braces, adaptive devices, locomotion devices, and therapy.
>   - Coordinate multidisciplinary care needs (PT, OT, speech therapy, recreation therapy, primary care provider, home health, school nurse and psychologist as needed).
> - Important nursing diagnoses (actual and potential) are:
>   - Impaired physical mobility
>   - Risk for injury
>   - Self-care deficit
>   - Ineffective airway clearance, ineffective breathing pattern
>   - Constipation or other bowel dysfunctions
>   - Impaired verbal communication
>   - Altered nutrition: Less than body requirements
>   - Altered growth and development
>   - Ineffective family coping
>   - Ineffective individual coping
>   - Impaired home maintenance management

Nursing Management of the Child with Muscular Dystrophies

- Social isolation
- Altered body image
- **Key Terms/Concepts**: Duchenne, pseudohypertrophic, Becker's, facioscapulohumeral, X-linked recessive, Gowers' sign, and waddling gait

Overview

Muscular dystrophies (MD) are a genetically-acquired group of disorders that lead to a progressive degeneration of muscle fibers. It causes muscle tissue atrophy in which muscle fibers are replaced with fatty deposits and connective tissue.

Gradual weakness and muscle wasting leads to symmetric deformity and disability in the child with muscular dystrophies. Eventually, the diaphragm and accessory muscles for breathing are affected and death usually results from cardiorespiratory failure or pneumonia. The insidious loss of strength is related to the origin of the disease, age of onset and rate of progression. It is important to maintain the unaffected muscles as long as possible. Continuing to be active keeps the child out of the wheelchair longer. Once the child is in the wheelchair the weakness accelerates and contractures begin to develop. Swimming is a good activity for these clients. It is not stressful to the joints and provides range of motion to the upper and lower extremities, hips and neck while it strengthens the muscles in much of the body. The parents should be alert to the special safety needs of the client in the pool relative to the level of disability and the age of the child. The major types of MD are Duchenne, Becker's, facioscapulohumeral, limb-girdle, and ocular. Duchenne MD (pseudohypertrophic) is the most common form and usually occurs in males between ages three and five. It is due to an X-linked recessive pattern of inheritance (mother to son).

Risk Factors

- Duchenne: X-linked inherited disorder usually manifests in boys, females are usually carriers
- Other types: Autosomal recessive (can affect males or females)

Signs and Symptoms

- Onset between two and six years
- Delayed motor development as an infant and toddler, slow walk and run, frank mental deficits in 25% of cases
- Frequent falls
- Clumsiness
- Waddling, wide-based gait
- Gowers' sign: Using hands on legs to brace the legs when rising from the floor (hip girdle weakness)
- Enlarged muscles (especially in calves) that feel unusually firm or woody on palpation
- Contractures of ankles, knees, and hips
- Loss of mobility (usually wheelchair dependent by age 10-12)
- Progressive respiratory weakness (many need a tracheostomy and mechanical ventilation by late adolescence)

- Weak, ineffective cough reflex; pneumonia
- Scoliosis or lordosis
- Tachycardia and enlarged heart (if cardiomyopathy)
- Obesity
- Atrophy related to disuse of muscles

Diagnostic Tests and Labs

- History and physical
- Creatinine phosphokinase (CPK), SGOT/AST, and aldolase extremely high in the first 2-3 years of life
- Muscle biopsy reveals degenerative muscle fibers
- EMG show decrease in amplitude and duration of motor unit potential
- Genetic testing to identify carriers, genetic counseling and prenatal diagnosis
- CXR, ECG: Cardiac and pulmonary complications
- CBC: Infection complications

Therapeutic Nursing Management

- Assess airway control; provide support as needed (percussion, postural drainage, suctioning, tracheostomy care, mechanical ventilation).
- Ensure appropriate posture using braces and wheelchair as needed.
- Maintain skin integrity; provide frequent skin care, turning, positioning, assess for pressure areas with assistive devices and on pressure points in bed.
- Reposition frequently to prevent immobility-related complication (respiratory, skin, and gastrointestinal).
- Provide activities that require ROM and use of muscular movements.
- Provide adequate nutrition using enteral feeding as needed. Provide a high-fiber, low-fat diet with adequate fluid intake.
- Assist the child with communication as needed.
- Collaborate with family and team in providing physical, occupational, speech, and recreation therapies.
- Assist child in meeting social, education, and schooling needs.
- Assist the family in setting realistic long and short-term goals.
- Assist family in finding community resources for financial support, case management, home health, respite care, and emotional support.
- As with all teaching, the information should consider the client's age, readiness to learn, developmental or maturity level, and knowledge base. Advise the parents to educate the child at the child's individual pace.

Pharmacology

- Analgesia for pain
- Stool softeners for constipation
- Antibiotics for infection

Complications

- Pneumonia
- Contractures
- Skin breakdown
- Cardiopulmonary complications, cardiomyopathy
- Developmental delay
- Learning disabilities
- Mental retardation
- Decreased body image and self-esteem
- Caregiver role strain
- Shortened lifespan

Critical Thinking Exercise: Nursing Management of the Child with Muscular Dystrophies

Situation: A 4-year-old male presents with an arm laceration that he received after falling off his tricycle. His mother tells the nurse that he is clumsy and seems to be weaker than her other children especially when he tries to get up from the floor. Diagnostic tests are scheduled to determine if the child has muscular dystrophy (MD).

1. What additional history questions should the nurse ask the child's mother?

2. What assessments are important for this child?

3. What type of muscular dystrophy most resembles the child's symptoms?

4. Matching:

Gowers' sign	a. Tracheostomy and mechanical ventilation by late adolescence
Delayed motor development	b. Uses hands on legs to brace the legs when rising from the floor
Duchenne muscular dystrophy	c. Muscle replaced with fatty and connective tissue
Progressive respiratory weakness	d. Manifests in boys
Pseudohypertrophy of the calf	e. Infants and toddlers

Integumentary System   CHAPTER 35

Nursing Management of the Child with Burns

> **Key Points**
>
> - Burns result from thermal, chemical, electrical or radioactive agents.
> - Severe burns result in multisystem involvement requiring airway support, fluid management, nutritional intervention, and protection from infection, pain management, and emotional support.
> - Mortality and morbidity from burn injuries are based on the burn extent and depth, related injuries, and the complications experienced.
> - Burns in children are considered a preventable accident. Education is directed toward removing risks based on developmental level.
> - Goals of collaborative management:
>   - Maintain a patent airway and adequate oxygenation.
>   - Maintain fluid and electrolyte balance.
>   - Prevent and treat infection.
>   - Control pain.
>   - Promote adequate nutrition.
>   - Provide education and support to child and family.
>   - Educate child and family regarding treatment and prevention of recurrence.
>   - Prevent complications related to pulmonary involvement, fluid and electrolyte imbalance, infection, nutritional deficits, and emotional response.
>   - Provide rehabilitation to restore mobility and functioning.
> - Important nursing diagnoses (actual or potential) are:
>   - Impaired tissue integrity
>   - Fluid volume deficit
>   - Altered nutrition: less than body requirements
>   - Risk for altered protection
>   - Impaired gas exchange
>   - Risk for injury
>   - Pain management
>   - Body image disturbance
>   - Sleep pattern disturbance
>   - Altered growth and development
>   - Altered family processes
>   - Caregiver role strain
>   - Activity intolerance

Nursing Management of the Child with Burns

- **Key Terms and Concepts:** First degree, superficial, second degree, partial thickness, third degree, fourth degree, full thickness, minor, moderate, major, necrosis, Rule of 9's, contracture, skin graft, debridement, intravascular fluid loss, secondary infection

Overview

Extensive or severe burn injuries account for some of the most difficult nursing care in the pediatric age group. Children who have suffered serious burn trauma must undergo prolonged, painful, and often restrictive hospitalizations. Thermal, electrical, and chemical agents cause burns. Burns occur in children of all ages after infancy and are the second leading cause of injury to children 1-4 years old. Typically, toddlers sustain hot water scalds, while older children are most likely to suffer flame-related burns. Approximately ten percent of burn injuries can be attributed to child abuse, most frequently by submersion in hot water. Children with severe burns have rapid fluid and electrolyte shifts in the first 24 hours resulting in hypovolemia, hypoproteinemia, hyponatremia, and hyperkalemia. Because of the high risk for hypovolemia and electrolyte imbalance, once the client has an airway, establishing and maintaining intravenous access is a priority. Other priorities should be given to prevention of infection, maintenance of the airway, and proactive administration of pain medications to decrease the suffering of the child (pain is more difficult to control once it peaks; early and continuous administration of pain medications following the orders is essential).

Risk Factors

- Water heaters with temperature set too high
- Access to very hot liquids (coffee, soup, etc.)
- Room heaters with pans of water for humidity
- Children with access to stovetops or electrical appliances (especially curling irons)
- Unguarded bathroom faucets
- Young children left unattended in bathtubs or showers
- Cooking without supervision
- Playing with fire or matches
- Child abuse

Signs and Symptoms

Burn Type	Description
Superficial (first-degree)	Involves epidermis, tender, slightly swollen, red, like a sunburn
Partial thickness (second-degree)	Involves epidermis and dermis. Blister formation or reddened discolored region with moist weeping surface
Full thickness (third-degree)	Involves entire dermis and portions of subcutaneous tissue. Leathery brown with little surface moisture
Full thickness (fourth-degree)	Involves subcutaneous, fascia, muscle and bone

Burn Type	Description
Minor burns	Superficial and partial thickness, first- and second-degree, covering <15% of body surface area (BSA) and not involving face, hands, feet, or genitalia
Moderate burns	Partial thickness, second-degree, covering >15% but <30% BSA or full thickness involving <10% BSA
Major (severe) burns	Partial thickness, second-degree, involving 30% BSA or full thickness involving >10% BSA or face, hands, feet, or genitalia

Diagnostic Tests & Labs

- History and physical
- Rule of "nines" may be used in older children (misleading in infants)
- Pediatric Estimated Distribution of Burns assessment tool
- Arterial blood gases
- CBC and electrolytes, serum glucose
- BUN, creatinine
- Serum protein levels
- Blood type and cross
- Chest x-ray

Therapeutic Nursing Management

- Minor burns
  - Immerse area in cold water to reduce pain and edema.
  - Cleanse with mild soap and water (iodophor).
  - Cover with fine mesh gauze lightly lubricated with water-soluble antimicrobial ointment.
  - Update tetanus if indicated.
  - Provide analgesia as needed.
- Emergency care
  - Stop the burning process.
  - Assess the victim's condition.
  - Cover the burn with clean dressing.
  - Transport the victim to medical facility or call for EMS transport.
  - Provide analgesia if possible.
  - Reassure and comfort the child.
- Moderate/major burns
  - Maintain airway.
  - Prevent shock.
  - Provide humidified oxygen and/or ventilator, as ordered.
  - Insert nasogastric tube to prevent paralytic ileus, gastric dilation, and vomiting, as ordered.

- Provide fluid replacement with Lactated Ringer's solution via central line, as ordered.
- Transfuse with blood products, as ordered.
- Insert indwelling catheter, as ordered.
- Maintain daily weights, intake, and output.
- Take frequent vital signs.
- Measure CVP measurements, as ordered.
- Administer intravenous pain medications.
- Assist with hydrotherapy and debridement.
- Provide increased caloric and protein intake after 24 hours.
- Provide emotional care and support to child and family.
- Administer antibiotics.
- Wound care
    - Shave hair adjacent to wound.
    - Cleanse wound with soap, an iodophor soap or saline.
    - Debride in hydrotherapy tub.
    - Apply silver nitrate 0.5% (AgNO4) or silver sulfadiazine 1% (Silvadene) topical preparation.
    - Apply topical antibiotic ointment for bactericidal and bacteriostatic properties.
    - Apply dressing using sterile technique.
    - Prepare skin for grafting.
- Rehabilitation
    - Splinting, traction, and frequent position changes
    - Plastic surgery
    - Educate the family on the importance of having working smoke detectors in the home. New batteries should be put in annually and the batteries should be checked each month.

Pharmacology

- Analgesics
- Antibiotics (IV)
- Antibiotics (topical)
    - Mafenide cream 10% Sulfamylon
    - Silver sulfadiazine 1% Silvadene
- Cimetidine (Tagamet)
- Antacids

Complications

- Fluid and electrolyte imbalance
- Respiratory injury secondary to smoke inhalation or carbon monoxide
- Pulmonary edema
- Infection/pneumonia

Nursing Management of the Child with Burns

- Stress ulcer
- Contracture deformities
- Mucosal erosion resulting in gastrointestinal bleeding
- Anemia due to cell destruction and hemolysis
- Metabolic acidosis
- Scarring
- Body image changes
- Shock
- Third spacing

Critical Thinking Exercise: Nursing Management of the Child with Burns

Situation: A nurse is working in the Emergency Department at a community hospital when the staff is notified of a day care center fire with explosion, probably in the kitchen. Several children are being transported to the Emergency Department with varying degrees of burns.

1. Matching:

Reddened, discolored area with a moist weeping surface	a. Superficial (first degree)
Sunburn	b. Partial thickness (second degree)
Deep burn to the muscle, bone and fascia	c. Full thickness (third degree)
Tender, slightly swollen, and red skin	d. Full thickness (fourth degree)
Leathery brown with little surface moisture	
Open blisters and reddened burns	

2. Identify each of the following burns as minor, moderate, or major (severe).

	Partial and full thickness burns on face, neck, torso, arms and hands
	First- and second-degree burns on legs covering 5% of the body surface
	Full thickness burn on calf involving 3% of the body surface
	Full thickness burns (third-and-fourth degree) on 50% of the body surface
	Partial thickness burn on the back covering 25% of the body surface
	Small, red, tender area on the forearm after being burned by the tip of an iron

Integumentary System CHAPTER 36

Nursing Management of the Child with Eczema

Key Points

- Infantile eczema is an atopic dermatitis considered to be partly an allergic reaction to an irritant.
- Common allergens include:
    - Foods- egg white, cow's milk, wheat products, orange juice, tomato juice
    - Inhalants- house dust, pollens, animal dander
    - Materials- wool, nylon, plastic
- Eczema is an acute or chronic cutaneous inflammation.
- Usually begins on the cheeks and spreads to the extensor surfaces of the arms and legs. Eventually it may affect the entire trunk.
- Eczema frequently leads to a hemolytic streptococci or staphylococci infection due to the client's scratching which opens the skin surface.
- Goals of Treatment:
    - Identify allergen/irritant.
    - Hydrate the skin.
    - Relieve pruritus.
    - Reduce flare-ups or inflammation.
    - Restore skin surface.
    - Eliminate scales and crusts.
    - Prevent and control secondary infections.
- Diagnostic Association (NANDA) nursing diagnosis:
    - Impaired skin integrity related to open areas on skin surface
    - Disturbed body image related to skin erythema, papules, and pustules
    - Impaired comfort related to burning and itching
    - Risk from infection related to break in skin integrity, secondary to scratching
- **Key Terms/Concepts**: Allergens/irritants, crusts, lesions, erythema, scales, papules, pustules, vesicles

Overview

Eczema or eczematous inflammation of the skin refers to a descriptive category of dermatologic diseases and not to a specific etiology. Atopic dermatitis or infantile eczema is a type of pruritic eczema that usually begins in infancy and is associated with an allergy. Eczema presents in three forms based on the age of the child and distribution of lesions:

- Infantile- 2 - 6 months with spontaneous remission by 3 years of age

- Childhood- Follows the infantile form; 2- 3 years of age with most manifesting symptoms by 5 years of age
- Preadolescent/adolescent- Begins at about 12 years of age and may continue into adulthood.

Signs and Symptoms

- Erythema, papules, vesicles, pustules, scales, crusts, or scabs alone or in combination.
- Dry or watery discharge with itching or burning.

Diagnostic Tests

- Skin testing
- Elimination of allergens by trial and error

Treatment

- Hypoallergenic diet consisting of a milk substitute such as soy formula
- Hypoallergenic foods
- Begin new foods slowly, introducing one food at a time.
- Oral antibiotics if secondary infection present
- Oral antihistamines to relieve itching
- Topical hydrocortisone ointment or other topical steroids
- Wet soaks or colloid baths
- Emollients containing lanolin or petrolatum, cream or ointment preferable to lotion

Therapeutic Management

- Maintain hydration of the skin by utilizing a tepid bath with a mild soap, no soap or emulsifying oil followed by an application of an emollient within three minutes.
- Cover with soft cotton clothing or wrap lightly to avoid the child scratching the skin surface. Keep the child cool and free of perspiration.
- Colloid baths such as warm water and cornstarch or oatmeal may relieve itching.
- Maintain short nails to prevent opening the skin or depositing bacteria into a wound from under the nails. Cotton gloves or socks may need to be placed over the hands.
- Administer medications to relieve itching or burning. Utilize topical medicated ointments to decrease inflammation and prevent infection.

Pharmacology

- Oral antibiotics for secondary infections
- Oral and topical antihistamines
- Topical anti-inflammatory
- Emollients

Complications

- Secondary skin infections

Critical Thinking Exercise: Nursing Management of the Child with Eczema

Situation: A mother has brought her 9-month-old daughter to a rural clinic. The daughter is diagnosed with eczema of the cheeks, knees, and elbows. The mother and nurse discuss strategies for care and troubleshoot any potential problem situations.

1. From the list below, select correct interventions. Identify the rationale for all interventions.
    a. Use a mild detergent in the laundry.
    b. Stay in a warm environment.
    c. Utilize latex gloves during care.
    d. Utilize a room humidifier.
    e. Apply topical steroids.
    f. Administer lotions with pleasing scents.
    g. Obtain adequate rest/naps.
    h. Bathe 3-4 times a day.
    i. Allow child to play in bubble bath.
    j. Assess for secondary skin infections.
    k. Administer an antihistamine.
    l. Bathe in a tepid bath with mild soap.
    m. Clip nails to prevent scratching.
    n. Place a thick layer of ointment on skin.
    o. Modify diet.
    p. Cover with a wool blanket.
    q. Soak in cornstarch and water.
    r. Wear cotton clothes.
    s. Utilize cool, wet compresses.
    t. Apply emollient following bath.

    Rationale for selections:
    1. To hydrate the skin:
    2. To relieve pruritus:
    3. Reduce inflammation:
    4. Prevent and control secondary skin infections:

Integumentary System CHAPTER 37

Nursing Management of the Child with Impetigo

> **Key Points**
>
> - Impetigo is a superficial bacterial skin infection most commonly affecting the face, including the nares, scalp, buttocks, and extremities.
> - Dissemination of the infection is caused by scratching an infected site or by contact with an infected individual or object (comb, brush, toy, etc.).
> - Topical and/or oral antibiotics should be initiated promptly to prevent spread of infection.
> - Goals of collaborative management:
>   - Promote skin healing.
>   - Prevent or minimize skin breakdown from itching and infection.
>   - Prevent the spread of infection.
>   - Provide comfort measures.
>   - Educate child and family regarding treatment and prevention of recurrence.
>   - Prevent complications associated with skin breakdown.
> - Important nursing diagnoses (actual or potential) are:
>   - Impaired tissue integrity
>   - Risk for injury
>   - Altered protection
>   - Altered comfort associated with itching
>   - Body image disturbance
>   - Sleep pattern disturbance
>   - Altered family processes
> - **Key Terms/Concepts**: Bacterial infection, flora, pathogen, contagious, staphylococci, streptococci, erythematous macular lesions, vesicles, pustules, erosions, pruritus, Burrow's solution 1:20

Overview

The function of the skin is to protect the body from invasive organisms. Normally, the skin harbors a variety of bacterial floras, including a variety of pathogenic types of staphylococci and streptococci. Impetigo begins in an area of broken skin, such as insect bite or dermatitis. Active infection depends on the combination of factors: the invasiveness and toxicity of the organism, the degree of compromise to the immunity of the host, and the skin integrity. Impetigo is highly contagious and spreads easily by direct contact. The incubation period is 7-10 days. It can be spread until the lesions are healed.

Nursing Management of the Child with Impetigo

Risk Factors
- Poor hygiene practices (common in young children)
- Insect bites or scabies
- Large community gatherings such as sports activities, swimming pools, summer camps
- Toddler and preschool-age groups

Signs and Symptoms
- Inflamed and erythematous macular lesions develop into small vesicles
- Vesicles rupture, leaving moist erosions
- Exudate dries and forms honey-colored lesions
- Lesions are pruritic
- Lesions tend to spread peripherally with sharply marginated, irregular outlines
- Lesions usually heal without scarring unless a secondary infection develops

Diagnostic Tests & Labs
- History and physical
- Culture of lesions

Therapeutic Nursing Management
- Practice diligent hand washing and universal precautions when handling child or objects which come into contact with the child.
- Cleanse and remove crusts.
- Soften lesions with 1:20 Burrow's solution compresses before removal of the crust.
- Apply topical antibiotics.
- Administer oral antibiotics, as ordered for severe infection.
- Instruct parents to keep child's fingernails short and clean.
- Instruct family use good hand washing and skin care.

Pharmacology
- Burow's solution 1:20 compresses
- Mupirocin ointment 2% (Bactroban), Bacitracin, Polysporin, Neosporin
- Penicillin, erythromycin, dicloxacillin, cephalexin, or other systemic antibiotics may be used for severe or extensive lesions.

Complications
- Secondary infections
- Scarring

Critical Thinking Exercise: Nursing Management of the Child with Impetigo

Identify each of the following statements regarding impetigo as **TRUE** or **FALSE**. Explain the rationale for each response.

1. Impetigo is a noncontagious autoimmune disease causing skin irritation when exposed to the sun.

2. Impetigo can be spread from one child to another by sharing the same brush.

3. Reddened macular lesions develop into small vesicles that become pustules and rupture leaving moist erosions. The dried exudate forms honey-colored lesions.

4. Rubbing alcohol solution in a tepid bath is used to dry and heal the lesions.

5. Topical antibiotic ointment may be used to treat infected skin lesions.

6. Providing interventions for pruritus will help the child with impetigo feel more comfortable.

Integumentary System **CHAPTER 38**

Nursing Management of the Child with Diaper Rash

> **Key Points**
>
> - Diaper rash is common in infancy, causing the baby discomfort and fussiness.
> - Diaper rash is common due to decomposing urine which produces ammonia, which is irritating to the baby's skin.
> - Disease processes producing diarrhea stools causes erythema and excoriation to the anal area.
> - The peak age for diaper rash is between 9 - 12 months of age and may be associated with the frequency of diaper changes and the addition of new foods in the diet.
> - The incidence of diaper rash is greater in bottle fed infants than in breast-fed infants.
> - Goals of Treatment:
>   - Heal skin in the diaper region.
>   - Prevent reoccurrence of diaper rash.
>   - Assess for secondary infections.
> - Diagnostic Association (NANDA) nursing diagnosis:
>   - Impaired skin integrity related to diaper area rash/excoriation
>   - Risk for infection related to skin breaks, redness and rash
>   - Knowledge deficit related to care of the diaper region
> - **Key Terms/Concepts:** Excoriation, diaper rash, increased pH, glucocorticoid preparations, hydrocortisone creams

Overview

Diaper rash is encountered frequently by pediatric nurses. Prolonged contact of the skin with wet diapers affects skin properties; therefore, prolonged and repeated contact with irritants like urine, feces, soap, detergents, and ointments, causes friction and skin breakdown. This contact produces greater abrasion damage, increased transepidermal permeability, and increased microbial counts.

Risk Factors

- Insufficient parental knowledge of diaper care
- Disease processes with increased excretion of urine and stool
- Allergic reactions
- Increased perspiration, temperature and humidity
- Altered immune status

Signs and Symptoms

- Irritation, redness and excoriation of the skin in the diaper region and gluteal folds
- Blotchy red rash, warm to touch
- Beefy red central erythema with satellite pustules
- Fussiness of the child, especially following urination or bowel movement
- Areas most commonly affected are the convex surface of the buttocks, inner thighs, mons pubis, and scrotum

Diagnostic Tests

- Inspection

Treatment

- Wash skin with mild soap and water.
- Keep diaper area clean and dry.
- Promptly remove diapers soiled with urine and stool.
- Utilize superabsorbent diapers to pull wetness away from the skin.
- Apply ointment in thick layers to protect skin.
- Apply topical ointments such as glucocorticoids or hydrocortisones.

Therapeutic Nursing Management

- Directed toward altering wetness, pH, and fecal irritants
- If using cloth diapers, use only over wraps that allow air to circulate; avoid rubber pants.
- Avoid fastening diapers too tightly.
- Expose skin only slightly irritated to air.
- Apply ointment, such as zinc oxide or petrolatum, in a thick layer to protect the skin.
- To completely remove ointment and cleanse the skin, use mineral oil.
- Rinse all the baby's clothes thoroughly to eliminate detergent residue.
- Utilize a cool, wet cloth placed over the diaper rash three or four times daily.
- Dry diaper area thoroughly before re-diapering.

Pharmacology

- Steroids such as hydrocortisone cream
- Antifungal/topical steroids agents (Lotrisone and Mycolog)
- Antifungals such as nystatin, clotrimazole
- Protective skin barriers with zinc oxide

Complications

- Secondary infections

Critical Thinking Exercise: Nursing Management for the Child with Diaper Rash

Situation: A 9-month-old is brought to the clinic for a regular check up. Upon physical examination, redness and excoriation of the diaper area is noted. The mother states that the child has had reddened areas for approximately two weeks.

1. The nurse recognizes that this is the first child of a young mother, and infant care instruction is necessary. Regarding general skin care, as well as specific care of diaper rash, what instruction would be essential?

2. Create and evaluate a care plan selecting nursing diagnoses, interventions, goals and outcomes to evaluate the effectiveness of care.

    Nursing diagnosis:

    Nursing interventions:

    Outcome:

    Goal:

    Evaluation:

Integumentary System CHAPTER 39

Nursing Management of the Child with Head Lice (Pediculosis Capitis)

Key Points

- Pediculosis capitis (head lice) is a parasitic infection of the scalp.
- It most commonly occurs in preschool-age children and school-age children in daycare due to close contact.
- The insects crawling and salivating on the skin causes itching.
- Head lice eggs may be mistaken for dandruff, hair spray or other small white objects in the hair.
- Goals of collaborative management:
    - Identify the presence of the organisms.
    - Treat the child and family by removing the nits (eggs) and applying pediculicides.
    - Prevent recurrence and/or spread.
    - Educate child and family regarding treatment and prevention of recurrence.
    - Prevent complications associated with itching and skin breakdown.
- Important nursing diagnoses (actual or potential) are:
    - Impaired tissue integrity
    - Risk for injury
    - Altered protection
    - Sleep pattern disturbance
    - Altered comfort associated with itching
    - Body image disturbance
    - Noncompliance with treatment plan
- **Key Terms/Concepts:** Parasitic infection, nits, louse, papules, pediculicides, contagious, and pruritus

Overview

Head lice (pediculosis capitis) are an infestation of the scalp with a grayish white parasite. Lice lay eggs, called nits, onto the shafts of the hair follicles. The adult louse lives for 48 hours when away from the human host and the average female can have a lifespan of one month when on a human host. The incubation period, in optimal conditions, is 7-10 days from the laying of eggs to the hatching of the lice. Pediculosis capitis occurs most frequently in school-age children or preschool children who attend day care centers, and is found in all socioeconomic groups.

Risk Factors

- Attending day care or school

Nursing Management of the Child with Head Lice (Pediculosis Capitis)

- Sharing hats, combs or hairbrushes
- Poor hygiene

Signs and Symptoms

- Severe itching of scalp
- Hair may become matted
- Pustules and excoriation around the face
- Foul hair odor
- Nits somewhat resemble dandruff but cannot be brushed off and is most easily seen in part of hair, nape of neck and behind the ears
- Secondary infection

Diagnostic Tests and Lab

- History and physical
- Direct visualization of hair for presence of lice and nits

Therapeutic Nursing Management

- Treat with medicated shampoo or cream rinse (with direction of primary care provider).
- Remove nits by combing with fine-toothed comb dipped in a 1:1 vinegar and water rinse.
- Wash clothing and bedding with hot water; then use hot dryer.
- Vacuum upholstery, mattresses, car seats and pillow.
- Seal clothing, linens, and other items such as stuffed animals that cannot be washed or dry cleaned in plastic bags for 14 days.
- Keep nails trimmed and cleaned.
- Examine close family and close contacts.
- Collaborate with school or day care to treat contact groups.
- Provide child and family education regarding the risk of sharing of personal items such as combs, brushes, hats, bedding, clothing, etc.
- Provide emotional support to the child and family.

Pharmacology

- Permethrin (Nix) creme rinse after shampooing: treatment of choice for infants and young children
- Pyrethrum shampoo (A-200 Pyrinate, RID)
- Lindane (Kwell) lotion or shampoo

Complications

- Secondary infections
- Itching

Other Parasitic Infestations of the Integumentary System

Pediculus pubis

Pediculus pubis stays in the pubic hair, axillary hair, eyelashes and eyebrows. The pubic crab louse has red legs. Pubic lice, like head lice, lay eggs or nits on the hairs. The eggs are white and stick to the hair shaft. They may appear to be dandruff-like.

Pediculus corporis (body lice)

Pediculus corporis (body lice) tends to cling to clothing. Lice are very small, grayish-white and difficult to see. Body lice in the clothing may not be present when the clothing is removed. These lice suck blood from the person and lay eggs in the clothing.

Signs and symptoms

Pediculus corporis may be suspected if: the client habitually scratches, the client has scratches on the skin, or there are hemorrhagic spots on the skin where the lice have sucked blood (blood is necessary for the louses' survival).

Pediculus pubis will present with itching.

Treatment

With pubic or body lice the client showers or bathes, dries, and applies the lotion or cream, (to the entire body for body lice, to the pubic area and adjacent areas for pubic lice). The lotion or cream is washed off after 12-24 hours and clean clothing and linens are used.

Scabies

Scabies is a contagious skin infestation by a mite. The lesion is a burrow made by the female mite penetrating the top layers of the skin.

Signs and symptoms

The borrows are short, wavy, brown or black threadlike lesions most common between the fingers and folds of the wrist and elbows. The mites cause severe itching, which is generally worse at night.

The warming of the areas stimulates the mites. Secondary lesions may be caused by the itching: scratches, vesicles, papules, pustules, crusting, and excoriation.

Treatment

Treatment includes bathing the entire body with soap and water to remove the scales and debris from the lesions. After bathing the client should apply a scabicide. All linens and clothing should be washed in very hot or boiling water.

Critical Thinking Exercise: Nursing Management of the Child with Head Lice (Pediculosis Capitis)

1. Fill in the blank:

    Head lice occur in children in _____ socioeconomic groups.

    Head lice are spread through _____ contact with infected objects.

    The feeling of the lice crawling and the saliva on the skin causes _____.

2. Matching:

Permethrin	a. One month
Pyrethrin shampoo	b. Eggs
Lindane	c. Kwell
Nits	d. Treats Itching
Louse	e. Treatment of choice for infants and young children
Incubation period of eggs	f. 7-10 days
Diphenhydramine (Benadryl)	g. Adult organism
Female adult life span	h. 48 hours
Lifespan if away from host	i. RID

3. Answer the following questions:
    a. How should families be instructed to look for signs of the organisms?

    b. How should families be instructed to treat head lice?

    c. What should the nurse teach the family to prevent the spread or reinfection of head lice?

Integumentary System **CHAPTER 40**

Nursing Management of the Child with Dermatophytosis (Ringworm)

Key Points

- Dermatophytosis, more commonly known as ringworm, is a fungal infection of the superficial skin, hair, and nails.
- The rapidly multiplying fungi cannot live in the deeper layers of the skin and will only survive on the dead keratin layer.
- Ringworm of the scalp is called tinea capitis or tinea tonsurans.
- Ringworm begins with a small papule on the scalp and spreads leaving scaly patches of baldness.
- Tinea corporis is ringworm of the body which affects the epidermis and may appear on any body surface.
- Tinea pedis is ringworm of the feet or most commonly known as athlete's foot.
- Tinea cruris is ringworm of the inner thighs and inguinal area or commonly known as jock itch.
- Goals of Treatment:
    - Eliminate the fungal infection.
    - Stop pruritus.
    - Restore hair growth.
    - Maintain skin surface.
- Diagnostic Association (NANDA) nursing diagnosis:
    - Disturbed body image related to bald spot in hairline, skin condition
    - Impaired skin integrity related to itchy scaly patches of the skin
    - Risk for infection related to disrupted skin integrity
    - Knowledge deficit related to disease process
- **Key Terms/Concepts:** Fungal infection, alopecia, tinea capitis, tinea corporis, tinea cruris, tinea pedis, ringworm, selenium sulfide shampoos, oral griseofulvin, topical tolnaftate

Overview

Ringworm is the popular term for dermatophytosis caused by various species of fungi. The various species infect body surfaces of the head, skin and nails. The condition is marked by a red-ringed patch of vesicles with itching, pain, and scaling. Treatment varies with each condition. The prescribed treatment is only successful if completed fully. Diagnosis for all types of fungal infections is made through microscopic examination of a scraping of the area.

Nursing Management of the Child with Dermatophytosis (Ringworm)

Risk Factors
- Poor personal hygiene
- Sharing of personal belongings during times of infection
- Infected household pets

Tinea Capitis
- Fungal infection of the scalp

Signs and Symptoms
- Lesions are itchy, scaly patches that often cause areas of alopecia.
- Patches are circular in nature.
- Vesicles can be noted.

Treatment
- Oral antifungals
- Selenium sulfide shampoos
- Oral systemic therapy

Tinea Corporis
- Fungal infection of the nail or skin
- Most often transmitted from an animal

Signs and Symptoms
- Round, red, scaly patch of the nails
- Round, red, scaly patch involving the arms, legs, and trunk
- Pruritus

Treatment
- Administer oral antifungals for extensive or unresponsive lesions.
- Apply topical antifungals.
- Maintain clean, dry site.
- Have pets examined for a fungal infection.

Tinea Cruris
- Fungal infections of the groin area and upper thighs
- Often seen in the adolescent/teen years, especially in males

Signs and Symptoms
- Itchy, scaly area around the groin
- Pinkish circular area
- Scratch marks on the skin surface

Nursing Management of the Child with Dermatophytosis (Ringworm)

Treatment

- Topical tolnaftate (Tinactin)
- Good personal hygiene
- Loose fitting, clean underclothes
- Absorbent powder

Tinea Pedis

- Fungal infection of the feet
- Develops frequently in adolescents/teens and adults
- Often acquired in pools, locker rooms and shower rooms

Signs and Symptoms

- Peeling of the top layers of the skin
- Fissures and vesicles on the surface of the foot
- Pruritus
- May affect toenails

Treatment

- Administer oral antifungals.
- Apply topical antifungals.
- Keep the feet clean, dry and free of perspiration.
- Maintain cotton absorbent socks during exercise.
- Wear shoes that are well ventilated.

Therapeutic Nursing Management

- Assess areas for resolving scaly, itchy patches.
- Inspect for further spread of fungal infection.
- Monitor hair regrowth.
- Observe for secondary infection.
- Instruct on personal hygiene practices.
- Monitor completion of antifungal therapy.
- Provide emotional support and teaching for child and family.
- Obtain liver and renal function studies during oral systemic therapy.
- Administer with a large, fatty meal for best medication absorption.

Complications

- Relapse of disease process
- Further spread of fungal infection
- Leukopenia

Critical Thinking Exercise: Nursing Management of the Child with Dermatophytosis (Ringworm)

Situation: A student nurse is teaching a junior high health class about ringworm. To illustrate the point, the student nurses made a drawing on poster board and utilized a mapping perspective concept. Placing the tinea in the center of the poster board, what other information is a priority to be included regarding each of the areas of infection? Specifically and creatively relate the information to the junior high class.

1. Creatively depict information of each of the fungal infections:

    a. Tinea Capitis

    b. Tinea Corporis

    c. Tinea Pedis

    d. Tinea Cruris

Lymphatic/Infectious/Immune System **CHAPTER 41**

Nursing Management of a Child's Immunizations

> **Key Points**
>
> - Childhood immunization has been credited with the elimination (or near elimination) of many infectious diseases.
> - The most current schedule and guidelines for childhood immunization are intended to be used by all practitioners providing vaccination to children in the United States.
> - Effective vaccination depends upon correct technique according to the recommended immunization schedule. Alternative immunization guidelines are available to "catch-up" with the missed vaccinations.
> - Nurses responsible for monitoring vaccination status and/or providing vaccines need to determine if prior vaccines have been given according to guidelines, assess for a history of prior reactions, and determine the current health status before administering vaccines.
> - Mild illness is not a contraindication for vaccination.
> - Goals of collaborative management:
>   - Eliminate preventable disease through widespread vaccination programs.
>   - Administer vaccines according to the published guidelines and schedule.
>   - Prevent complications associated with vaccination.
>   - Provide "catch-up" vaccination to children who have missed prior doses.
>   - Prevent recurrence.
> - Important nursing diagnoses (actual or potential) are:
>   - Pain related to intramuscular (IM), or subcutaneous (SQ) injections
>   - Infection related to missed or incorrectly administered vaccines
>   - Risk for injury related to incorrect technique and/or complications associated with contraindications/precautions
>   - Anxiety and fear related to IM injections and/or immunization side effects
>   - Knowledge deficit related to lack of awareness of guidelines, schedules, immunization benefits, or vaccine side effects
>   - Noncompliance related to missed vaccines
> - **Key Terms/Concepts:** Immunization, vaccination, cellular immunity, inborn immunity, acquired immunity, live attenuated vaccine, inactivated vaccine, acellular pertussis vaccine, diphtheria, tetanus, polio, hepatitis B, hepatitis A, rubella, measles, mumps

Nursing Management of a Child's Immunizations

Overview

Immunizations provide the body with a mechanism of defense against disease. The decline of infectious diseases in the pediatric population is related to the widespread administration of selected vaccines. There are two types of immunity: inborn (which is inherited) and acquired. Acquired immunity can result from exposure to an infectious disease or the artificial exposure by immunization.

Therapeutic Nursing Management

- Obtain a detailed history of prior immunizations received and any side effects experienced.
- Identify children who should not receive vaccine due to contraindications (vary with specific vaccination):
    - General for all vaccines
        - Contraindications
    - Anaphylactic reaction to a vaccine contraindicates further doses of that vaccine.
    - Anaphylactic reaction to a vaccine constituent contraindicates the use of vaccines containing that substance.
    - Moderate or severe illnesses with or without a fever
    - DTaP
        - Contraindication
    - Encephalopathy within 7 days of administration of previous dose of DTaP
        - Precautions
    - Fever of 40.5° C or 105° F or higher within 48 hours after vaccination with a prior dose of DTaP
    - Collapse or shock-like state (hypotonic-hyporesponsive episode) within 48 hours of receiving a prior dose of DTaP
    - Seizures within 3 days of receiving a prior dose of DTaP
    - Persistent, inconsolable crying lasting 3 hours within 48 hours of receiving a prior dose of DTaP
    - IPV
        - Contraindication
    - Anaphylactic reaction to neomycin or streptomycin
        - Precaution
    - Pregnancy
    - MMR
        - Contraindications
    - Anaphylactic reactions to egg ingestion or to neomycin
    - Pregnancy
    - Known altered immunodeficiency (hematologic and solid tumors; congenital immunodeficiency; and long-term immunosuppressive therapy)
        - Precaution
    - Recent (within 3 months) immune globulin administration
    - HIB: No contraindications identified.

- HBV: No contraindications identified.
- Vaccines may be administered if:
    - General for all vaccines
        - Mild-to-moderate local reaction (soreness, redness, swelling) following a dose of injectable antigen
        - Mild acute illness with or without low-grade fever
        - Current antimicrobial therapy
        - Convalescent phase of illnesses
        - Prematurity (same dosage and indications as for normal, full-term infants)
        - Recent exposure to an infectious disease
        - History of penicillin or other nonspecific allergies or family history of such allergies
    - DTaP
        - Temperature of 40.5° C or 105° F following a previous dose of DTaP
        - Family history of seizures
        - Family history of sudden infant death syndrome (SIDS)
        - Family history of an adverse event following DTaP administration
    - MMR
        - Tuberculosis or positive skin test
        - Simultaneous TB skin testing
        - Breastfeeding
        - Pregnancy of mother or recipient
        - Immunodeficient family member or household contact
        - Infection with HIV
        - Non-anaphylactic reactions to eggs or neomycin
    - HBV
        - Pregnancy
- Provide child/parents education for the following:
    - Benefits of the immunization/risks of the disease if immunizations are not given
    - The current immunization recommendations and schedule
    - Potential side effects from the vaccines (teach families what to assess during the next few days after immunization)
    - Developmentally appropriate information, support, and medical play to assist the child in coping with the trauma associated with IM injection
    - Need to return for future vaccination and to keep vaccination records current
- Understand and recognize the following immunization considerations:
    - Polio: Inactivated Polio Vaccination (IPV) is the recommended type to be administered. The use of oral poliovirus vaccine is not recommended due to the risk of vaccine-associated paralytic poliomyelitis. It is no longer recommended for routine use in the United States.

Nursing Management of a Child's Immunizations

- Diphtheria and tetanus boosters should be given every 10 years after last dose in adolescence.
- Pertussis: Acellular pertussis vaccination is the recommended type to be administered. The fourth pertussis can be given as early as 12 months if all other doses have been given and at least 6 months has lapsed since the third dose.
- Varicella: Administer vaccination after first birthday unless the child has had the illness (as reported by a reliable historian). If needed, administer 2 doses at least 4 weeks apart to susceptible adolescents aged 13 or older.

- Administer vaccines according to guidelines. Refer to CDC guidelines and manufacturer's recommendations before administering:
  - Store vaccines at the appropriate temperature.
  - Reconstitute and/or dilute solutions according to manufacturer's recommendations.
  - Only mix medications in the same syringe when appropriate. Combination of some vaccinations in the same injection and/or during the same office visit may render them ineffective for some infants/children.
  - IM injections - inject at a 90-degree angle using a 22 to 25 gauge, 0.625 to 1" needle; The vastus lateralis site is recommended for infants and children under 2; after which the ventral gluteal site can be used.
  - SQ injections: Inject at a 45-or 90-degree angle with a 25 gauge, 5/8-inch needle. Do not reuse the same needle or same site for multiple injections during the same visit.
  - Administering vaccines too early may decrease their effectiveness. Follow the most current immunization schedule.
  - Administer make-up vaccinations if previous doses were missed or given before the recommended ages (*Refer to grid).

Department of Health and Human Services
Centers for Disease Control and Prevention
2005 Childhood Immunization Schedule for the United States

Age Vaccine	Birth	Months							Years		
		1	2	4	6	12	15	18	24	4-6	11-12	13-18
Hepatitis B	HepB #1					HepB #3				HepB Catch-up Series		
		HepB #2										
Diphtheria, Tetanus, Pertussis (DTaP)			DTaP	DTaP	DTaP		DTaP			DTaP	Td	Td Catch-up
Haemophilus influenzae type b			Hib	Hib	Hib	Hib						
Inactivated Poliovirus			IPV	IPV		IPV				IPV		
Measles, Mumps, Rubella						MMR #1				MMR #2	MMR#2 Catch-up	
Varicella						Varicella				Varicella Catch-up		
Pneumococcal Conjugate			PCV	PCV	PCV	PCV				PCV		
Influenza						Influenza (Yearly)				Influenza (Yearly)		
Varicella							X				Make-up	
Hepatitis A										Hepatitis A Series		

Critical Thinking Exercise: Nursing Management of a Child's Immunizations

1. Match the immunizations that are on the schedule for a child of each the following ages:

Birth	a. DPT, HIB, polio & Pneumococcal vaccine & Hepatitis B #2
4 months old	b. DPT, Polio, & MMR
6 months old	c. Hepatitis B #1
2 months old	d. DPT, HIB, Polio, Pneumococcal vaccine & Hepatitis B #3
5 years old	e. Make up vaccinations
11 years old	f. HIB, Polio, Pneumococcal vaccine, Varicella, MMR, & Hepatitis B #3 (if not already administered)

2. The mother of a 3-week-old infant is concerned because her baby has only had one immunization since birth. Has the infant missed any scheduled immunizations?

3. The father of a 15-month-old asks the nurse to give the IM vaccination in his daughter's buttocks so she does not have to see the needle. What should the nurse tell the father?

4. A 4-month-old child presents for routine immunization with lethargy, tachycardia, fever of 104° F, and decreased urine output over the past 24 hours. Should the nurse give the immunization? Why or why not?

Lymphatic/Infectious/Immune System **CHAPTER 42**

Nursing Management of the Child with Oral Candidiasis (Thrush)

> **Key Points**
>
> - Thrush is an infection of the mouth and throat caused by *Candida albicans*.
> - Thrush, commonly seen in infants that are nursing or bottle feeding and young children, is a specific form of oral candidiasis.
> - Cancer clients, immunosuppressed clients and children with AIDS have a high incidence of thrush.
> - Thrush can also be the result of medication therapy.
> - Thrush can be spread down the gastrointestinal and respiratory tracts.
> - Goals of Treatment:
>   - Prevent the spread of the fungal infection.
>   - Provide antibiotic therapy to eliminate the fungal infection.
>   - Teach proper hygiene practices.
>   - Manage side effects from the infection.
> - Diagnostic Association (NANDA) nursing diagnosis:
>   - Risk for aspiration related to ineffective sucking secondary to oral infection
>   - Interrupted breast feeding related to discomfort during sucking
>   - Impaired comfort related to discomfort of the oral cavity
>   - Risk for impaired parenting related to baby/child fussiness
> - **Key terms/Concepts:** *Candida albicans*, oral candidiasis, immunosuppression, oral nystatin

Overview

Oral candidiasis, more commonly known as thrush, is a yeast-like fungal infection of the oral cavity. Thrush is often the result of antibiotic therapy decreasing the protective flora of the oral cavity. It can be spread by caretakers who utilize poor handwashing technique after caring for an infected child. Oral candidiasis is generally self limiting but may take up to eight weeks to resolve. The priority for care is to prevent transmission of the infection.

Risk Factors

- Immunosuppressed children
- Recent antibiotic therapy
- Poor cleaning of bottles and nipples

Signs and Symptoms

- Fussiness, discomfort or pulling away when eating, drinking or sucking
- White patches on the tongue, palate or inside the cheeks
- White patches that adhere to mucous membranes
- White patches that are difficult to remove and may bleed when scraped

Diagnostic Tests

- Oral scraping to assess status of white patches

Treatment

- Oral antifungal agent, commonly oral nystatin
- Administer antifungal to oral cavity and allow the infant/child to swallow the medication to treat any candidiasis in the throat, stomach and intestines.
- Breastfeeding mother of infected infant should apply antifungal to nipples
- Boil pacifiers and bottle daily

Therapeutic Nursing Management

- Instruct on good handwashing techniques to prevent transmission or reoccurrences
- Administer antifungal as prescribed
- Treatment should be continued for a few days after resolution of the oral lesions
- Follow feedings with water or by rinsing the child's mouth
- Meticulous hygiene is the best way to prevent and limit this infection

Complications

- Pain
- Feeding disorder
- Weight loss
- Spread of infection to other body systems
- Spread of infection to others

Critical Thinking Exercise: Nursing Management of the Child with Oral Candidiasis (Thrush)

Situation: A 12-week-old is brought to the pediatricians' office for a follow up visit. The nurse brings the infant into the room and questions the mother about the recent upper respiratory infection and antibiotic completion. The mother states that the infant's symptoms have improved; he is sleeping better, but is not eating well.

The physician examines the oral cavity and discovers white patches on the tongue, palate and inner aspect of the cheek.

1. Correlate the past history of the infant with the symptoms described. How is it best to explain the occurrence to the mother?

2. In what other instances would it be a priority to complete teaching related to thrush?

3. What instruction is most effective in providing treatment for thrush?

Lymphatic/Infectious/Immune System **CHAPTER 43**

Nursing Management of the Child with Human Immunodeficiency Virus (HIV) and Acquired Immunodeficiency Syndrome (AIDS)

Key Points

- HIV is an infectious disease that is spread to infants and children by direct contact with infected blood and body fluids through IV drug use, unprotected sexual contact, perinatal blood exposure, and breastfeeding.
- AIDS is the most severe disease produced by HIV infection.
- There is no cure for HIV infection or AIDS. Current treatments and medication protocols have improved the quality of life for children with AIDS.
- Goals of collaborative management:
    - Prevent the spread of HIV infection through education of high-risk populations (adolescents).
    - Provide early diagnosis and treatment.
    - Prevent further transmission of the disease.
    - Maintain optimal immune function.
    - Prevent and/or treat opportunistic infections.
    - Promote optimal nutritional status.
    - Promote optimal growth and development.
    - Support the child and family during the end-of-life process.
- Important nursing diagnoses (actual or potential) are:
    - Infection related to immune suppression
    - Fluid volume deficit
    - Altered nutrition, Less than body requirements
    - Injury related to complications (failure to thrive, opportunistic infections)
    - Ineffective airway clearance related to pulmonary complications
    - Altered growth and development
    - Fatigue, activity intolerance related to illness
    - Fear, anxiety related to serious life-threatening disease
    - Caregiver role strain related to chronic illness
    - Ineffective individual/family coping
    - Social isolation related to stigma and disease effects
    - Hopelessness, powerlessness related to terminal disease with no cure
    - Ineffective management of therapeutic regimen
    - Grieving related to loss of "normal" child and/or end-of-life process
- **Key Terms/Concepts:** Immune deficiency, immune modulator, T-suppressor cells, CD4 helper lymphocytes, cell mediated immunity, opportunistic infection, failure to thrive, lymphadenopathy, hepatosplenomegaly, thrush, maternal-infant transmission

Human Immunodeficiency Virus (HIV) and Acquired Immunodeficiency Syndrome (AIDS)

Overview

Acquired immune deficiency syndrome (AIDS) is the most severe manifestation of a human immunodeficiency virus (HIV) infection. AIDS is caused by a retrovirus which attacks the T-helper cells that support immune function. T-suppressor cells that shut down the immune system are not altered. HIV targets and destroys CD4 helper lymphocytes (cell-mediated immunity). This leads to vulnerability to opportunistic infection.

HIV is currently believed to be spread by exposure to infected blood, semen, and breast milk. This most commonly occurs through direct sexual contact and/or exposure to contaminated needles during illicit drug use. There is no evidence at the current time that casual contact between infected and uninfected individuals leads to virus transmission. Most of the cases of maternal-infant HIV transmission result from perinatal exposure of a fetus or infant by an infected mother. The current testing procedure enables identification of the infection early in infancy. Infants with HIV infection usually develop symptoms by age 9 months. Advances in diagnostics and treatment have resulted in decreased maternal-infant HIV transmission and decreased AIDS-related symptoms.

Risk Factors

- Exposure to contaminated blood or body fluids
- Unprotected vaginal, anal, or oral intercourse
- Sexual abuse
- Intravenous drug use with contaminated needles
- HIV-infected mother (intrauterine, intrapartum or postpartum exposure)
- Bisexual males (adolescents and adults) and homosexual
- Haitian or African origin
- Exposure from contaminated blood and blood products (rarely occurs since routine testing)

Signs and Symptoms

- Generalized lymphadenopathy
- Weight loss
- Failure to thrive
- Chronic diarrhea
- Oral candidiasis (thrush)
- Hepatosplenomegaly (enlarged liver and spleen)
- Developmental delay, loss of developmental milestones
- Progressive encephalopathy
- Repeated respiratory infections
- Sinusitis
- Opportunistic infections (PCP, EBV, etc.)
- Fever
- Night sweats

Human Immunodeficiency Virus (HIV) and Acquired Immunodeficiency Syndrome (AIDS)

- Weakness
- Fatigue
- Malaise
- Anemia
- Thrombocytopenia
- Myalgia

Diagnostic Tests and Labs

- History and physical
- Enzyme-linked immunosorbent assay (ELISA)
- Western Blot assay if ELISA is positive
- HIV culture
- HIV antigen test
- CD4 cell count (reduced)
- CD4/CD8 ratio
- HIV/RNA cell count
- Polymerase chain reaction (PCR)
- CBC
- Chest x-ray
- Cultures

Therapeutic Nursing Management

- Assess child and family's knowledge of HIV/AIDS.
- Provide education and support during diagnostic process and on an ongoing basis.
- Educate regarding the need for repeat testing if risk factors are present and initial diagnostic tests are negative.
- Administer medication according to current protocol recommendations.
- Prevent the spread of infection.
    - Use universal precautions for potential contact with blood and body fluids.
    - Assess for signs of infection.
    - Teach child and family about risk factors and transmission (use protection with sexual contact, avoid contact with infected blood and needle sticks, and do not breast feed if there is a possibility of HIV infection).
- Protect the child from infection.
    - Maintain good hand washing.
    - Avoid others with colds, viruses or other infectious illnesses.
    - Assess for signs of infection.
    - Administer antibiotics and antiviral agents as needed.
    - Instruct parents that immunizations should be kept up to date.
    - Monitor for signs and symptoms of opportunistic infections (oral lesions, dyspnea, cough, seizures, skin lesions, and fever).

Human Immunodeficiency Virus (HIV) and Acquired Immunodeficiency Syndrome (AIDS)

- Monitor skin for signs of breakdown and treat as indicated.
- Promote adequate nutrition and hydration.
  - Assess intake and output.
  - Monitor nutritional status and weight.
  - Identify factors that may interfere with nutrition (anorexia, nausea, vomiting, oral lesions, and dysphagia).
  - Provide high-protein, high-calorie foods that the child is most likely to eat.
  - Provide frequent, small meals.
  - Monitor for fluid or electrolyte imbalance.
- Provide rest with monitored periods of activity.
- Monitor respiratory status and provide support as needed.
- Assess for pain status, provide pain relief measures as needed.
- Monitor developmental milestones and neurological status.
- Provide education regarding home medication administration: dose, route, schedule, and side effects.
- Emphasize the importance of compliance with therapeutic protocols.
- Monitor laboratory values to determine current status.
- Teach family the importance of reporting signs/symptoms of infection immediately.
- Collaborate with case manager, home health agency, social services, support groups, and other community agencies to address medical, psychological, financial, and other support needs.

Pharmacology

- Zidovudine (ZDV, AZT)
- Didanosine-dideoxyinosine (DDI)
- Lamivudine (3TC)
- Intravenous immunoglobulin
- Protease inhibitors (ritonavir, nelfinavir)
- Trimethoprim sulfamethoxazole (Bactrim, Septra) for treatment of Pneumocystis Carinii pneumonia
- Inactivated polio vaccination
- Antibiotics to prevent or treat bacterial infection
- Antifungal agents as needed
- Antidiarrheal agents as needed

Complications

- Diarrhea
- Opportunistic infections
  - *Pneumocystis carinii* pneumonia (cough, dyspnea, chest pain)
  - Candidiasis (white patches on the tongue and inner cheeks, painful swallowing, diaper rash)

- *Mycobacterium avium* complex (cough, dyspnea, chest pain)
- *Toxoplasma gondii* (seizures, dementia)
- Tuberculosis (cough, fever, dyspnea)
- Epstein Barr (fatigue, fever, sore throat, lymphadenopathy)
- Cytomegalovirus (fever, hepatosplenomegaly)
- *Cryptococcal neoformans* (fever, stiff neck, nausea, vomiting, seizures)
* Anemia
* Failure to thrive, weight loss
* Developmental delay
* Skin diseases
* Progressive encephalopathy
* Lymphoma
* Kaposi sarcoma (rare in children)
* Decreased self-esteem
* Depression
* Death

Critical Thinking Exercise: Nursing Management of the Child with Human Immunodeficiency Virus (HIV) and Acquired Immunodeficiency Syndrome (AIDS)

Situation: A 17-year-old client presents with a recurrent upper respiratory tract infection, cough, fever, enlarged lymph nodes, and weight loss. She tells the nurse that she has been sleeping more than usual and has been sweaty at night. She admits to participating in sexual partner trading games at 2-3 parties during the past year. She did not remember using a condom during intercourse.

1. How is HIV most commonly spread?

2. What typical adolescent beliefs and behaviors increase their risk of becoming infected with the HIV virus?

3. Identify the factors in the 17-year-old female's history and presentation that are associated with HIV infection.

4. Tests reveal that the adolescent does have an HIV infection. What nursing interventions are needed at this time?

Lymphatic/Infectious/Immune System **CHAPTER 44**

Nursing Management of the Child with Otitis Media

> **Key Points**
>
> - Infants and young children are at increased risk for otitis media (OM) because their eustachian tubes are shorter, more horizontal, and more cartilaginous than older children and adults.
> - By preschool-age, most children will have had at least one episode of OM.
> - Acute otitis media is an infectious process characterized by red tympanic membranes, fever, ear pain, and poor feeding.
> - Myringotomy or pressure-equalizing tubes (PE tubes) may be needed for negative pressure relief and fluid drainage in children with chronic OM.
> - The goals of collaborative management:
>   - Provide prompt recognition, diagnosis, and treatment.
>   - Administer antibiotics when needed.
>   - Place PE tubes by myringotomy as needed.
>   - Provide comfort measures.
>   - Prevent recurrence.
>   - Prevent complications (hearing loss, tympanic membrane rupture, meningitis, etc.).
>   - Provide education and support to the child and family.
> - Important nursing diagnoses (actual or potential) are:
>   - Hyperthermia related to infection
>   - Pain related to inner ear pressure and/or myringotomy procedure
>   - Fluid volume deficit related to fever and/or decreased intake
>   - Altered nutrition: Less than body requirements related to decreased intake
>   - Sleep pattern disturbance related to discomfort
>   - Altered auditory sensory perception due to fluid in middle ear
>   - Impaired protection related to frequent antibiotic use
>   - Potential for injury related to damage to inner ear structures
>   - Knowledge deficit related to illness
> - **Key Terms/Concepts:** Acute otitis media, otitis media with effusion, bacterial infection, antibiotics, PE tubes, myringotomy, tympanic membrane rupture, hearing

Overview

Otitis media (OM) is defined as the inflammation of the structures of the middle ear. The condition may result from the anatomical structure and position of the eustachian tube in young children and is triggered by a bacterial or viral

Nursing Management of the Child with Otitis Media

infection, allergies, or enlarged tonsils. Acute otitis media is frequently caused by a variety of organisms, especially *Streptococcus pneumoniae*, *H. influenzae* and *Moraxella*. It may also be caused by a viral infection and/or may occur after an upper respiratory infection. Otitis media with effusion is a condition of fluid in the middle ear without signs of infection. It most frequently occurs with allergies, viral illness, or after acute otitis media. OM is most commonly seen in children between three months and three years of age. The incidence of OM is highest in the winter and spring, primarily due to the frequency of the common cold during this time.

Risk Factors

- Bottle feeding in supine position
- Parental smoking
- Respiratory tract infection
- Male gender
- Craniofacial abnormalities (cleft lip/palate, Down's syndrome, etc.)
- Prior ear infections, particularly if occurring at a young age
- Exposure to other sick children (large group day care)

Signs and Symptoms

- Acute otitis media
  - Red, bulging tympanic membranes
  - Decreased or no tympanic movement with pneumatic otoscopy
  - Purulent material in middle ear, or drainage from external canal if tympanic membrane ruptures
  - Irritability, fussiness
  - Pulling on ears
  - Description of the pain as severe, sharp, or constant
  - Fever up to 104°
  - Decreased oral intake
  - Inability to sleep
  - Ringing in the ears (tinnitus)
  - Sudden, transient hearing loss
  - Persistent rhinorrhea
  - Vomiting
  - Nasal congestion
  - Signs and symptoms of upper respiratory or pharyngeal infection
  - Lymphadenopathy of the neck and head
  - Anorexia
- Otitis media with effusion
  - Feeling of fullness in the ear
  - Dull gray or yellowish coloration of the tympanic membrane

- Decreased tympanic movement
- Transient hearing loss
- Balance disturbances

Diagnostic Tests and Labs

- History and physical
- Visualization of tympanic membrane (TM) and adjacent structures. For a child under 3 years of age, gently pull the pinna down and back to visualize the TM; for the child over 3 years of age, gently pull the pinna up and back to visualize the TM.
- Pneumatic otoscopy (pulse of positive or negative pressure using the bulb insufflator attachment of the otoscope)

Therapeutic Nursing Management

- Administer antibiotics as appropriate. Observation may be used prior to antibiotics for some cases.
- Address comfort needs: analgesics, warm or cold compresses to the ear, diversional activities etc.
- Administer antipyretics for fever as needed.
- Provide child and family education.
  - Avoid risk factors (smoking, positioning during feeding, large group day care, etc.).
  - Home medications: dose, schedule, potential side effects, and the need to give all doses
  - Comfort measures
  - Follow-up appointments and hearing assessment
- Care for the child receiving myringotomy and PE tubes placement.
  - Prepare child and family for a surgical procedure (medical play, tour, etc.).
  - Assess for recovery from anesthetic agents.
  - Monitor for ear drainage. Small amount of reddish drainage usually occurs for a few days.
  - Teach family to follow healthcare provider's instructions regarding the need to keep the ears dry.
  - Instruct parents that the tubes will usually fall out in 6-12 months.

Pharmacology

- Antibiotics
  - Amoxicillin: drug of choice
  - Pediazole not used as often with otitis media (erythromycin and sulfa)
  - Trimethoprim-sulfamethoxazole (Septra, Bactrim)
  - Cephalosporins
  - Augmentin for organisms resistant to amoxicillin

Nursing Management of the Child with Otitis Media

- Antipyretics/Analgesics
    - Acetaminophen (the most common medication used for fever in children)
    - Children's ibuprofen best for pain relief and antipyretic effects
    - Ear drops

Complications

- Hearing loss: some children have conductive hearing loss up to six months after an infection
- Tympanic membrane rupture
- Mastoiditis
- Chronic otitis media
- Meningitis
- Brain abscess
- Speech difficulties
- Labyrinthitis

Critical Thinking Exercise: Nursing Management of the Child with Otitis Media

Situation: A 7-month-old infant is brought to the clinic with a fever of 102° F. The infant's mother reports that her baby has had a "runny nose" and cough for the last three days. The infant is crying and is irritable. The primary care provider assesses red, bulging tympanic membranes and diagnoses bilateral otitis media. Amoxicillin is to be given at home every six hours for ten days.

1. The child's mother asks the nurse what she can do to prevent additional ear infections. What should the nurse tell the parent about risk factors associated with otitis media?

2. The child's mother then asks the nurse if her baby will suffer any damage from the infection. What should the nurse tell her?

3. What instructions should the nurse give the mother regarding the antibiotics?

Lymphatic/Infectious/Immune System **CHAPTER 45**

Nursing Management of a Child's Varicella-Zoster Infection (Chickenpox and Shingles)

Key Points

- Chickenpox is a primary, and shingles is a secondary infection of the varicella-zoster virus.
- Transmission of chickenpox occurs through respiratory droplets, airborne particles, and direct contact.
- Although most children who contract chickenpox will have mild illness, immunocompromised children are at risk for developing severe complications from the disease.
- Chickenpox manifests as a macular rash progressing to draining lesions that cause severe itching.
- Shingles produces painful, unilateral skin lesions caused by activation of a latent varicella infection.
- The goals of collaborative management:
    - Provide prompt recognition of the illness and isolation of the client.
    - Prevent exposure of the virus.
    - Provide comfort measures (pain relief, pruritus relief, diversional activities).
    - Maintain adequate hydration.
    - Prevent secondary infection.
    - Prevent complications (CNS damage, pneumonia, corneal damage, etc.).
    - Provide education and support to child and family.
- Important nursing diagnoses (actual or potential) are:
    - Hyperthermia
    - Altered comfort/pain related to skin lesions
    - Fluid volume deficit related to fever and/or decreased intake
    - Altered nutrition: Less than body requirements related to decreased intake
    - Impaired protection related to open skin lesions and/or immunocompromised state
    - Potential for injury related to CNS infection, respiratory infection, skin infection, dehydration
    - Knowledge deficit related to acute illness
    - Altered body image related to skin lesions
    - Anxiety related to skin lesions, itching, and isolation
    - Diversional activity deficit related to isolation
- **Key Terms/Concepts:** Exposure, incubation, macular rash, vesicles, papules, strict isolation, varicella-zoster immune globulin (VZIG), passive immunity, immune compromise, anti-viral, varicella-zoster

Nursing Management of a Child's Varicella-Zoster Infection (Chickenpox and Shingles)

Overview

Chickenpox is an acute, viral infection caused by the varicella-zoster virus. Shingles (zoster) is a secondary varicella-zoster infection caused by activation of the latent infection in the dorsal root ganglion that usually occurs in the elderly but can also affect children, adolescents, and young adults. Chickenpox typically affects children from 5 - 9 years old, or children entering day care or school (due to exposure to other children). It is highly contagious and is spread by direct contact or air droplet routes. It is contagious from 1-2 days before a rash develops until the vesicles have crusted over, which usually takes about a week. The incubation period is 10-21 days. Once contracted, if immunologic markers are elevated, there is usually a lasting natural immunity.

Administration of varicella-zoster immune globulin (VZIG) can assist the child to develop a passive immunity up to 96 hours after exposure. It is often given to high-risk children to prevent them from developing severe varicella.

Risk Factors

- Exposure to other children: day care centers and schools
- Family member with varicella
- Immunocompromise

Signs and Symptoms

- Chickenpox
    - General malaise
    - Slight fever
    - Anorexia
    - Successive crops of maculae, papules, vesicles and crusts occurring 24-48 hours after the fever
    - Severe itching of skin
    - Generalized lymphadenopathy
    - Greatest concentration of lesions occurs on the trunk, face, and neck progressing to sparse appearance on the extremities
- Shingles
    - Pain, tenderness, itching, tingling, or burning along peripheral sensory nerve of trunk, thorax, or face (may be present for approximately 2 weeks before the rash appears)
    - Unilateral skin lesions along sensory nerve tracts
    - Paresthesia
    - Pruritus
    - Fever

Diagnostic Tests and Lab

- History and physical
- Varicella titers (rare)
- CBC, WBC count (assess for bacterial infection)

Therapeutic Nursing Management

- Place hospitalized children in strict isolation from 8-21 days after exposure to a child with chickenpox.
- Protect all immunosuppressed children from inadvertent exposure (screen visitors who may have been recently exposed, promptly isolate children with suspected disease and/or exposure).
- Assess skin, eyes, and mucous membranes for rashes and lesions.
- Monitor for the presence of secondary infection.
- Assess neurological status for varicella CNS infection (behavior change, ataxia, tremor, nystagmus, and seizures).
- Assess respiratory status for varicella pneumonia (rare in children)
- Prevent scratching: cut fingernails short, cover hands with soft cotton mittens if needed, provide diversion activities that involve the use of the hands.
- Apply topical lotions for itching.
- Administer oral antihistamines.
- Administer non aspirin antipyretics for fever.
- Administer analgesics for discomfort.
- Use comfort measures such as a tepid, oatmeal bath.
- Maintain hydration status with oral fluids (as tolerated) and/or IV fluids.
- Monitor intake and output.
- Administer antiviral medications as ordered.
- Provide diversional activities, especially for children who must remain in isolation.
- Dispose of infected linen in proper container.
- Teach parents to care for child as described above when managing at home.
- Teach parents to avoid aspirin-containing products to minimize the risk of Reye's syndrome.
- Teach child to cover his/her mouth when sneezing and/or coughing.
- Teach parents it is safe for the child to be around others and/or return to school after all the vesicles have dried.
- Report occurrence to area health department (It is a reportable disease in some states).

Pharmacology

- Calamine lotion
- Oral antihistamines
- Antipyretics
- Acyclovir: used with immunocompromised child
- Antibiotics if secondary infection (Zovirax)
- Vaccination
- Varicella-zoster immune globulin (VZIG) after exposure of high-risk child to varicella

Complications

- Bacterial superinfection from skin lesions
- Hemorrhagic lesions
- Varicella encephalitis (seizures, brain damage, mental retardation, behavioral disorders, death)
- Varicella pneumonia (rare in children)
- Corneal damage (Vesicular lesions on eyelids common leading to corneal damage is rare.)
- Reye's syndrome (associated with aspirin use and viral infection)

Critical Thinking Exercise: Nursing Management of a Child's Varicella-Zoster Infection (Chickenpox and Shingles)

1. Matching:

Contagious period begins	a. Provides passive immunity 92 hours after exposure
Most commonly infected	b. 1-2 days after the rash develops
Time for vesicles to crust	c. One week
Crusting usually begins	d. 10-21 days
Shingles infection	e. 5-9 year olds
Contagious period ends	f. Infants and immunocompromised children
Incubation period	g. Elderly adults
VZIG	h. When lesions have dried
Increased risk for complications	i. 24-48 hours after the fever

2. Fill in the blank:

   a. The typical chickenpox rash lesions progress from a _____ to _____ rash, then forms _____ before erupting into _____ lesions.

   b. Children with varicella may have a slight fever and malaise _____ to _____ hours before the rash appears.

   c. A nurse should wear a _____, _____, and a _____ when bathing a child with draining varicella lesions.

   d. _____ is a secondary varicella-zoster infection caused by activation of the latent infection in the dorsal root ganglion.

Lymphatic/Infectious/Immune System **CHAPTER 46**

Nursing Management of the Child with Rubeola (Measles)

Key Points

- The incidence of rubeola infection in the United States has greatly decreased because of routine childhood vaccinations.
- Rubeola typically manifests with Koplik spots, fever, cough, runny nose, and a maculopapular rash beginning on the head and neck and traveling downward.
- Transmission is through airborne particles and by direct contact with droplets.
- The goals of collaborative management:
  - Provide prompt recognition of the illness and isolation of the client.
  - Prevent exposing others to the virus.
  - Support the child's airway and breathing; and manage the cough and runny nose.
  - Control hyperthermia.
  - Maintain adequate hydration.
  - Provide comfort measures (pain relief, pruritus relief, diversional activities).
  - Prevent complications (CNS damage, pneumonia, corneal damage, etc.).
  - Provide education and support to the child and family.
- Important nursing diagnoses (actual or potential) are:
  - Hyperthermia related to measles infection
  - Impaired sensory perception related to conjunctivitis
  - Altered comfort related to photophobia, conjunctivitis, and acute illness
  - Fluid volume deficit related to fever and/or decreased intake
  - Altered respiratory status related to cough, coryza, and/or pneumonia
  - Potential for injury related to complications (respiratory infection or other complications)
  - Knowledge deficit related to acute illness
  - Altered body image related to skin lesions and/or conjunctivitis
  - Diversional activity deficit related to isolation
- **Key Terms/Concepts**: Exposure, incubation, immunity, vaccination, Koplik spots, coryza, maculopapular rash, conjunctivitis, photophobia, hyperthermia

Overview

Rubeola is an infection caused by the measles virus. It is spread by droplet contact and once acquired, provides lasting natural immunity. Rubeola is sometimes called the "Seven Day Measles." The incubation period is 7-14 days; the period of communicability is from 1-2 days before the rash is apparent until 4 days after the appearance of the rash. It occurs most often in the winter and early spring.

Nursing Management of the Child with Rubeola (Measles)

> The presence of Koplik spots helps differentiate this type of measles from other viral infections. The incidence of measles in the United States has dramatically decreased due to routine childhood immunizations. Current outbreaks usually occur in populations that have not been vaccinated (recent immigrants, toddlers, unimmunized home schooled children, etc.).

Risk Factors

- Exposure to the virus: day care centers, schools, colleges, crowded living environments
- Lack of immunization for the virus: recent immigrants, toddlers before 12-15 month immunization, home schooled children who have not been immunized, etc.

Signs and Symptoms

- Symptoms peak on the second and third day and last 5-7 days
- Coryza (severe runny nose)
- Cough
- Malaise
- Conjunctivitis
- Photophobia
- Koplik spots: Small, bright red spots with a blue-white center on buccal mucosa (occurs approximately 2 days before the rash develops)
- High fever
- Enlarged lymph nodes
- Rash
  - Proceeded by fever and Koplik spots
  - Red maculopapular
  - Begins behind ears, at the hairline, on the forehead or neck
  - Progresses downward to extremities
  - Lasts about five days
  - Changes from red to brown after several days

Diagnostic Tests and Lab

- History and physical
- Viral culture from nasopharyngeal secretions, blood, urine, conjunctiva
- Serum measles antibody test (acute specimen titers and convalescent titers 2-4 weeks later)
- Serum IgM antibodies

Therapeutic Nursing Management

- Place hospitalized children in isolation during contagious period.
- Assess eyes for conjunctivitis and corneal ulceration.

- Assess oral mucous membranes for Koplik spots.
- Assess for enlarged lymph nodes.
- Maintain bedrest during acute phase of illness.
- Administer cooling measures and non aspirin antipyretics for fever.
- Assess respiratory status (related to impaired airway management due to runny nose, cough, and potential for pneumonia).
- Use comfort measures: tepid bath, topical lotions, positioning.
- Remove secretions from eyes by gently cleaning with warm normal saline. Saline eye drops to relieve itching (ineffective due to viral cause of conjunctivitis).
- Remind the child to keep his/her hands away from his/her eyes.
- Provide a quiet, dimly lit room for child with photophobia and/or headache.
- Administer analgesics as needed for discomfort.
- Maintain hydration status with oral fluids (as tolerated) and/or IV fluids. Monitor intake and output.
- Provide diversional activities especially for children who must remain in isolation.
- Dispose of infected linen in proper container.
- Teach parents to care for the child as described above when managing at home.
- Teach parents to avoid aspirin-containing products to minimize the risk of Reye's syndrome.
- Teach child to cover his/her mouth when sneezing and/or coughing.
- Teach parents when it is safe for the child to be exposed to others and/or return to school.
- Report occurrence to local health department

Pharmacology

- Immunizations
- Antipyretics, as needed
- Antibacterial for complications

Complications

- Otitis media
- Pneumonia
- Mastoiditis
- Tracheobronchitis
- Encephalitis
- Acute encephalitis - often resulting in permanent brain damage in 1/1000 cases
- Death in 1-3/1000 cases

Critical Thinking Exercise: Nursing Management of a Child with Rubeola (Measles)

1. List the following rubeola symptoms in the order in which they occur.

    _____ Fever, Koplik spots, photophobia, no rash

    _____ Red rash on the face, trunk, and legs

    _____ Positive convalescent serum measles titers

    _____ Brown rash over entire body

    _____ Maculopapular rash along on the head and neck

    _____ Fever, cough, and a runny nose without a rash or Koplik spots

2. A 5-year-old with rubeola is admitted to the hospital. What should the nurse do for the following symptoms?
    a. Cough and upper respiratory congestion

    b. Fever

    c. Photophobia and headache

    d. Eye irritation from conjunctivitis

    e. Rash

    f. Emotional distress

Lymphatic/Infectious/Immune System **CHAPTER 47**

Nursing Management of the Child with Rubella (German Measles)

Key Points

- The incidence of rubella infection in the United States has greatly decreased because of routine childhood vaccination.
- Transmission is through airborne particles and through direct contact with droplets.
- The goals of collaborative management:
  - Provide prompt recognition of the illness and isolation.
  - Prevent exposing others to the virus.
  - Support the child's airway and breathing; manage a runny nose.
  - Control hyperthermia.
  - Maintain adequate hydration.
  - Provide comfort measures (pain relief, pruritus relief, diversional activities).
  - Prevent complications (arthritis in adolescents, encephalitis.) Complications are rare.
  - Provide education and support to child and family.
- Important nursing diagnoses (actual or potential) are:
  - Hyperthermia related to measles infection
  - Altered comfort related to acute illness
  - Fluid volume deficit related to fever and/or decreased intake
  - Altered respiratory status
  - Potential for injury related to complications (arthritis or encephalitis)
  - Knowledge deficit related to acute illness
  - Altered body image related to skin lesions and/or conjunctivitis
  - Diversional activity deficit related to isolation
- **Key Terms/Concepts:** Exposure, incubation, immunity, vaccination, maculopapular rash, hyperthermia

Overview

Rubella, also called German or 3-day measles, is caused by the rubella virus. It is spread by direct and indirect contact with droplets. The incubation period is 14-21 days; the period of communicability is seven days before and five days after the appearance of the rash. Once it is acquired, there is lasting natural immunity. The incidence of rubella has decreased because of immunizations.

If rubella is acquired during the first trimester of pregnancy, there is a risk of spontaneous abortion, birth defects, or mental retardation. It occurs most frequently during the spring and affects school-age and adolescent children most often.

Nursing Management of the Child with Rubella (German Measles)

Risk Factors

- Exposure to the virus: day care centers, schools, crowded living environments
- Lack of immunization for the virus: recent immigrants, toddlers before 12-15 month immunization, home schooled children who have not been immunized, etc.

Signs and Symptoms

- Young children have no symptoms until the rash appears.
- Nasal drainage
- Low-grade fever
- Headache
- Malaise
- Anorexia
- Enlarged lymph nodes
- Petechiae (reddish pinpoint spots) on the soft palate: Forchheimer's sign
- Rash
  - Appears within five days of incubation
  - Pink-red maculopapular
  - Begins on the face, scalp and neck
  - Fades as it spreads downward to the trunk and legs
  - Disappears on the third day
- Transient polyarthralgia and polyarthritis may occur in teens and adults (especially females)

Diagnostic Tests and Lab

- History and physical
- Rubella antibody titer

Therapeutic Nursing Management

- Administer non-aspirin antipyretics as needed.
- Provide bed rest for 2-3 days.
- Place hospitalized children in isolation during contagious period.
- Assess for rash, Forchheimer's sign, and symptoms associated with rubella.
- Provide supportive care for discomfort (analgesics and nonpharmacologic interventions).
- Administer cooling measures and antipyretics for fever.
- Maintain hydration status with oral fluids (as tolerated) and/or IV fluids. Monitor intake and output.
- Provide diversional activities, especially for children who must remain in isolation.
- Dispose of infected linen in proper container.

- Provide child and family education.
- Avoid aspirin-containing products to minimize the risk of Reye's syndrome.
- Identify when the child is no longer infective and is safe to be exposed to others and/or return to school.
- Report occurrence to local health department.

Pharmacology

- Immunizations
- Antipyretics as needed
- Analgesics as needed

Complications

- Few complications are associated with rubella unless acquired during pregnancy.
- Arthritis, arthralgia: Occurs most frequently in adults and teens, especially females
- Thrombocytopenia: Self-limiting
- Encephalitis: Rare
- Congenital rubella: Growth retardation, deafness, cardiac defects, retinopathy, cataracts, mental retardation, encephalitis, diabetes, and thyroid disorders

Critical Thinking Exercise: Nursing Management of the Child with Rubella (German Measles)

1. Explain why each of the children listed below is at risk for acquiring rubella.

   a. A 7-year-old child attending home school:

   b. A 10-year-old child from a family visiting from a foreign country:

   c. A 1-year-old healthy infant:

   d. A 2-year-old with chronic respiratory illness and frequent hospitalizations:

   e. A 3-year-old child from a family without medical care who is sharing a small one bedroom apartment with 2 other families:

2. Identify which of the following children with rubella is at greatest risk for serious complication associated with the disease. Explain your rationale. Discuss the risk of complications associated with rubella for the remaining children.

   a. A 7-year-old male with fever, nasal drainage, enlarged lymph nodes, and a rash on his face
   b. A 16-year-old female with diarrhea, nausea, and positive Forchheimer's sign
   c. A 1-year-old female with a rash on her head and neck, irritability, decreased appetite, and sleep disturbance
   d. A 3-year-old male with chills, joint pain, vomiting, diarrhea, anorexia, and a rash over entire body

   Answer:

Lymphatic/Infectious/Immune System **CHAPTER 48**

Nursing Management of a Child with Epstein-Barr Viral Infection (Mononucleosis)

> **Key Points**
>
> - Epstein-Barr viral infection (EBV), mononucleosis, is most commonly transmitted in adolescents through kissing.
> - EBV typically manifests with a sore throat, fever, enlarged lymph nodes, fatigue, headache, and enlarged spleen. Symptoms may occur acutely or gradually over 1-2 months.
> - Child isolation is not needed with Epstein-Barr viral infection (EBV) infection.
> - The goals of collaborative management:
>   - Provide prompt recognition of the illness; and prevent exposure of the virus to others.
>   - Provide supportive care for the associated symptoms (fever, sore throat, and headache).
>   - Maintain adequate airway control (associated with throat swelling).
>   - Maintain adequate hydration and nutrition.
>   - Provide adequate rest periods.
>   - Prevent complications (respiratory compromise, splenic rupture, and overexertion).
>   - Provide education and support to the child and family.
> - Important nursing diagnoses (actual or potential) are:
>   - Hyperthermia
>   - Altered comfort related to the sore throat, headache, and acute illness
>   - Ineffective airway clearance related to soft tissue swelling
>   - Fluid volume deficit related to fever and/or decreased intake
>   - Altered nutrition: less than body requirements related to decreased intake from sore throat
>   - Fatigue, activity intolerance related to disease process
>   - Potential for injury related to complications
>   - Knowledge deficit related to illness
>   - Impaired social interaction related to chronic fatigue and missed school
>   - Diversional activity deficit related to fatigue and activity intolerance
>   - Anxiety related to missed school, activities, and disease process
>   - Self-concept deficit related to length of illness, fatigue, and social isolation
> - **Key Terms/Concepts:** Oral-salivary transmission, incubation, lymphadenopathy, exudative pharyngitis, splenomegaly, immunocompromise, atypical lymphocytes

Nursing Management of a Child with Epstein-Barr Viral Infection (Mononucleosis)

Overview

Epstein-Barr viral infection (EBV) causes mononucleosis or "kissing disease," a disease most commonly affecting adolescents and young adults. This acute, self-limiting infectious disease is characterized by an increase in the mononuclear elements in the blood. The infection can be mild or complicated by a secondarily-acquired infection. The incubation period is four to six weeks after exposure. Transmission occurs primarily by contact with saliva. Close, intimate contact and/or blood contact may also lead to EBV infection. Acute symptoms usually resolve in one to two weeks, although the fatigue may last for one to two months. EBV infection is also associated with some types of cancer and autoimmune diseases.

Risk Factors

- Eating and/or drinking after others (sharing utensils, drinking glasses)
- Adolescents and young adults with close, intimate contact
- Immunocompromise (cancer, autoimmune disorders, etc.)

Signs and Symptoms

- Symptoms may occur acutely or over several weeks
- Fever
- Severe sore throat
- Exudative pharyngitis
- Lymphadenopathy
- Headache
- Fatigue: May last up to eight weeks after recovery of the disease
- Splenomegaly
- Abdominal pain
- Anorexia
- Skin rash
- Malaise
- Jaundice (with hepatitis)

Diagnostic Tests and Labs

- History and physical
- WBC shows atypical lymphocytes
- Epstein-Barr virus (EBV) antigen tests (Monospot)
- Heterophil antibody (a titer of 1:160 considered diagnostic)
- Viral cultures from saliva, blood or lymphatic tissue (may take 6-8 weeks for results)
- Elevated LFT with hepatic complications

Nursing Management of a Child with Epstein-Barr Viral Infection (Mononucleosis)

Therapeutic Nursing Management

- Assess for presence of symptoms that may lead to complications (airway obstruction, dehydration, splenic rupture, etc.).
- Obtain blood test by finger puncture for diagnostic purposes. The Monospot is rapid, inexpensive, easy to perform, and highly specific.
- Provide bedrest during acute illness. Gradually increase activity as tolerated.
- Administer non-aspirin antipyretics for fever.
- Address comfort needs (analgesics and nonpharmacologic interventions).
- Monitor hydration status. Encourage adequate oral intake and/or administer intravenous fluids as needed.
- Provide gargles with warm saline for pharyngitis.
- Provide cool, soft, bland, non-acidic foods when the child's throat is sore.
- Provide diversional activities that require minimal energy expenditure (videos, books, etc.).
- Collaborate with school to arrange make-up schoolwork assignments.
- Instruct parents and child to avoid heavy lifting, trauma to the abdomen, and vigorous athletics to decrease the risk of splenic rupture.
- Monitor for signs of hepatitis (jaundice, elevated LFT, etc.).

Pharmacology

- Antipyretics
- Analgesics
- Antibiotics for secondary infection
- Corticosteroids for severe throat swelling

Complications

- Respiratory compromise related to severe throat swelling or secondary infection
- Ruptured spleen
- Hepatitis
- Depression

Critical Thinking Exercise: Nursing Management of a Child with Epstein-Barr Viral Infection (Mononucleosis)

1. Discuss why each of the following children may be at risk for acquiring EBV. Identify which of the following children is at greatest risk for acquiring this disease. Explain your rationale.

    a. 4-year old twins imitating kissing seen on television:

    b. A 16-year old male who tells the nurse he enjoys "making out" with his 16-year-old girlfriend:

    c. A 1-year-old infant who puts a pacifier in his mouth after picking it up off the carpet:

    d. A 7-year-old who shares a bedroom with his parents and two younger siblings:

2. A 15-year-old with EBV tells her nurse that her disease is really upsetting her. Describe five or more reasons why an adolescent with EBV might be distressed.

Lymphatic/Infectious/Immune System **CHAPTER 49**

Nursing Management of a Child with Rheumatic Fever

> **Key Points**
>
> - Rheumatic fever is an autoimmune response to group A, beta-hemolytic streptococci.
> - Rheumatic fever is the result of inadequate treatment of streptococcal pharyngitis.
> - Rheumatic fever is a self-limiting disease and if not for the potential for heart valve damage (known as rheumatic heart disease) would be a fairly benign childhood illness.
> - Diagnosis is made not by one conclusive test but through presentation of major and minor symptoms and positive laboratory tests defined by the American Heart Association and known as the Jones Criteria.
> - The nurse should encourage the client and parents of any child with streptococcal pharyngitis to complete the prescribed antibiotic therapy.
> - The nurse should encourage all clients and parents of clients with typical signs and symptoms of streptococcal pharyngitis or those who exposed without symptoms, to be seen by a health care provider and be screened with a throat culture.
> - The goals of collaborative management:
>   - Provide complete treatment of strep pharyngitis in all diagnosed.
>   - Provide prompt recognition and treatment of rheumatic fever.
>   - Prevent complications (rheumatic heart disease most particularly).
>   - Educate the child and family about the need for close follow-up and treatment of any recurrence of symptoms.
>   - Educate the child and family on the need for antibiotic prophylaxis for dental work and some invasive procedures with rheumatic heart disease (ask the primary care provider).
>   - Provide adequate bedrest during the acute febrile phase.
>   - Provide adequate fluid and nutrition.
>   - Support care for relief of associated symptoms (fever, arthralgia, and chorea).
> - Important nursing diagnoses (actual or potential) are:
>   - Hyperthermia related to the disease process:
>   - Pain in the joints related to the disease process
>   - Knowledge deficit related to the need for adequate rest, fluids, and nutrition during the illness
>   - Knowledge deficit related to the need for antibiotic prophylaxis for dental procedures and some invasive procedures
>   - Potential for life-threatening complications related to the disease process
>   - Potential for impaired social interaction related to the complications (chorea) and absence from school and inability to complete ADLs independently

Nursing Management of a Child with Rheumatic Fever

Overview

Rheumatic fever is the result of inadequately-treated streptococcal pharyngitis, commonly know as strep throat. If it were not for the potential of dangerous cardiac complications, rheumatic fever would be of little consequence for most victims. The cardiac complications (known as rheumatic heart disease) involve: inflammation of the endocardium, pericardium, and myocardium, with damage to the valve(s) of the heart being the most common major complication. The symptoms of rheumatic fever stem from Aschoff bodies/nodules: inflammatory, hemorrhagic, bullous lesions known as Aschoff bodies or nodules. These nodules are vegetative growth that causes swelling and other changes in the connective tissue. Aschoff bodies are found in the brain, on joint surfaces, in blood vessels, on pleura surfaces, and in the heart. These areas can develop small spots of necrosis. As these areas heal, scarring develops, with the most common complication being thickening and deformity of the heart valves. This, then, results in heart valve stenosis and insufficiency and, depending upon the severity, may require valve replacement surgery.

Terms and Definitions

Antistreptolysin-O (ASO) titers: Measures the concentration of antibodies formed in the blood against streptomycin-O (O means it is oxygen labile), a streptococcal extracellular component that produces lysis of the red blood cells. ASO inhibits or prevents the effects of streptomycin O by group A strep. A rise in the titer shown by at least two ASO test is the most reliable indicator of recent strep infection. Norms are 0-to-120 Todd units. Results over 333 Todd units are positive for recent strep infection in children.

Aschoff bodies or nodules: Inflammatory hemorrhagic bullous lesions that cause swelling and changes in connective tissue; found of all patients with clinical rheumatic fever in the heart, blood vessels, brain, and surfaces of the pleura and joints

Carditis: Inflammation of the tissue in and around the heart

Chorea: Involuntary spasmodic movements of the limbs and face

Erythema marginatum: Transient macule with a clear center; wavy, well-defined border; generally found on the trunk and proximally on the extremities

Polyarthritis: Inflammation and pain in multiple joints; acutely present during the febrile phase and can persist for weeks in the untreated client

Rheumatic heart disease: Heart disease associated with rheumatic fever

Subcutaneous nodules: Small, non-tender nodules that persist for a long period; are rare and found over bony areas

St. Vitus dance or Sydenham chorea: Acute chorea associated with rheumatic fever

Risk Factors

- Exposure to groups of children – day care and school
- Exposure to a family member or peer with streptococcal pharyngitis
- Immunocompromised

Signs and Symptoms
- Major manifestations
  - Carditis
  - Polyarthritis
  - Chorea (transient), acute
  - Erythema marginatum
  - Subcutaneous nodules
- Minor manifestations
  - Arthralgia
  - Fever

Diagnostic Tests and Lab
- Elevated antistreptolysin-O (ASO) titers (minor manifestation)
- Elevated erythrocyte sedimentation rate (ESR) (minor manifestation)
- Elevated C-reactive protein (minor manifestation)
- Positive throat culture or rapid strep test (supporting evidence of a antecedent group A streptococcal infection)
- Elevated or rising strep antibody titer (supporting evidence of a antecedent group A streptococcal infection)
- Elevated white blood cell count

Therapeutic Nursing Management
- Encourage and educate the client and family in the importance of maintaining bedrest status during the acute febrile phase.
- Encourage and educate the client and parents on the importance of taking the prescribed antibiotic therapy for the duration of the illness (for strep throat, rheumatic fever, or the prescribed long-term therapy for prevention of recurrent rheumatic fever or complications of rheumatic heart disease).
- Educate the client and family regarding the importance of antibiotic prophylaxis prior to dental work, some invasive procedures, and other active infection.
- Educate the client and family regarding the need for close follow-up for five years following the illness and susceptibility to recurrence of rheumatic fever throughout the life of the client.
- If the child has developed chorea (spasmodic involuntary movements of the limbs or face) provide education and support to the family and school staff. Advise them that this is a transient complication of rheumatic fever (it can occur months after diagnosis) and the symptoms should completely resolve.
- Advise the parents and child to follow activity restrictions; generally once the fever resolves the child can resume moderate physical activity.
- If there is joint involvement, positioning is important to minimize pain.
- Provide emotional support to the child and family.

Nursing Management of a Child with Rheumatic Fever

- Encourage and educate the child and family on the importance of adequate fluids and good, balanced nutrition.
- Offer analgesics, anti-inflammatories, and moist heat to painful joints.

Pharmacology

- Penicillin is the first-line drug.
- Erythromycin is recommended for those with penicillin sensitivity.
- Salicylates or NSAIDS may be used to control inflammation, fever, and pain.
- Prophylaxis against recurrent rheumatic fever begins once acute therapy is complete, and can be one of the following:
    - IM benzathine penicillin G, 1.2 million units, monthly
    - Penicillin, 200,000 units, orally twice a day
    - Sulfadiazine, 1 gram, orally each day if greater than 60 pounds; 500mg if less than 60 pounds

Complications

- Carditis
- Polyarthritis
- Erythema marginatum
- St. Vitus dance or Sydenham chorea
- Subcutaneous nodules

Critical Thinking Exercise: Nursing Management of a Child with Rheumatic Fever

Fill in the blank:

1. Rheumatic fever is a complication of _____ pharyngitis and is self-limiting.

2. The dangerous complication associated with rheumatic fever is _____.

3. The inflammatory, hemorrhagic, bullous lesions that result from rheumatic fever are known as _____.

4. Rheumatic heart disease may require _____ surgery due to the thickening and deformity of the _____.

5. Minor manifestations of rheumatic fever noted on the Jones Criteria from 1992 include _____ and _____.

6. The gold standard in treating rheumatic fever is _____.

7. The best way to prevent rheumatic fever is to ensure _____ streptococcal pharyngitis.

Identify 5 teaching points for the family of a child with rheumatic fever.

1.

2.

3.

4.

5.

Gastrointestinal/Hepatic System CHAPTER 50

Nursing Management of the Child with Gastroenteritis/Diarrhea

Key Points

- The onset of gastroenteritis is often abrupt with rapid loss of fluids and electrolytes from persistent vomiting and diarrhea.
- Rotavirus is the most common cause of gastroenteritis in the United Sates and throughout the world.
- Hypokalemia and hyponatremia, acidosis or alkalosis may develop during the acute period of the disease.
- Organisms that cause gastroenteritis spread via personal contact. Sources of gastroenteritis include lack of clean water, poor hygiene, poor sanitation, recent exposure to infectious microorganisms, exposure to pathogens, and ingestion of contaminated food.
- Goals of Treatment:
  - Identify source of gastroenteritis.
  - Maintain fluid and electrolyte balance.
  - Reintroduce fluids and food.
  - Return to pre-illness state.
- Diagnostic Association (NANDA) nursing diagnosis:
  - Activity intolerance related to fatigue and dizziness secondary to progression of disease process
  - Impaired comfort related to abdominal pain
  - Diarrhea related to progression of disease process
  - Deficient fluid volume related to fluid loss from vomiting and diarrhea
  - Nausea related to progression of disease process
  - Imbalanced nutrition: less than body requirements related to anorexia
- **Key Terms/Concepts:** rehydration therapy, enterotoxins, lactose intolerance, anorexia

Overview

Gastroenteritis is the inflammation of the stomach and intestines accompanying numerous gastrointestinal disorders with symptoms including anorexia, nausea, vomiting, abdominal discomfort and diarrhea. Gastroenteritis may be attributed to bacterial enterotoxins, bacterial or viral invasions, chemical toxins or miscellaneous conditions such as lactose intolerance.

Signs and Symptoms

- Nausea, vomiting, diarrhea
- Abdominal cramping, pain, fever

- Anorexia, weight loss

Diagnostic Tests

- Stool sample
- General chemistry
- History and physical exam

Treatment

- Oral rehydration therapy
- Intravenous therapy
- Reintroduce diet with age-appropriate foods.

Therapeutic Nursing Management

- Weigh the child and compare to the pre-illness weight.
- Monitor for signs of dehydration: dry, pale, cool lips; dry mucous membranes; decreased skin turgor; diminished urinary output; concentrated urine; thirst; increased pulse; and decreased blood pressure; sunken eyes.
- Monitor laboratory studies such as: electrolytes, BUN/creatinine, hemoglobin and hematocrit, urine-specific gravity.
- Assess for signs of irritation or skin breakdown from passing stools frequently.
- Once dehydration has been corrected, offer age appropriate diet plus breast milk, formula or cow's milk.
- Maintain strict intake and output.
- Instruct parents to change diapers frequently.
- Wash diaper area with water and mild soap.
- Utilize soothing ointment, if skin excoriation is noted.
- Enforce strict handwashing practices.

Complications

- Dehydration
- Excoriated skin integrity in the diaper area

Critical Thinking Exercise: Nursing Management of the Child with Gastroenteritis/Diarrhea

Situation: A 6-month-old male is admitted to the hospital with diagnosis of gastroenteritis/diarrhea. He is alert but listless. The child is pale with sunken eyes. VS-101.6 - 146 - 42. The child is refusing all oral food and fluids. The parent reports that the child has vomited 6 times and has had numerous diarrhea stools. Currently watery diarrhea is noted. Abdomen is soft with hyperactive bowel sounds. The nurse notes that the child cries and pulls his legs to the abdomen.

Following a detailed health history and physical assessment, the nurse begins to formulate a plan of care with nursing diagnosis. The nurse has started with the following NANDA approved nursing diagnosis. Enter the symptoms, both from the scenario above and your knowledge of the disease process that could complete the nursing diagnosis statement. Explain rationale for the choices.

Risk for impaired parent/infant attachment related to:

    Rationale:

Risk for caregiver role strain related to:

    Rationale:

Impaired comfort related to:

    Rationale:

Interrupted family processes related to:

    Rationale:

Fluid volume: Deficient related to:

    Rationale:

Hyperthermia related to:

    Rationale:

Ineffective infant feeding pattern related to:

    Rationale:

Knowledge: Deficient related to:

    Rationale:

Nausea related to:

    Rationale:

Nutrition: Less than body requirements:

Risk for impaired skin integrity related to:

    Rationale:

Identify the 3 nursing diagnosis (2 physical and 1 psychosocial) that are priorities. Justify your answer.

1.

2.

3.

Gastrointestinal/Hepatic System CHAPTER 51

Nursing Management of the Child with Cleft Lip and Palate

Key Points

- Cleft lip and palate occur because maxillary and nasal tissue failed to fuse during embryonic development. They can result in an abnormal opening in the lip, palate, and/or nose.
- Preoperative care focuses on promoting parent-infant bonding, preventing pulmonary complications from aspiration while providing adequate nutritional intake.
- Postoperative care focuses on promoting healing of surgical site and preventing complications.
- Goals of collaborative management:
    - Promote family involvement in the infant's care.
    - Provide adequate nutrition.
    - Maintain a patent airway and prevent aspiration.
    - Correct defect surgically.
    - Provide pain relief.
    - Prevent infection of or trauma to the surgical site.
    - Prevent complications (aspiration, failure to thrive, speech difficulties, otitis media, and body image disturbance).
- Important nursing diagnoses (actual or potential) are:
    - Altered nutrition: Less than body requirements
    - Altered growth and development
    - Fluid volume deficit
    - Ineffective airway clearance
    - Pain (related to surgical intervention)
    - Altered parent/infant attachment
    - Altered family processes
    - Impaired home maintenance management
- **Key Terms/Concepts**: Embryonic development, feeding difficulty, failure to thrive, cleft palate feeding devices, corrective surgical repair, Z-plasty surgery, elbow restraints

Overview

Cleft lip and palate are facial malformations that occur during embryonic development (6-12 weeks gestation) causing a failure of the maxillary and median nasal structures to fuse. Cleft lip is more common in males. Cleft palate is more common in females. The etiology is unknown. Cleft lip and palate may also occur as a part of a genetic disorder or environmental factors.

Risk Factors

- Exposure to teratogens
- Familial tendency
- Increased incidence in Asians and Native Americans
- Lowest incidence in African-Americans

Signs and Symptoms

- Cleft lip
    - May be unilateral or bilateral
    - Varies from simple notching of vermilion border of the lip to a deep cleft, extending through the lip or into the nose
- Cleft palate: Midline fissure or opening in the hard and/or soft palate areas
- Difficulty forming a seal for sucking
- Coughing and choking with feeding
- Nasal distortion
- Congestion
- Failure to thrive (in unrepaired defect with persistent feeding difficulties)

Diagnostic Tests and Lab

- History and physical
- Prenatal ultrasound
- Preoperative laboratory data: CBC, electrolytes
- Wound and sputum cultures if infection is suspected

Therapeutic Nursing Management

- **Preoperative**:
    - Encourage parents to hold, touch, and kiss the infant and to participate in the care to promote bonding and acceptance.
    - Allow family members to work through emotional issues associated with loss of "perfect baby."
    - Offer information regarding support groups and community resource agencies.
    - Offer information regarding corrective surgeries.
    - Provide oral care and suctioning as needed.
    - Instruct parent regarding use of feeding devices: Cleft palate nipple, syringe with soft rubber tubing, or soft nipple with enlarged hole.
    - Feed upright, directing fluid to the back of the mouth. Burp frequently.
    - Position on side with the head of bed elevated.
    - Use of orthodontic appliance to prevent speech problems.
    - Teach family to use bulb suction as needed to clear the airway.
    - Prepare for surgery.

- **Postoperative**:
  - Address pain management needs.
  - Use elbow restraints to prevent trauma to incision.
  - Avoid placing hard items in mouth (suction catheters, straws, spoons, ice chips, etc.).
  - Clean lip area per protocol.
  - Rinse mouth with water after feedings.
  - Monitor for signs of bleeding, infection, or breakdown near the surgical site.
  - Provide information regarding long-term management and resources for speech, hearing and dental needs.
  - Use a cup for drinking to avoid placing anything in the mouth.

Complications

- Surgical site bleeding, infection or rupture
- Otitis media and hearing loss
- Speech difficulties
- Failure to thrive
- Pulmonary complications from aspiration
- Impaired bonding due to loss of perfect baby and multiple surgeries
- Malocclusion due to abnormal teeth eruption
- Altered body image

Critical Thinking Exercise: Nursing Management of the Child with Cleft Lip and Palate

Identify each of the following statements regarding **preoperative care** of an infant with cleft lip and palate as **TRUE** or **FALSE**.

1. Family members should be encouraged to participate in cares as soon as possible after birth.

2. Keep the infant flat and in the prone position to prevent aspiration.

3. Feeding best done by nurses who can ensure the child's safety.

4. Feed by holding the infant parallel to arm. Direct nipple towards the gums. Allow the child to suck until the seal is broken.

5. Use an orthodontic appliance to promote alignment of the maxilla.

Nursing Management of the Child with Cleft Lip and Palate

Identify each of the following statements regarding **postoperative care** of a child with cleft lip and palate as **TRUE** or **FALSE**.

6. The child will have a smooth, straight incision to prevent the lip from notching.

7. The child will need to wear elbow restraints after surgery to prevent injury to the surgical site.

8. The child will be encouraged to sip water slowly through a straw.

9. A medicated pacifier will be used to decrease postoperative pain.

Gastrointestinal/Hepatic System **CHAPTER 52**

Nursing Management of the Child with Pinworm Infection (Enterobiasis)

> **Key Points**
>
> - Infestation of pinworms most frequently occur in children in school and day care.
> - Rectal itching and irritation (hallmark signs of the disorder) are due to female pinworms laying their eggs in the perianal area at night.
> - Infection and reinfection occurs because the disease is transmitted via the oral-fecal route. This usually occurs as a result of scratching with subsequent nail biting or thumb sucking.
> - Goals of collaborative management:
>   - Identify the presence of pinworms.
>   - Treat the child and family with anthelmintic medication.
>   - Prevent recurrence and/or spread of infestation.
>   - Educate the child and family regarding treatment and prevention of recurrence.
>   - Prevent complications.
> - Important nursing diagnoses (actual or potential) are:
>   - Impaired tissue integrity
>   - Risk for injury
>   - Altered protection
>   - Sleep pattern disturbance
>   - Noncompliance with treatment plan
> - **Key Terms/Concepts:** Parasitic infection, eggs, enterobiasis vermicularis, oral-fecal route, autoinoculation, anthelmintic medication

Overview

Enterobiasis (pinworms) is caused by the nematode, which is a small, white, threadlike worm approximately 1/3-1/2 inch long. Pinworms infest the lower intestine after ingestion of the egg via the oral-fecal route. This usually occurs from the child scratching and placing his or her hand in the mouth (thumb sucking, nail biting). The female pinworms come out of the anus at night to lay eggs in the perianal region. This leads to intense pruritus and scratching in the rectal area. Eggs can survive for up to 2-3 weeks. Migrant female worms can cause vaginitis, salpingitis, or pelvic peritonitis in girls.

Risk Factors

- Crowded conditions (schools and day care)
- Handling contaminated toys or soiled linen
- Fingers in mouth after rectal contact

Signs and Symptoms
- Scratching the anal area, particularly at night
- Perianal and rectal area irritated from scratching
- Irritability and restlessness
- Poor appetite
- Stomachache

Diagnostic Tests and Labs
- Pinworm diagnostic tape or tongue blade covered with transparent tape (parent may obtain as child awakens in a.m. before toileting or bathing)
- Microscopic exam of specimen obtained on tape

Therapeutic Nursing Management
- Administer anthelmintic medications.
- Inform schools and/or day care center regarding need for treatment.
- Treat family members and those with close contact if they manifest symptoms.
- Promote good hand washing.
- Treat bed linen and underwear by washing in hot water.
- Teach that fingernails should be short and clean.
- Teach child and family to discourage nail biting and thumb sucking.
- Provide education regarding importance of proper hygiene and cleaning: Bathe daily, change underwear daily, clean toilet seat and diaper change area, wash bedding each day for several days, etc.
- Provide education to family, schools, and day care centers to reduce anxiety and spread of infection.

Pharmacology
- Pyrantel pamoate: Single dose, repeat in 2 weeks
- Mebendazole (Vermox): Chewable tablet, may need to repeat in 2 weeks

Complications
- Secondary infections
  - Urethritis
  - Vaginitis, salpingitis, or pelvic peritonitis in girls

Critical Thinking Exercise: Nursing Management of the Child with Pinworm Infection (Enterobiasis)

Situation: A 5-year-old male presents to the health care provider's office with a one-week history of rectal itching, restlessness, and perianal irritation. Pinworms are suspected.

1. What causes the rectal itching and perianal irritation in children with pinworm infections?

2. What factors are associated with the spread of pinworms?

3. How should the nurse instruct the family to obtain a pinworm specimen?

4. What instructions should the nurse give the family regarding treatment of a pinworm infection?

5. What instructions should the nurse give the family regarding prevention of recurrent pinworm infections?

Genitourinary/Reproductive System CHAPTER 53

Nursing Management of the Child with Hypospadias

Key Points

- Hypospadias refers to a condition in which the urethral opening is located below the glans penis or anywhere along the ventral surface (underside) of the penile shaft.
- Chordee or ventral curvature of the penis results from the replacement of normal skin with a fibrous band of tissue and usually accompanies more severe forms of hypospadias.
- The foreskin can also be absent ventrally and when combined with chordee gives the penis a hooded and crooked appearance.
- Surgical correction is completed to improve the physical appearance of the genitalia for psychological reasons, enhance the child's ability to void in the standing position with a straight stream and preserve the sexual ability of the organ.
- The exact type of surgical correction depends on the severity of the defect and the presence of associated anomalies. Some surgical procedures require the approximation of non-joined urethral opening with the lengthening of the urethra. Other procedures create a ventral flap to reach the tip of the penis. Commonly, the chordee that often coexists with a hypospadias defect is repaired by the release of the ventral skin.
- Improvements in surgical procedures have decreased the need for staged procedures.
- The preferred time for surgical repair is 6 - 18 months of age, before the child has developed body image and castration anxiety.
- Goals of Treatment:
    - Improve the physical appearance of the penis.
    - Enable the child to have usual urinary function.
    - Allow the child to have sexual ability as an adult.
- Diagnostic Association (NANDA) nursing diagnosis
    - Impaired urinary elimination related to misplaced urethral meatus
    - Impaired skin integrity related to surgical incision
    - Acute pain related to surgical procedure
- **Key Terms/Concepts**: Chordee, hypospadias, glans penis

Overview

Hypospadias is a congenital defect of the penis in which the urinary meatus is on the underside of the penis. Urinary difficulties do not occur because the sphincters are not defective. The opening of the urinary meatus may be off

Nursing Care of Children

Nursing Management of the Child with Hypospadias

center, along the under side of the penis or on the perineum. Surgical correction is performed as necessary for cosmetic, urologic or reproductive indications.

Risk Factors

- Sibling or father with the same condition

Signs and Symptoms

- Misplaced urinary meatus

Treatment

- Frequent diapering
- Surgical repair

Therapeutic Nursing Management

- Examine every male newborn
- Prepare parents for type of treatment to be performed and the expected cosmetic results
- Instruct on the need for a silicone stent or feeding tube as a urinary diversion to promote optimum healing following surgery
- Maintain position and patency of newly formed urethra
- Administer pain medication
- Sponge bathe until stent is removed
- Encourage increased fluid intake

Pharmacology

- Apply antibacterial ointment to the penis daily for infection control
- Pain medication

Complications

- Post operative incisional infection
- Urinary tract infection
- Blocked catheter or urethra

Critical Thinking Exercise: Nursing Management of the Child with Hypospadias

Situation: A nursery room nurse is completing an admission assessment on a newborn. Upon review of systems, it is noted that the child has hypospadias.

1. What anatomical changes would the nurse document in the admission assessment and identify the nursing responsibilities.

2. If the family declines surgical repair of the hypospadias, what difficulties could be anticipated in the future?

3. What post operative education following repair is necessary for the parents?

Genitourinary/Reproductive System **CHAPTER 54**

Nursing Management of the Child with Wilms' Tumor (Nephroblastoma)

> **Key Points**
>
> - Wilms' tumor is a rapidly-growing, solid malignant tumor arising from the renal parenchyma.
> - Factors associated with Wilms' tumor include: Congenital urinary malformations, cardiac anomalies, and neurofibromatosis.
> - Wilms' tumors are encapsulated and should NOT be palpated.
> - Goals of collaborative management:
>   - Prevent injury caused by palpation of the tumor (preoperatively).
>   - Maintain fluid and electrolyte balance.
>   - Assess and manage pain.
>   - Maintain a patent airway and promote adequate oxygenation (postoperative).
>   - Promote wound healing.
>   - Prevent infection.
>   - Provide the child/family education and support.
>   - Promote optimal growth and development.
>   - Prevent complications from disease process, surgical intervention, and treatment (bleeding, infection, gastrointestinal complications, renal failure, and hypertension).
> - Important nursing diagnoses (actual and potential) are:
>   - Risk for injury
>   - Impaired tissue integrity
>   - Alteration in fluid and electrolyte balance
>   - Impaired gas exchange
>   - Risk of infection
>   - Anxiety and fear
>   - Pain management
>   - Body image disturbance
>   - Altered growth and development
>   - Knowledge deficit
>   - Ineffective family and individual coping
>   - Altered family process
> - **Key Terms/Concepts:** Histology, staging, prognosis, metastasis, chemotherapy, radiation

Nursing Management of the Child with Wilms' Tumor (Nephroblastoma)

Overview

Wilms' tumor (nephroblastoma) is the most common primary malignant tumor of the kidney in children. It may be genetically inherited; however, no identifying gene markers have been located at this time. The tumor is most common in boys. The peak incidence is 3-4 years of age. Treatment is based on the tumor stage and type. Surgery with chemotherapy and radiation is commonly used for treatment. Prognosis for Wilms' tumor without metastasis and with favorable histology is 90%. Metastasis occurs through the bloodstream and is most commonly found in the lungs, liver, contralateral kidney, and bone marrow.

Diagnostic Tests and Lab

- Abdominal ultrasound
- Intravenous pyelogram (IVP)
- Serum labs: CBC (anemia), BUN/creatinine (renal function), erythropoietin levels (metastasis), liver function studies
- Urine labs: Urinalysis (hematuria)
- Imaging studies: Liver scan, CT scan, chest x-ray (metastasis)
- Bone marrow aspiration (metastasis)

Signs and Symptoms

- Abdominal mass. Mass may be on either side of the abdomen or bilateral (classic sign)
- Abdominal swelling (occasionally)
- Pain (occasionally)
- Hematuria (occasionally)
- Hypertension (occasionally)
- Weight loss (occasionally)
- Fever (occasionally)
- Fatigue/malaise (occasionally)

Therapeutic Nursing Management

- **Preoperative care**
  - Prepare child and family for surgery and treatment.
  - Avoid palpation of the abdomen.
- **Postoperative care**
  - Assess and manage pain.
  - Monitor and support respiratory status.
  - Support gastrointestinal functioning.
    - Maintain patent NG tube.
    - Monitor bowel sounds.
    - Assess for signs of complications (adhesions, bowel obstruction, and infection).

- Maintain fluid and electrolyte balance.
- Promote wound healing.

Ongoing care
- Administer chemotherapy as ordered.
- Monitor for side effects of radiation therapy.
- Protect child from infection.
- Promote adequate nutritional intake.
- Monitor and support renal function.

- **Child and family education**
    - Preoperative teaching
    - Postoperative plan and progress
    - Skin, wound and central line care (as applicable)
    - Preventing infection
- **Signs and symptoms of infection**
    - Side effects of chemotherapy and radiation
    - Importance of following plan and keeping appointments with health care provider
    - Coping with illness and altered body image

Pharmacology

- Analgesics
- Chemotherapy agents
- Antiemetics

Complications

- Infection
- Renal failure
- Gastrointestinal complications related to chemotherapy
- Intestinal obstruction related to chemotherapy and surgical procedure
- Metastasis

Critical Thinking Exercise: Nursing Management of the Child with Wilms' Tumor

Situation: A 4-year-old female is admitted with a Wilms' tumor. The child's mother tells the nurse that her daughter has been fussy and her clothing seems too tight around her enlarged abdomen. The nurse's initial assessment reveals the following: pronounced abdominal distention and low-grade fever with an increased respiratory rate, heart rate, and blood pressure. The child cries and pulls away when her abdomen is approached.

1. Which of the child's symptoms are characteristic of Wilms' tumors?

2. What preoperative interventions are indicated for a child with a Wilms' tumor?

3. What are the priority postoperative interventions for a child who has had a Wilms' tumor removed?

Genitourinary/Reproductive System **CHAPTER 55**

Nursing Management of the Child with Nephrotic Syndrome

> **Key Points**
>
> - Nephrotic syndrome is a manifestation of glomerular damage and altered glomerular permeability.
> - The clinical presentation of nephrotic syndrome is characterized by proteinuria, hypoalbuminemia, hyperlipidemia, and edema.
> - Nephrotic syndrome may exhibit as a primary event (minimal change nephrotic syndrome, congenital, or inherited) or secondary to a systemic disease (drug toxicity, systemic lupus erythematosus, heavy metal poisoning, allergic response, stings, venom, infectious disease, hepatitis, cancer, or renal vein thrombosis).
> - Minimal change nephrotic syndrome (MCNS) is the most common type in children.
> - Goals of collaborative management:
>   - Maintain fluid and electrolyte balance.
>   - Assess and manage protein loss and nutritional status.
>   - Assess and manage cardiovascular functioning.
>   - Maintain a patent airway and promote adequate oxygenation.
>   - Prevent skin breakdown.
>   - Prevent infection.
>   - Assess and manage pain.
>   - Educate and support child and family.
> - Important nursing diagnoses (actual and potential) are:
>   - Altered pattern of urinary elimination
>   - Fluid volume excess related to impaired renal function
>   - Fluid volume deficit related to impaired renal function
>   - Altered respiratory function
>   - Altered nutrition: Less than body requirements related to anorexia, nausea, and dietary restrictions secondary to renal failure
>   - Activity intolerance
>   - Impaired tissue integrity
>   - Infection, risk related to presence of indwelling catheter and instillation of dialysate (if required)
>   - Altered comfort, acute pain
>   - Sleep pattern disturbance
>   - Body image disturbance
>   - Knowledge deficit related to disease process and its treatment

- Ineffective family and individual coping
- Pain related to instillation of dialysate (if required)
- Constipation related to medications, fluid and dietary restrictions, and decreased activity level
- **Key Terms/Concepts**: Glomerular filtration, proteinuria, hypoalbuminemia, hyperlipidemia, fluid volume shift, edema, hypertension, pallor, corticosteroids, and immunosuppressive agents

Overview

Nephrotic syndrome (nephrosis) is a disorder that most commonly affects toddlers and preschool-age children. The cause may be idiopathic, congenital or a secondary disorder resulting from glomerular damage. The pathophysiologic mechanism of this disorder is the abnormal permeability of the glomerular basement membrane to protein molecules, particularly albumin. These proteins are excessively filtered through the renal tubules and excreted in the urine. The process results in pressure changes to the kidney, causing edema and progressive renal failure. Complications that can occur may be: severe hypovolemia, thromboembolism, thyroid and aldosterone activity, osteomalacia, and increased risk for infection.

Signs and Symptoms

- Edema: first around the eyes and ankles; later generalized edema/ascites
- Weight gain secondary to edema
- Normal or slightly hypotensive blood pressure
- Dark and frothy urine
- Decreased urinary output
- Poor appetite
- Irritability
- Listlessness and activity intolerance
- Pallor
- Vomiting
- Diarrhea
- Weight loss due to anorexia (may be obscured due to edema)
- Skin breakdown
- Muehrcke bands (white lines on nails associated with prolonged hypoalbuminemia)

Diagnostic Tests and Labs

- History and physical
- Urinalysis: Proteinuria, increased specific gravity, hyaline casts
- Serum levels: Hypoalbuminemia (<2.5 g/dL), hyperlipidemia, increased cholesterol, increased hematocrit and hemoglobin, increased platelet count, hyponatremia
- Renal biopsy to determine type of nephrotic syndrome, status and response to therapy

Nursing Management of the Child with Nephrotic Syndrome

Therapeutic Nursing Management

- Administer corticosteroid/immunosuppressive therapy.
  - Administer corticosteroids (prednisone) according to treatment schedule.
  - Administer immunosuppressive agents if the disease is resistant to steroids (Cytoxan or chlorambucil).
  - Monitor for side effects and complications related to medications.
- Maintain fluid, electrolyte balance, and control edema.
  - Record accurate intake and output.
  - Measure and record daily weights.
  - Monitor abdominal girth.
  - Monitor urine protein, specific gravity, color, and amount.
  - Monitor vital signs for hypotension and tachycardia indicating fluid volume deficit.
  - Administer diuretics as ordered.
  - Administer fluids as ordered for fluid volume deficit.
  - Monitor for pulmonary involvement (crackles, increased work of breathing, cough).
- Provide appropriate nutritional intake.
  - Provide a well-balanced, regular diet with no added table salt during the edematous phase. Also do not provide highly salt foods.
  - Work with child's individual dietary preferences to promote intake.
  - Allow normal amounts of fluid intake.
- Provide skin care and appropriate positioning.
  - Turn frequently to prevent respiratory complication and skin breakdown.
  - Use meticulous skin care techniques (bathing, pressure relief, etc.).
  - Assess for genital edema; provide diaper area care if not toilet trained.
  - Use a protective pressure-equalizing mattress with high-risk children.
  - Position with pillow between pressure areas (knees, elbows, etc.).
  - Elevate head to reduce facial edema.
  - Avoid use of donuts or ring-type pressure devices (can lead to breakdown along ring).
- Prevent infection.
  - Examine skin carefully for signs of breakdown.
  - Monitor vital signs for temperature variations.
  - Always use careful hand washing and infection control procedures.
  - Administer antibiotics to prevent or treat infection as ordered.
  - Avoid immunizations/vaccines during active disease.
- Provide support to the child and family.
  - Teach family home care.
  - Support the family when dealing with emotional issues related to coping with a child with a serious medical condition.
  - Assist the family in problem-solving issues related to the disease process and treatment (edema, skin care, dietary restrictions, activity tolerance, etc.).

- Identify and collaborate with support resources as appropriate.

Complications

- Renal failure
- Infection, sepsis
- Peritonitis
- Cellulitis
- Pneumonia
- Prolonged course of illness with relapse

Critical Thinking Exercise: Nursing Management of the Child with Nephrotic Syndrome

Identify the reason each of the following interventions is important when caring for the child described in the case study.

Situation: A 2-year-old boy has been admitted to the pediatric unit with a diagnosis of nephrotic syndrome. His mother states that he has had a five-day history of irritability, poor appetite, and vomiting and woke up today with swelling around the eyes. She also says his urine output has decreased significantly in the past 24 hours, even though he has gained 4 pounds.

Intervention	Rationale
Elevate head of bed to semi-Fowler position.	
Obtain urine for urinalysis.	
Assess for signs of infection.	
Measure abdominal girth.	
Administer prednisone per order.	
Assess for skin breakdown	
Daily weights	
Take the vital signs q 4 h.	
Provide high-protein, low-salt, high- potassium diet.	
Monitor I and O.	

Genitourinary/Reproductive System CHAPTER 56

Nursing Management of the Child with Acute Glomerulonephritis

> **Key Points**
>
> - Acute glomerulonephritis is caused by an inflammation injury resulting in glomerular damage.
> - The most common type of acute glomerulonephritis is preceded by an upper respiratory tract streptococcal infection.
> - The clinical presentation is characterized by hematuria, hypertension, and edema.
> - Goals of collaborative management:
>   - Monitor and support renal function.
>   - Maintain fluid and electrolyte balance.
>   - Manage cardiovascular functioning and control hypertension.
>   - Maintain a patent airway and promote adequate oxygenation.
>   - Assess and manage pain.
>   - Prevent complications.
>   - Educate and support the child and family.
> - Important nursing diagnoses (actual and potential) are:
>   - Altered pattern of urinary elimination
>   - Fluid volume excess
>   - Altered respiratory function
>   - Altered nutrition: Less than body requirements
>   - Altered tissue perfusion
>   - Activity intolerance
>   - Impaired tissue integrity
>   - Risk of infection
>   - Altered comfort, due to acute pain
>   - Knowledge deficit
>   - Ineffective family and individual coping
> - **Key Terms/Concepts**: Streptococcal infection, glomerular filtration, hematuria, fluid volume shift, edema, hypertension

Overview

Acute glomerulonephritis may be a primary event or a manifestation of a systemic disorder. This inflammatory disease of the glomeruli occurs as a post-infectious condition, usually related to a streptococcal organism.

The proposed mechanism of injury is related to an antigen-antibody reaction from the streptococcal infection. The immune complexes become trapped in the glomerular capillary loop, causing obstruction, edema, and vasospasm.

The renal damage and decreased glomerular filtration leads to hematuria, volume retention, and decreased urinary output. Due to the risk for neurological complications related to hypertension, the nurse should assess the child frequently for signs of neurological involvement (changes due to the illness). The condition most often affects school-age children and is rare in those younger than two years. Acute glomerulonephritis usually lasts for one to two weeks. Almost all children correctly diagnosed will recover completely. Recurrences are relatively rare.

Risk Factors

- Antecedent streptococcal infection
- History of respiratory infection or pharyngitis
- Impetigo

Signs and Symptoms

- Sudden onset of brown "tea colored" or smoke-colored urine
- Decreased urine output
- Edema–periorbital and facial edema in the morning spreading to extremities during the day
- Hypertension
- Low-grade fever
- Weakness
- Fatigue, activity intolerance
- Irritability
- Headache, abdominal discomfort
- Anorexia

Diagnostic Tests and Labs

- History and physical
- Urinalysis
  - Hematuria: Red blood cells in the urine
  - Proteinuria: Protein in the urine
  - Specific gravity increased
- Blood tests
  - Streptococcal antibody titers (ASO, Streptozyme, etc.): increased
  - Potassium: normal or increased
  - Albumin: mild decrease
  - C3 compliment level: decreased initially, returns to normal 8-10 weeks after onset
  - Hematocrit and hemoglobin: slightly decreased due to hemodilution
  - BUN and Creatinine: increased with renal failure

- Throat culture may be positive for streptococcus
- Chest x-ray (with complications): pulmonary congestion, pleural effusion, cardiac enlargement
- Renal biopsy: Rarely used, but may be indicated for an atypical presentation or when the child fails to respond to treatment

Therapeutic Nursing Management

- Maintain fluid balance and adequate nutritional intake.
  - Assess and record accurate intake and output.
  - Measure and record daily weights.
  - Monitor urine protein, specific gravity and color.
  - Monitor vital signs for hypertension.
  - Administer antihypertensives as indicated.
  - Maintain fluid limit as ordered.
  - Administer diuretics as ordered.
  - Monitor for pulmonary involvement (crackles, dyspnea, retractions, and cough).
  - Provide a regular diet, "no added salt" diet or moderate sodium diet as ordered.
  - Consult with the dietary department regarding appetizing foods that comply with dietary restrictions.
- Provide skin care, positioning, and activity as tolerated.
  - Provide skin care to prevent break-down (bathing, pressure relief, etc.).
  - Use a protective pressure-equalizing mattress with high-risk children.
  - Position with pillow between pressure areas (knees, elbows, etc.).
  - Elevate body parts most affected by edema (head elevated, pillows under feet, etc.).
- Prevent infection.
  - Examine skin carefully for signs of breakdown.
  - Monitor vital signs for temperature variations.
  - Always use careful hand washing and infection control procedures.
  - Administer antibiotics to prevent and/or treat infection as indicated.
- Provide support to the child and family.
  - Teach family home care and assessment.
  - Encourage the child and family to identify issues related to the disease process and care (emotional and practical).
  - Identify and collaborate with resources for supportive care.
  - Support child and families coping with issues associated with complications from the disease.

Complications

- Renal failure
- Infection, sepsis

- Seizures
- Hypertensive encephalopathy
- Hypertension
- Pulmonary congestion
- Cardiac congestion
- Prolonged course of illness

Critical Thinking Exercise: Nursing Management of the Child with Acute Glomerulonephritis

1. Describe how the following symptoms manifest in acute glomerulonephritis and nephrotic syndrome.

Symptom	Acute Glomerulonephritis	Nephrotic Syndrome
Edema		
Hematuria		
Proteinuria		
Blood pressure		
Anorexia		
Pain, discomfort		
Fatigue, activity intolerance		
Serum albumin/protein levels		
Serum lipid levels		
Serum electrolyte levels		
Hemoglobin and hematocrit		
Serum creatinine and BUN		
Serum streptococcal antibody titers		
Age at onset		

Nursing Management of the Child with Acute Glomerulonephritis

2. Compare and contrast nursing interventions appropriate when caring children with acute glomerulonephritis and nephrotic syndrome.

Nursing Intervention	Acute Glomerulonephritis	Nephrotic Syndrome
Intake and Output		
Weight Measurement		
Diet		
Fluids		
Positioning		
Skin care		
Medications		

Genitourinary/Reproductive System **CHAPTER 57**

Nursing Management of the Child with Urinary Tract Infections

Key Points

- Urinary tract infection (UTI) is a common disorder in children. It is caused by bacterial invasion of the sterile urinary tract.
- Symptoms in infants may be vague and difficult to detect.
- Antibiotic treatment is based on the sensitivity of the invading organism.
- If untreated, infected urine may reflux back to the kidney, causing pyelonephritis and kidney damage.
- Goals of collaborative management:
    - Identify the presence of a UTI and type of invading organism and sensitivity of the organism to different antibiotics.
    - Provide antibiotic therapy.
    - Assess for the presence of structural abnormalities associated with UTI.
    - Prevent recurrent infection.
    - Assess and manage pain.
    - Provide the child and family with education and support.
- Important nursing diagnoses (actual and potential) are:
    - Altered pattern of urinary elimination
    - Hyperthermia
    - Altered comfort, acute pain
    - Altered nutrition (related to abdominal pain, vomiting, diarrhea, and poor feeding)
    - Knowledge deficit
- **Key Terms/Concepts:** Bacterial invasion, hematuria, pyuria, dysuria, neurogenic bladder, circumcision, vesicoureteral reflux, urinalysis, urine culture, clean catch, intermittent catheterization, suprapubic aspiration, urine Chemstrip, voiding cystourethrogram, intravenous pyelogram

Overview

Infection of the genitourinary tract is one of the most common infections in childhood. A urinary tract infection (UTI) occurs when the organism count exceeds 100,000 colonies/ mL. UTI may involve the lower urinary tract (urethra or bladder) or upper kidney structures (renal pelvis and renal parenchyma). The single, most important factor influencing the occurrence of a UTI is the presence of urinary stasis, which provides a medium for bacterial growth.

Altered urine and bladder chemistry (alkaline pH) may also play a role in the development of an infection. *Escherichia coli* (*E. coli*) is the most common

Nursing Management of the Child with Urinary Tract Infections

bacterium causing the infection. UTIs are more frequent in females than males. UTI should be ruled out in infants and toddlers with a fever of unknown origin.

Risk Factors

- Congenital malformations of urinary tract
- Vesicoureteral reflux
- Ignoring urge to void (stasis)
- Neurogenic bladder (stasis)
- Uncircumcised male
- Mechanical factors (tight diapers or underwear, bubble baths, incorrect wiping methods)
- Sexual abuse

Signs and Symptoms

- May be vague and nonspecific in infants
- Abrupt and severe onset
- Fever up to 104° F
- Pallor
- Anorexia, decreased feeding
- Vomiting, diarrhea
- Abdominal pain
- Sharp or dull, flank pain
- Hematuria
- Pyuria
- Dysuria
- Frequency, urgency and burning (urinary)
- Fever and chills
- Fussiness/irritability
- Foul-smelling urine
- Incontinence if previously toilet-trained or holding urine

Diagnostic Tests and Lab

- History and physical
- Urinalysis
- Urine culture: clean catch, intermittent catheterization, suprapubic aspiration
- Urine Chemstrip
- Complete blood count (CBC)
- Renal ultrasound
- Voiding cystourethrogram (VCUG)
- Intravenous pyelogram (IVP)

- Cystometer

Therapeutic Nursing Management

- Administer appropriate antibiotic therapy.
- Obtain follow-up urine culture 2-3 days after finishing antibiotics.
- Administer antipyretics.
- Light clothing and minimum of blankets.
- Prevent dehydration.
- Increase fluids as tolerated.
- IV fluids as ordered.
- Provide nutritious diet.
- Child and family education: Identifying signs of UTI, completing course of antibiotics, providing proper hygiene and perianal cleaning, avoiding bubble baths, maintaining adequate hydration, and encouraging frequent bladder emptying.

Complications

- Pyelonephritis
- Re-infection
- Renal scarring
- Hypertension (related to renal damage)

Critical Thinking Exercise: Nursing Management of the Child with Urinary Tract Infections

1. Matching:

Intravenous pyelogram	a. Invasion of a bacterial pathogen
Bacterial infection	b. Blood in the urine
Urinalysis	c. White blood cells in the urine
Neurogenic bladder	d. Stopping and starting of the urinary stream
Stranguria	e. Radiocontrast is used to assess the kidney, ureters and bladder
Vesicoureteral reflux	f. Bedside urine test for blood, protein, glucose and pH
Suprapubic aspiration	g. Urine test for white blood cells, hematuria, and organisms
Hematuria	h. Urine sample obtained directly from the bladder using a needle
Urine culture	i. Back flow of urine into the ureter and kidney.
Hematuria	j. Urine test for bacterial infection
Clean catch	k. Incomplete bladder emptying due to inadequate innervation
Pyuria	l. Non-invasive method of collecting a urine sample

2. Answer the following questions:
   a. Why are uncircumcised males more prone to urinary tract infections than circumcised males?

   a. Why are children with spina bifida and spinal cord injury prone to urinary tract infections?

   a. Why should children be taught go to the bathroom and not to ignore the urge to urinate?

Genitourinary/Reproductive System CHAPTER 58

Nursing Management of the Child with Sexually Transmitted Disease

Key Points

- Sexually transmitted diseases (infections) are preventable and treatable.
- Adolescents need honest information, a safe environment for questions and access to condoms if sexually active.
- Goals of collaborative management include:
  - Provide early recognition and treatment.
  - Eradicate the pathogenic organism.
  - Prevent transmission from one person to another.
  - Prevent recurrence.
- Important nursing diagnoses (actual or potential) are:
  - Pain management
  - Risk for infection
  - Risk for injury
  - Anxiety and fear
  - Altered health maintenance
  - Knowledge deficit (how disease is contracted, symptoms, treatment)
- **Key Terms/Concepts**: Transmission, multiple sex partners, prevention

Overview

Sexually transmitted disease (STD) is a description of a classification of infections that are spread through direct sexual activity. Sexually active adolescents are at increased risk for STDs when there is more than one sexual partner and they delay seeking treatment. There are over twenty types of STDs; the most common are herpes, gonorrhea, and chlamydia infections. Effective treatment for both partners is mandatory to eradicate the infection. The nurse plays a vital role in educating the adolescent about prevention, transmission, and complications that can occur as a result of STDs.

Risk Factors

- Increased risk in teenagers and young adults
- Adolescent thought process, the "Personal fable" ("I can't get an STD even though other people can.")
- Increased risk with drug and alcohol use
- Lack of use of condoms
- Urban settings
- Limited access to health care

- Multiple sexual partners
- Victims of sexual assault, incest, sexual abuse

Signs and Symptoms

- Chlamydia
  - Asymptomatic in some cases
  - Most common symptoms in males: Urethral discharge, dysuria
  - Most common symptoms in females: Vaginal discharge, dysuria. Later: alteration in menses and abdominal pain
- Gonorrhea
  - Males experience: Dysuria, urinary frequency and purulent urethral discharge
  - Females experience: Abnormal menses, abdominal pain, purulent vaginal discharge. Later: pelvic inflammatory disease or may be asymptomatic
- Syphilis: Three stages
  - Stage 1
    - Open lesions (chancre)
    - Enlarged lymph nodes
  - Stage 2
    - Skin rash on palms of hands
    - Mucous patches in mouth
    - Sore throat
    - Generalized lymph node enlargement
    - Papules on labia, anus
    - Flu-like symptoms
    - After stage 2, there is a long period of time where the client is asymptomatic
  - Stage 3
    - Tumors in skin, bones and liver
    - CNS damage is irreversible

Diagnostic Tests and Labs

- History and physical
- Blood tests (HIV, AIDS, HBV, VDRL-Venereal disease laboratory test)
- Vaginal/cervical culture (gonorrhea, Chlamydia)
- Urethral drainage culture
- VDRL (Venereal disease laboratory test)

Therapeutic Nursing Management

- Administer medication specific to the disease as prescribed.
- Report STDs according to county health department policy.
- Identify and treat sexual partners whenever possible.

- Educate about STDs and their transmission.
  - Explain the risks and signs of STDS.
  - Advise sexually active teens of the need for annual screenings for sexually transmitted diseases and a PAP smear (in females), and prompt examination of any signs or symptoms of disease(s).
  - Provide instructional material regarding use of condoms, safe sex.
  - Encourage abstinence or the use of condoms to prevent disease transmission.
  - Provide safe environment for questions and access to condoms if sexually active.
- Teach client regarding drug therapy and need for medical compliance.
- Encourage client to abstain from sexual activities while receiving treatment or when lesions are present.
- Collaborate with multidisciplinary team regarding related psychosocial and family issues.
- If an STD is diagnosed in a child, the nurse needs to report to SRS for possible abuse.
- Advise client of potential complications, infertility, etc.

Pharmacology

- Chlamydia: Doxycycline, azithromycin, erythromycin
- Gonorrhea: Ceftriaxone, doxycycline, erythromycin
- Syphilis: Penicillin G
- Herpes: Acyclovir

Complications

- Chlamydia: Chronic pelvic inflammatory disease (PID), infertility, ectopic pregnancy
- Gonorrhea: PID, urethral strictures, epididymitis, infertility, abscesses
- Syphilis: Blindness, paralysis, mental illness, brain damage, death

Critical Thinking Exercise: Nursing Management of the Child with Sexually Transmitted Disease

Situation: A 16-year-old female is admitted with abdominal pain and purulent vaginal discharge. After conversing privately with the nurse, the child revealed that she participated in a sexual activity with several different partners in the past two months. She told the nurse that she did not use condoms during sexual intercourse. The child also hinted that she had been sexually abused as a child but refused to divulge any additional information on this subject.

1. What aspects of the child's history put her at risk for contracting a sexually transmitted disease (STD)?

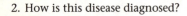

2. How is this disease diagnosed?

3. What are the appropriate interventions for this child?

4. The child asks the nurse if there will be any long-term problems because of this disease. How should the nurse respond?

Special Pediatric Emergencies CHAPTER 59

Nursing Management of the Child with Sudden Infant Death Syndrome

> **Key Points**
>
> - Sudden infant death syndrome (SIDS) is the sudden, unpredictable death of an infant with no detectable cause.
> - The incidence of SIDS in the United States has decreased significantly.
> - The introduction of widespread education for the prevention of SIDS has increased.
> - Goals of collaborative management:
>   - Support the family.
>   - Correct the underlying cause.
>   - Restore respiratory function and stability.
>   - Prevent recurrence.
> - Important nursing diagnoses (actual or potential) are:
>   - Fear and anxiety
>   - Powerlessness and hopelessness
>   - Grieving and loss
>   - Altered family processes
>   - Ineffective family coping
>   - Knowledge deficit
> - **Key Terms/Concepts**: Hypoxia, hypercarbia, acid-base imbalance

Overview

Sudden infant death syndrome (SIDS) is defined as the sudden, unexpected death of an apparently healthy infant at less than 1 year of age. The death remains unexplained after a complete post-mortem examination, review of the case history, and investigation of the death scene. In some communities the medical examiner may not correctly identify SIDS from other etiologic factors; therefore, the incidence of SIDS can vary in different regions. Peak age for SIDS is 2-4 months of age. American Academy of Pediatrics (AAP) recommends the supine sleep position for healthy infants. Infants with breathing problems or excessive vomiting should sleep prone on a firm mattress, preferably with the head of the bed elevated.

Risk Factors

Infants
- Prematurity
- Small for gestational age

- Intrauterine drug exposure
- Central hypoventilations
- Persistent apnea of prematurity > 45 post conceptual weeks
- Twin gestation
- Bronchopulmonary dysplasia (BPD)
- Male gender

Maternal/Family
- Two or more SIDS victims in family
- Heavy alcohol consumption or tobacco use
- Illicit drug use
- Adolescent mother

Environmental
- Impoverished home surroundings
- Crowded living conditions
- Winter months
- Use of soft pillows, sheep skin mattress covers or moldable sleep surface, blanket in crib
- Prone position while asleep
- Side-lying position while asleep
- Co-sleeping

Signs and Symptoms
- Cannot be predicted
- Death occurs during sleep for unknown reason.

Therapeutic Nursing Management
- Home monitoring is indicated for any subsequent siblings in a high-risk category.
- Avoid soft, moldable mattresses and pillows, blankets, toys/stuffed animals in crib.
- Prevent overheating during sleep.
- Provide emotional support to the grieving family.
- Educate family on importance of putting baby to sleep on his/her back.

Diagnostic Tests and Labs
- There are no diagnostic tests at the present time that successfully identify or predict which infants will survive or die. Home monitoring is no guarantee of survival or protection.

Critical Thinking Exercise: Nursing Management of the Child with Sudden Infant Death Syndrome

1. Identify which of the following sleeping conditions follows the current SIDS prevention recommendations.
    a. Infant in a home where both parents are smokers
    b. Prone positioning on a quilted blanket
    c. Infant sleeping in hot room and covered with a heavy blanket
    d. Supine positioning on a sheepskin with small stuffed animals at the foot of the bed
    e. Side-lying on a firm mattress and covered with a thick blanket
    f. Use of a small pillow under an infant's head during sleep
    g. None of the above responses are correct.

2. What things should the nurse tell the family to DO to prevent SIDS?

3. What things should the nurse instruct the family to AVOID to prevent SIDS?

Special Pediatric Emergencies CHAPTER 60

Nursing Management of the Abused Child

> **Key Points**
>
> - Child abuse is a non-accidental trauma that leads to physical injury, emotional harm, and/or sexual violation of the child.
> - Neglect is the failure to provide a safe environment for the child that supports his/her basic needs.
> - The most common forms of child abuse are physical abuse, emotional abuse, neglect, and sexual abuse.
> - Child maltreatment occurs from a combination of family, child, and environmental characteristics.
> - Abuse occurs across all socioeconomic, cultural, religious, and professional groups.
> - Children of low-income and adolescent parents are in the highest risk group.
> - Goals of collaborative management:
>   - Provide resuscitation and treat injuries.
>   - Preserve evidence and document assessment findings.
>   - Identify and report suspected cases of child abuse and/or neglect.
>   - Protect the child and other family members from additional harm.
>   - Provide crisis intervention and support the child.
>   - Connect with community resources as appropriate (child protective services, crisis intervention, counseling, educational programs, home nursing, financial support, and support groups, etc.).
>   - Collaborate with services that provide family support: counseling, parenting skills education, promotion of parent-child attachment, coping strategies, and positive role modeling.
> - Important nursing diagnoses (actual or potential) are:
>   - Injury related to intentional trauma and/or lack of parental supervision
>   - Altered nutrition: Less than body requirements related to inadequate intake
>   - Altered skin integrity related to trauma and/or poor hygiene
>   - Altered protection
>   - Altered growth and development
>   - Pain management
>   - Fear and anxiety
>   - Hopelessness and powerlessness
>   - Risk for self-harm or suicide
>   - Self-concept disturbance
>   - Impaired social interaction

- Ineffective family coping, ineffective individual coping
- Altered family processes
- Altered parenting
- Impaired home management
- Violence and lack of self-control

• **Key Terms/Concepts:** Non-accidental trauma, suspected abuse and neglect, mandatory reporting, suspicious injuries, altered parenting, physical abuse, emotional abuse, sexual abuse, neglect, shaken baby syndrome, Münchhausen Syndrome by Proxy, prevention programs

Overview

Child maltreatment refers to the non-accidental infliction of physical or emotional injury or neglect of the needs of a child. It usually results from the action of a caregiver or family member. Abuse is evidenced in a variety of ways: physical harm, sexual abuse, emotional abuse, and neglect. Child abuse is frequently associated with stress and the inability of the family to handle internal and external stressors. Parental characteristics (poor coping skills, lack of parenting skills, poor impulse control, aggressiveness, anger control issues, family violence patterns, substance abuse, etc.); child characteristics (chronic illness, behavioral problems, etc.); and/or environmental characteristics (lack of resources, substance availability, violence, environmental stressors, etc.) can lead to child maltreatment. Children who are abused can have immediate and long-term effects. For example, abused children may develop aggressive and/or antisocial behavior. They may also become passive and fearful, have poor self-esteem, lack self-control, suffer from chronic depression, become socially isolated, feel guilty, and/or have difficulty maintaining relationships. It is critical that health care providers promptly identify potentially abusive situations and report findings to the appropriate authorities. Münchhausen syndrome by proxy is a form of child abuse that is characterized by deliberate infliction or falsification of injury to child by caretaker. This is most frequently manifested as decreased LOC, bleeding, infection, apnea, seizures, diarrhea, vomiting, fever, and/or rash. Shaken baby syndrome (SBS) is a result of vigorous shaking of a baby leading to a severe whiplash-type injury. SBS causes intracranial damage (cerebral edema and increased ICP) and intraocular damage (retinal hemorrhage), which often leads to vision loss, severe brain damage and brain death.

Risk Factors

- **Families**
  - Poor parenting skills
  - Frustration and poor coping skills
  - Isolation from community/social groups
  - Competition for emotional resources (affection, attention, nurturing)
  - Altered family roles
  - Lack of trust (inside and outside family)
  - Altered family processes (substance abuse, mental illness, etc.)
  - Aggression used for conflict resolution

- Altered communication patterns (threats, mixed messages, nonverbal expression)
- Rigid, traditional family rules and roles
- Dominant family member who controls with manipulation, intimidation, aggression
- Financial strain
- Family history of abuse
- **Children**
  - Premature infants: altered bonding
  - Chronic illness, developmental delay
  - Frustrating behaviors
  - Infants with irritability, poor feeding and/or high pitched cry, GERD, colic
  - Children with ADHD, learning disabilities
  - Emotional disturbances
  - Birth order
  - Stepchildren
  - Gender
- **Environment**
  - Poverty
  - Lack of positive role models
  - Lack of education
  - Crowded living conditions
  - Availability of substances of abuse

Signs and Symptoms

- **Physical Abuse**
  - Behavioral signs
    - History or report of injury that does not match physical injuries
    - Inconsistent story of how injuries occurred
    - Distant from parent, does not cry or protest physical exam or strangers (per developmental level)
    - Withdrawn, apathetic, vacant stare
    - Aggressive behavior
    - Inappropriate attention seeking behaviors
    - Difficulty with relationships
  - Physical signs
    - Cuts, bruises or fractures in various stages of healing
    - Infected wounds (may be from a delay in seeking treatment)
    - Fractures: spiral fractures, facial trauma multiple fractures, infants with fractures
    - Burns: circular cigarette burns, geographic burns (iron, scalding, sock or glove burns), burns on buttocks, donut-shaped burns
    - Skin: bruises, cuts, slap marks, welts, or scars on face, neck, shoulders, back or buttocks

- **Neglect**
  - Behavioral signs
    - Unsuitable clothing for season (no coat, socks, shoes, etc.)
    - Poor caregiver supervision, failure to recognize or protect from dangerous conditions
    - Poor concentration, poor school performance
  - Physical signs
    - Failure to thrive/malnutrition
    - Poor hygiene
    - Sparse hair with bald patches
    - Infections
    - Skin breakdown
- **Emotional abuse**
  - Behavioral signs
    - Social isolation, withdrawal
    - Aggression
    - Hyperactive or disruptive behavior
    - Poor self-esteem
    - Depression
    - Learning disorders
    - Sleep disturbances
    - Psychological problems
  - Physical signs
    - Speech or developmental delay
    - Failure to thrive
- **Sexual abuse**
  - Behavioral signs
    - Social isolation, withdrawal
    - Running away from home
    - Truancy, lateness, poor school performance
    - Inappropriate or bizarre behavior
    - Aggressive behavior
    - Promiscuity, unusual sexual behavior or knowledge
    - Eating disorders (anorexia, bulimia, obesity)
    - Sleep disturbance/nightmares
    - Substance abuse
    - Suicide threats or attempts
  - Physical signs
    - Sexually transmitted disease
    - UTI, painful urination
    - Difficulty walking
    - Stained underwear (blood, feces, etc.)
    - Trauma to genital or anal area (tears, bruises, bleeding, etc.)

Diagnostic Tests and Lab

- History and physical examination
- Photographs of injured areas
- Imaging studies (long bone X-rays, CT scan, MRI)
- Culture of vaginal or cervical secretions
- Ophthalmologic examination (retinal hemorrhages related to shaken baby syndrome)

Therapeutic Nursing Management

- Identify any signs of maltreatment in children at risk. Assess for characteristic signs of abuse.
- Report suspected child abuse to child protective services (nurses are mandatory reporters) and document detailed nursing notes (may be subpoenaed in court).
- Treat injuries.
- Provide comfort measures for physical pain.
- Provide emotional support to child and family. Be careful not to assign blame before all facts are known.
- Protect the child's safety (maintain police hold, visitation restrictions, etc.).
  - Assess family behavior patterns and report of injury.
  - Ask for an account for the injury: how did this happen (assess for how the story matches injury).
- Be alert for contradictions in the story of how the injury occurred.
- Collaborate with multidisciplinary team in meeting child and family needs (social services, healthcare provider, psychology, child life specialist, child protective services, law enforcement, support groups, etc.).
- All documentation should be done in exact quotes from the child, parent, or care provider. As with all documentation, no personal judgments should be reflected in the nurse's documentation.

Complications

- Death
- Permanent disability from injuries (brain damage, blindness, etc.)
- Psychological problems
- Developmental delay
- Learning problems
- Pregnancy
- Infection, sexually transmitted disease
- Continuing the family pattern of abuse (when abused child has a family)

Critical Thinking Exercise: Nursing Management of the Abused Child

Situation: A 9-year-old female presents in the emergency department with a spiral fracture of her left arm, dislocated right shoulder, and several small circular burns on her arms. The child's mother tells the nurse that the child was hurt when she fell out off her bed two days ago. When the nurse asks the child's mother about the presence of several old bruises and scars on the back of the child's arms and legs, the mother claims that the child is very clumsy. The mother also told the nurse that she had no idea how her daughter received the burns.

1. What parts of the child's presentation and history are suspicious for child maltreatment? Why?

2. What additional questions should the nurse ask the mother and the child?

3. What else should the nurse assess?

4. Identify nursing interventions that are appropriate for this child and family.

Special Pediatric Emergencies **CHAPTER 61**

Nursing Management of the Child with Lead Poisoning (Plumbism)

> **Key Points**
>
> - Lead poisoning, an accumulation of lead in the blood, can lead to excessive amounts in the blood, bones, and soft tissue.
> - Central nervous system damage and renal toxicity are the most serious complications.
> - Young children are at greatest risk because of their behavioral tendencies and greater absorption rate.
> - Treatment for lead poisoning is through the use of chelating drugs (EDTA, Chemet, and BAL).
> - Goals of collaborative management:
>   - Provide routine screening and risk reduction.
>   - Provide early identification and treatment.
>   - Monitor for complications.
>   - Provide family education and support.
> - Important nursing diagnoses (actual or potential) are:
>   - Risk for injury (encephalopathy, brain damage, anemia, renal damage)
>   - Knowledge deficit
>   - Altered nutrition: Less than body requirements
>   - Altered growth and development
>   - Impaired home maintenance management
> - **Key Terms/Concepts:** Plumbism, pica, encephalopathy, chelating agents

Overview

Repeated ingestion or inhalation of substances containing lead can lead to a condition called, plumbism, which can have detrimental effects on the developing central nervous system of a child. Lead toxicity results from the slow accumulation of lead in the systemic circulation and is very slowly excreted through the kidney. The most serious and irreversible effects are seen in the central nervous system. Low-dose accumulation can lead to hyperactivity, aggression, impulsivity, and irritability. Cognitive impairment can occur surfacing in the form of distractibility and learning difficulties. Additionally, lead interferes with the formation of red blood cells, resulting in anemia. Lead poisoning occurs most often in toddlers and preschoolers in the summer months. No economic or racial subgroup of children is free from the risk.

Lead encephalopathy is rarely seen today; however, many children have levels sufficient to lead to neurologic and intellectual damage. Developmentally, young

> children are at increased risk for lead toxicity because of the frequency of hand-to-mouth activity. Small children are closer in proximity to the ground where lead may be found. Younger children have a greater absorption rate because of their increased fat intake and deceased calcium and iron intake. Some children with plumbism may have pica, which is the habitual ingestion of non-food substances that may contain the toxin. Environmental sources of lead primarily include lead-based paint, auto exhaust, improperly-fired ceramic pottery used for food, water and air contaminated from the dust emitted from lead smelters.

Risk Factors

- Children in urban areas with homes containing lead-based paint (prior to 1960)
- Use of some glazed earthenware pottery and other lead-based surfaces
- Member of the household with occupation or hobby involving lead (construction, foundry work, repair work, painting contracting, mining, metal repair work, stained glass work, jewelry making, ceramics work)
- Renovation of an old house (lead dust)
- Use of cultural remedies (azarcon, greta, paylooah, surma and forms of ayurvedic)
- A diet high in fat, and low in iron and calcium increases lead absorption.

Signs and Symptoms

- **Mild** (serum level at 10 µg/dL or above)
  - Myalgia or paresthesia
  - Mild fatigue
  - Irritability
  - Lethargy
  - Occasional abdominal discomfort
- **Moderate** (serum level > 45 µg/dL)
  - Arthralgia
  - General fatigue
  - Difficulty concentrating
  - Muscular excitability
  - Tremor
  - Headache
  - Diffuse abdominal pain
  - Vomiting
  - Weight loss
  - Constipation
  - Anemia
  - Learning disabilities
- **Severe** (serum level at 100 µg/dL or greater)
  - Paresis or paralysis
  - Encephalopathy (seizures-coma-death)

Nursing Management of the Child with Lead Poisoning (Plumbism)

- Lead-line (blue-black) on gingival tissues
- Colic

Diagnostic Tests and Labs

- Blood lead level test; capillary testing if >10µg/dL, follow with venous sample
- Routine screening at 1 year, unless at risk, and then at 6 months
- CBC, iron levels (assess for anemia)
- BUN, creatinine, UA (assess for renal damage)
- Abdominal x-ray (positive with ingestion)
- Erythrocyte protoporphyrin (EP) test no longer recommended for routine screening because of low sensitivity for levels less than 25 µg/dL

Therapeutic Nursing Management

- Monitor vital signs.
- Assess neurological status and intervene as needed.
- With IV hydration, monitor renal function, accurate intake and output, and laboratory results.
- Administer chelating agents; monitor the child's response and side effects.
- Provide screening for other members of the household.
- Rotate injection sites if administering IM injections of chelating agents.
- Use therapeutic medical play with child.
- Provide child and family education regarding diagnosis, treatment, and possible lead sources.
- Report to local health department or appropriate agency to help with finding source and lead abatement.

Pharmacology

- Calcium disodium edentate (Ca EDTA): IV or IM
- British anti-lewisite (BAL or dimercaprol): deep IM
- Succimer-oral

Treatment for lead poisoning is through the use of chelating drugs (EDTA, Chemet, and BAL). These drugs are heavy metal antagonists. The drug is administered and blood levels are monitored for a decrease. There can be a rebound or an elevation after a decrease of the lead level. Rebound levels will be lower than the pre-chelation level. Many times the chelation is repeated, maybe several times, if the original level is very high. The labs are obtained to measure the effectiveness of the treatment.

Complications

- Metabolic acidosis
- Renal toxicity
- Encephalopathy, cerebral edema
- Permanent brain damage

- Attention deficit hyperactivity disorder
- Shock
- Seizures
- Coma
- Death

Critical Thinking Exercise: Nursing Management of the Child with Lead Poisoning (Plumbism)

Identify if each of following clients has a **high** or **low** likelihood of having lead poisoning or an increased lead level.

1. A 2-year-old female is seen in a clinic with a history of irritability, decreased appetite, vomiting, and weight loss over the past month. Her father tells the nurse she has not been as active as usual over the last several months. The child cries and guards when her abdomen is approached. The father works in a foundry where lead is used.

2. An 8-year-old male is brought to the health care provider's office with a two-week history of constipation. The boy's mother also reports that her child has been complaining about difficulty seeing the blackboard and often has a headache at school. The mother reports that the only possibility of lead exposure was a stained glass-making workshop she attended 2 days ago. The child did not attend the workshop with his mother.

3. A 4-year-old boy presents in a clinic with vomiting, muscle tremors, and lethargy. He has a history of attention deficit disorder and experienced unexplained weight loss and loss of developmental milestones over the past 6 months. When asked, his mother tells the nurse that she owns orange earthenware dishes she bought while traveling outside the United States one year ago. She also tells the nurse that these are her favorite dishes and has been routinely using them to prepare the family meals.

4. A 5-year-old girl presents with a 3-day history of fever, vomiting, nausea, diarrhea, and abdominal pain. Her brother and sister both had acute gastroenteritis the week prior. She lives in a house built in 1982.

Special Pediatric Emergencies **CHAPTER 62**

Nursing Management of the Child with Acetaminophen Poisoning

> **Key Points**
>
> - Toddlers, preschool-age children, and adolescents are at highest risk.
> - Acetaminophen is the most often used medication for fever in children and the most common type of drug overdose in children.
> - Hepatic involvement can last one week or be permanent.
> - Goals of collaborative management:
>   - Provide immediate gastric decontamination (charcoal, lavage).
>   - Administer antidote N-acetylcysteine.
>   - Monitor for hepatic involvement.
>   - Provide child/family teaching and counseling.
> - Important nursing diagnoses (actual or potential) are:
>   - Risk for injury (hepatic damage, encephalopathy, and hypoglycemia)
>   - Fluid volume deficit (vomiting, shock)
>   - Hypothermia
>   - Confusion
>   - Fear and anxiety
>   - Ineffective individual coping
>   - Altered family processes
> - **Key Terms/Concepts**: Hepatic damage, N-acetylcysteine

Overview

The ingestion of injurious agents or excessive doses of pharmacotherapeutic agents, such as acetaminophen, is a concern in toddler and preschool-age children. Adolescents attempting suicide may also ingest a toxic amount of acetaminophen. The most serious side effect is hepatic involvement. Ingestion of more than 150 mg/kg is potentially toxic.

Risk Factors

- Medication being referred to as "candy"
- Improper storage of medication
- Medications without child safety caps
- Adolescent depression and suicidal thoughts

Nursing Management of the Child with Acetaminophen Poisoning

Signs and Symptoms

Four stages in clinical course

- **Initial period** occurs within 2-4 hours after ingestion. The symptoms include: nausea, vomiting, malaise pallor, and diaphoresis. Young children may present with hypothermia, hypoglycemia, encephalopathy, and shock.
- **Latent period** occurs at 24 hours and lasts 36-48 hours. During this period the child appears to improve, but PT, bilirubin and hepatic enzymes are elevated.
- **Hepatic involvement** begins to appear at 72-96 hours. The effects last from seven days to permanently. Symptoms include: increased abnormal liver enzymes, jaundice, right upper quadrant pain, coagulation abnormalities, and confusion/stupor.
- **Terminal stage** of involving progressive liver dysfunction leading to death

Diagnostic Tests and Labs

- History and physical
- PT, bilirubin, ALT, AST
- Serum acetaminophen level

Therapeutic Nursing Management

- Obtain blood sample for serum acetaminophen level.
- Administer N-acetylcysteine according to the protocol. Consider administering in a covered cup, with juice or via NG tube due to strong odor.
- Assess baseline vital signs and monitor intake/output.
- Monitor liver function tests.
- Assess for jaundice and liver tenderness.
- Provide education and emotional support to child and family.

Pharmacology

- Syrup of ipecac may be administered at home (hospital use less common) to induce vomiting, if within 60 minutes of ingestion and only upon the direction of local poison control center or primary health care provider.
- N-acetylcysteine (Mucomyst) antidote given according to serum acetaminophen levels

Complications

- Hepatic damage
- Coma
- Death

Critical Thinking Exercise: Nursing Management of the Child with Acetaminophen Poisoning

Situation: A 2-year-old presents in the emergency department at 4 p.m. after ingesting 40–50 children's chewable acetaminophen tablets at approximately 3:15 p.m.

1. What initial symptoms should the nurse anticipate?

2. Rank the following interventions in order of priority. Explain the rationale for the rank order.

Intervention	Rank order	Rationale for rank order
Educate family regarding home safety needs.		
Gastric lavage		
Administer syrup of ipecac.		
Obtain a serum acetaminophen level.		
Administer N-acetylcysteine.		
Monitor liver function tests.		
Administer activated charcoal.		

3. The child's mother asks the nurse to explain the signs of liver damage. What should the nurse tell her?

Special Pediatric Emergencies — CHAPTER 63

Nursing Management of the Child with Substance Abuse

> **Key Points**

- Psychosocial, societal and developmental issues faced by adolescents make them more likely to experiment and/or abuse substances.
- Substance abuse often leads to physical and/or psychological addiction.
- Alcohol, tobacco, marijuana, and inhalant drugs are the most frequently abused substances by adolescents. The majority of teens less than 18 years of age have used alcohol at least once.
- Goals of collaborative management:
    - Identify disorder and initiating treatment.
    - Protect the child from harm while under the influence of substances.
    - Treat any injuries.
    - Provide detoxification and support through substance withdrawal.
    - Provide crisis intervention.
    - Initiate psychological/psychiatric counseling and/or drug rehabilitation.
    - Provide education and support to the child and family.
    - Prevent relapse into substance abuse pattern.
- Important nursing diagnoses (actual or potential) are:
    - Risk for self harm, suicide
    - Risk for injury related to substance use
    - Self-esteem disturbance
    - Impaired social interaction
    - Sleep pattern disturbance
    - Altered thought processes
    - Anxiety and fear
    - Ineffective individual coping
    - Ineffective family coping
    - Altered family processes
    - Noncompliance with treatment plan
    - Risk of violence related to altered thought process, paranoia, drug effects
    - Altered nutrition: Less than body requirements related to inadequate intake
    - Altered skin integrity related to needlestick
- **Key Terms/Concepts:** Self-esteem, peer pressure, physical addiction, psychological addiction, substance use, substance dependence, detoxification, drug rehabilitation, prevention programs

Nursing Management of the Child with Substance Abuse

Overview

Substance abuse is a growing social problem in the United States and worldwide. Substance abuse produces physical, psychological, and cognitive effects that vary according to the type of substance. The abuser is attracted to the altered sensorium changes in perception, pain reduction, anxiety reduction, relaxation, euphoria and/or a sense of well-being associated with various substances. The non-medical use of psychotherapeutic agents and illicit drugs can lead to dependence (tissue dependency, tolerance, withdrawal symptoms) and habituation. Adolescents are at risk for substance abuse.

Some of the common motives include rebellion, peer pressure, thrill seeking, poor judgment, experimentation, desire to escape from reality, enjoyment of substance-related sensations, poor self-esteem and family dysfunction.

Risk Factors

- Availability of abused substances
- Adolescent developmental level: need for rebellion, need for experimentation, conformity with peers (peer pressure), beliefs about invincibility/invulnerability
- Poor self-image
- Poor coping skills, delayed psychosocial maturation
- ADHD
- Ineffective family coping and communication: unrealistic expectations, inflexibility, overly permissive, parental disapproval or rejection, dysfunctional divorce
- Parents or role models who abuse alcohol/drugs
- Family genetic predisposition for addiction
- Child maltreatment: physical abuse, emotional abuse, sexual abuse, neglect

Signs and Symptoms

- Lack of personal grooming, change in appearance
- Inability to maintain normal activities of daily living
- Expresses craving for drugs or alcohol
- Expresses a need for drug or alcohol to cope or "get through the day"
- Legal difficulties, stealing, truancy, poor school performance
- Lethargy
- Paranoia, anxiety
- Mood disturbance: moodiness, nervousness, agitation, short temper
- Distortions of time, perceptions of colors and hearing
- Eyes: dilated pupils, redness, difficulty focusing, nystagmus
- Impaired memory and reaction time
- Gastrointestinal distress: nausea, vomiting, diarrhea, anorexia, dry mouth
- Cardiovascular: hypotension, tachycardia
- Other symptoms vary, based on individual reactions, and type and amount of drug used.

- Skin: flushing, rash, needle "track marks", skin breakdown or tissue damage from needlestick
- Musculoskeletal: poor coordination, clumsiness, unusual movement, tremors

Diagnostic Tests and Labs
- History and physical
- Blood levels
- Urine toxicology

Therapeutic Nursing Management
- Discover the type, amount, and time of the last substances taken.
- Obtain drug use history and pattern: drug of choice, frequency, amount, routes, combinations, and duration of addiction.
- Maintain child safety when under the influence of substances that alter mood, judgment, and LOC.
- Provide skin care as needed for wounds caused by IV drug abuse.
- Manage substance withdrawal symptoms.
- Collaborate with multidisciplinary team (social services, psychological services, rehabilitation, etc.).
- Provide information/referral to community treatment centers/programs, and/or community support agencies.
- Maintain non-threatening, nonjudgmental supportive approach.
- Communicate using active listening and other therapeutic techniques.
- Help child identify positive coping strategies.
- Plan educational programs for the prevention of substance abuse.
- Provide support/education to the child's family.

Complications
- Behavioral, personality disorders, developmental delays
- Memory loss, flashbacks
- Depression and suicide attempts
- Hepatic damage
- Pancreatitis
- Nutritional deficits, weight loss
- Cardiovascular complications: stroke, MI, arrhythmias, sudden cardiac arrest
- HIV infection
- Hepatitis infection
- Skin breakdown, tissue damage (from IV drug abuse)
- Increase incidence of teenage pregnancy

Critical Thinking Exercise: Nursing Management of the Child with Substance Abuse

1. Match the level of risk for substance abuse for each of the following adolescents.

    _____ 13-year-old male caught experimenting with inhalant drugs in his friend's garage. He claims he only occasionally uses inhalants. He begs the neighbor not to tell his parents because of fear of severe punishment.

    _____ 14-year-old girl who is described as "popular" at school. She was sexually abused when she was ten years old. She gives a vague answer when asked if she uses drugs or drinks alcohol. She does admit to smoking cigarettes.

    _____ 15-year-old female who reports having many friends and a good relationship with her parents. She admits to having tried alcohol once but denies current use because she doesn't like the way it made her feel.

    _____ 16-year-old male with a blood alcohol level above the legal limit after a recent auto accident. He recently received his driver's license and his own car. He reports that his parents don't care when he comes home at night.

    a. Low risk of substance abuse

    b. Moderate-to-high risk of substance abuse

2. What are the risk factors for substance abuse in the adolescents described above?

3. Identify interventions to assist families with members who are at risk for substance abuse.

Special Pediatric Emergencies **CHAPTER 64**

Nursing Management of the Child in a Suicidal Crisis

> **Key Points**
>
> - Suicide is one of the leading causes of death in adolescents. Adolescent males age 14 to 19 are at greatest risk.
> - Suicidal ideation can range from a passing thought about killing oneself to developing a plan for completion of suicide.
> - A variety of physical, emotional, psychological, environmental, and situational stressors can lead to suicide.
> - Goals of collaborative management:
>   - Identify disorder and initiate treatment.
>   - Treat any self-inflicted injuries.
>   - Provide crisis intervention.
>   - Initiate psychological/psychiatric counseling.
>   - Protect the child from self-harm while suicidal.
>   - Provide education and support to the child and family.
> - Important nursing diagnoses (actual or potential) are:
>   - Risk for self harm, suicide
>   - Risk for injury related to suicide attempts
>   - Self-esteem disturbance, chronic low self-esteem, and situational low self-esteem
>   - Impaired social interaction
>   - Sleep pattern disturbance
>   - Altered thought processes
>   - Anxiety and fear
>   - Loneliness and despair
>   - Hopelessness and powerlessness
>   - Ineffective individual coping
>   - Ineffective family coping
>   - Altered family processes
>   - Altered parenting
>   - Noncompliance with treatment plan
>   - Risk of violence related to murder-suicide behaviors
>   - Grieving and loss
> - **Key Terms/Concepts:** Self esteem, suicidal ideation

Nursing Management of the Child in a Suicidal Crisis

Overview

Suicide, the taking of one's own life, is one of the leading causes of death among 14-to-19-year-olds and ranks second as the cause of death for adolescents and college students. Most authorities distinguish among suicidal ideation, gestures, premeditated attempts, and impulsive acts. At least 90% of people that kill themselves have some type of mental or substance abuse disorder. It is felt that through screening and early recognition of these problems that some suicides can be prevented. Social and environmental factors must be considered. When there is a handgun in the home a teen is six times more likely to commit suicide (related to the teen's tendency to act impulsively).

Where there is a lack of social support systems, isolation, or few social, educational, or vocational opportunities the risk for suicide among teens increases. About 30% of all teens that commit suicide each year are gay, suggesting a need for support for this subgroup of teens.

Substance overdose (83%) and self-inflicted laceration are the most common means used in suicide attempts. Firearms are by far the most commonly used means in successful suicides among male and female adolescents. For adolescent males, hanging, followed by overdose, are the second and third most common means of successful suicide. For adolescent females overdose followed by strangulation are the second and third most common means of successful suicide.

Suicide among teens tends to happen in clusters and a single suicide should alert the community to a higher level of awareness of suicide education and prevention. Suicide rates have increased dramatically in the past 20 years and are explained by family disintegration, access to drugs, alcohol, and lethal weapons. Health care providers should continually screen adolescents on their coping ability and for depression related to a peer's suicide. Counselors and health care providers must work closely with survivors, including adolescent friends. The nurse's primary goal in working with those at risk for suicide is to ensure their safety.

Risk Factors

- Substance abuse, or alcoholism
- Child abuse, incest or sexual abuse
- Recent high profile suicides, "cluster suicides," "copycat suicides"
- Conflict with parents
- Poor communication/coping skills
- Poor problem-solving ability, impaired judgment
- Depression
- Chronically teased or bullied at school, not "fitting in" with peers
- Low self-esteem
- Social isolation from peers and family
- Crisis event (break up with girlfriend/boyfriend, death of loved one, etc.)
- Access to lethal weapons, guns
- Prior psychological problems and/or suicide attempts
- Dysfunctional family

Nursing Management of the Child in a Suicidal Crisis

Signs and Symptoms

- Depression
- Moodiness, sadness
- Quiet, withdrawn
- Expresses emptiness, loss or despair
- Inability to experience pleasure, serious
- Difficulty concentrating, difficulty with decision making, confusion
- Expresses that life is meaningless or purposeless, hopelessness about the future
- Low self-esteem
- Expresses feelings of being trapped, rejected or abandoned
- Difficulty with anger, aggressiveness, and/or acting out
- Behavioral problems (drop in school performance, sexual promiscuity, truancy)
- Sleep pattern disturbance: excess sleeping or insomnia
- Agitation, hyperactivity
- Gives away possessions
- Hints, jokes or talks about suicide
- Alcoholism/substance abuse
- Eating disorders, lack of appetite
- Social isolation, withdrawal from family and/or friends

Diagnostic Tests and Labs

- Psychological examination, history and physical
- Urine and blood toxicology screen

Therapeutic Nursing Management

- Identify children and adolescents who are at risk, based on risk factors, signs and symptoms; teach family and friends to watch for these signs in high-risk children.
- Immediately respond to suicidal threats, jokes, hints, and/or plans.
- Identify specificity of suicidal tendency (in general, specifying the details and plans indicate a greater threat than a vague comment).
- Identify and remove methods the client could use to carry out suicidal threats (knives, guns, pills, etc.).
- Provide close and constant supervision when suicidal.
- Connect child and family with crisis intervention team.
- Facilitate psychological/psychiatric counseling and intervention (individual, group, and family therapy).
- Maintain a nonjudgmental and supportive approach.
- Communicate using active listening and other therapeutic techniques.
- Provide community education for suicide prevention.

- Include the client in planning care. Adolescents and teens are more likely to participate and comply with the plan of care if they have been involved in the planning.

Pharmacology

- Antidepressants
- Sedatives/antianxiety medications for agitation
- Activated charcoal, reversal agents for intentional medication overdose

Complications

- Organ and tissue damage related to self-inflicted injuries
- Chronic unresolved suicidal tendencies and/or psychological illness
- Repeated attempts leading to death

Critical Thinking Exercise: Nursing Management of the Child in a Suicidal Crisis

1. Identify each of the following statements about suicide as a myth or reality.

Statement	Myth or Reality
Suicide is a disease that affects only adults and adolescents.	
Parental expectations that are high but realistic can serve as is associated with a low risk of suicide.	
An apparently happy teen involved in school activities that earns A's in school will not commit suicide.	
Past suicide attempts puts a teen at risk for future suicide attempts.	
It is best to ignore a child who has a tendency for fighting and truancy.	
A joke about suicide is not a serious threat.	
A person who describes specifics regarding how and where he would commit suicide is at high risk.	
If an adolescent is serious enough to make a suicide attempt, there is not much that can be done to prevent them from succeeding.	
Breaking up with a serious boyfriend can lead to a suicide attempt.	

2. Identify which of the following behaviors is associated with children who are at risk for suicide:

   a. Abuses alcohol
   b. Feels sad most of the time
   c. Popular among peers
   d. Gets in fights frequently
   e. From a large family
   f. Involved in sports
   g. Sleeps most of the time
   h. Feels that life is meaningless
   i. Has a low self esteem
   j. Inflexible parents with poor communication skills
   k. Doesn't have an interest in spending time with others
   l. Skips school and gets in trouble frequently
   m. Suddenly starts giving away prized possessions to friends
   n. Parents who are supportive and provide structure
   o. Chronically teased at school for a physical deformity

Developmental or Psychosocial Disorders CHAPTER 65

Nursing Management of the Child with Down Syndrome

> **Key Points**
>
> - Down syndrome is the most common chromosome abnormality, occurring in 1 in 800 to 1000 live births.
> - Approximately 95% of all cases of Down syndrome are attributed to an extra chromosome 21, hence the name trisomy 21. The level of physical and cognitive impairment is related to the percentage of abnormal cells present.
> - Because of the distinctive physical characteristics, the infant with Down syndrome is usually diagnosed at birth.
> - There is a wide variation in both physical characteristics and mental abilities of those diagnosed with Down syndrome.
> - Serious problems associated with Down syndrome include congenital heart defects, hypotonicity of the chest muscles, immune system dysfunction, hearing defects, congenital hypothyroidism, and an increased incidence of leukemia.
> - Genetic counseling is suggested for future pregnancies as parents with one child diagnosed with Down syndrome have an increased risk of 1 in 100 of having another child with Down syndrome. Prenatal diagnosis is available through amniocentesis or chorionic villi sampling.
> - More individuals with Down syndrome are living with family members or in group homes under supervision. Life expectancy has increased with more than 80% of individuals living past the age of 30. Cardiac and respiratory disorders are the major cause of death.
> - Goals of Treatment:
>   - Identify the syndrome.
>   - Educate the parents on the needs and care of the child.
>   - Stress the importance of regular care, stimulation, and medical attention.
>   - Encourage socialization.
>   - Offer genetic counseling.
> - Diagnostic Association (NANDA) nursing diagnosis:
>   - Impaired adjustment related to parental denial
>   - Caregiver role strain related to extended care of individual
>   - Risk for impaired parenting related to disappointment of imperfect child
>   - Ineffective tissue perfusion related to congenital heart defect
>   - Disturbed sensory perception related to deficits of sight and sound
>   - Impaired feeding (in infants) related to poor muscle tone
>   - Impaired growth related to congenital hypothyroidism

Nursing Management of the Child with Down Syndrome

Overview

The cause of Down syndrome is unknown; however, a genetic predisposition, radiation before conception, immunological problems, and infection may help trigger the improper cell division. Recent reports suggest cytogenetic and epidemiologic studies support a multiple causality. Maternal age over 35-40 and a paternal age over 55 are also possible factors.

Signs and Symptoms

- Smaller stature
- Slower mental development
- Delayed language and walking
- Flattening of the back of the head
- Slanting of the eyelids
- Epicanthal folds of the inner corner of the eyes
- Depressed nasal bridge
- Smaller ears
- Small mouth and jaw with large/protruding tongue
- Decreased muscle tone
- Loose ligaments
- Transverse palmar crease
- Small hands and feet
- Congenital heart defects
- Poor vision

Diagnostic Tests

- Inspection at birth
- A chromosomal analysis or karyotype

Treatment

- Supportive as there is no cure
- Early hearing and vision testing to identify deficits

Therapeutic Nursing Management

- Encourage bonding and promote acceptance of the infant.
- Anticipate feeling of grief and loss.
- Instruct parents on general health maintenance, immunizations, attending to medical emergencies.
- Emphasize holding the infant securely as hypotonic muscles and hyperextensible joints make the infant flaccid and limp.
- Teach the parents about respiratory problems and interventions such as using the bulb syringe, cool mist humidifier, changing positions and using chest percussion.

- Offer local support group information.
- Provide information on early intervention programs, preschools, and special education programs which foster developmental progress.
- Height and weight assessment, as well as, nutritional counseling should be provided as needed.

Critical Thinking Exercise: Nursing Management of the Child with Down Syndrome

Situation: The parents of a child diagnosed with Down syndrome are attending the first meeting of Parents of a Down Syndrome Child Support Group. The new parents are obviously overwhelmed with the diagnosis and seeking information regarding care.

1. Identify the myths associated with the diagnosis of Down syndrome.

2. Define the nurse's role in promoting the true character and abilities of those with Down syndrome.

3. How does a karyotype determine a person's genetic make-up? What differences in karyotype are seen in the Down syndrome client that are not present in the general population?

Developmental or Psychosocial Disorders **CHAPTER 66**

Nursing Management of the Child with Autism

> **Key Points**
>
> - Autism is not diagnosed conclusively until after a child is 12 months old.
> - Autistic children are totally self-centered and can not relate to others; they often exhibit bizarre behaviors and are destructive to themselves.
> - Current theories of the cause of autism include genetic and organic etiology and include: a disturbance in language comprehension, a biochemical problem involving neurotransmitters, or abnormalities in the central nervous system and probably brain metabolism.
> - The characteristics of autism are divided into three categories: inability to relate to others, inability to communicate with others, and obviously limited activities and interests.
> - Autistic children test in the mentally retarded range of standard intelligence tests; but may actually have good memories and good intellectual potential.
> - To confirm a diagnosis of autism, at least eight of sixteen identifying characteristics must be present and all three categories must be present.
> - Boys are four times as likely to be affected, although girls are more severely affected. The symptoms can have a wide range of severity, from mild forms requiring minimal supervision and intervention, to severe forms in which self abusive behavior is common.
> - Goals of Treatment:
>   - Identify specific characteristics related to the child's disease process.
>   - Educate the parents on specific signs and symptoms and correlate safety measures.
>   - Maintain current level of communication skills, social contact and participation in daily activities.
>   - Promote educational and social growth and development.
> - Diagnostic Association (NANDA) nursing diagnosis:
>   - Anxiety related to social situations
>   - Risk for impaired parent/infant/child interaction related to child's inability to relate to others
>   - Interrupted family processes related to behavioral characteristics
>   - Impaired parenting related to parental anxiety
>   - Self-mutilation related to characteristics of disease process

Nursing Management of the Child with Autism

Overview

Autism is referenced as a pervasive developmental disorder (PDD) with primary characteristics including severe behavioral disturbance that affects the practical use of language as a means of communication, interpersonal interaction, attention, perception, and motor activity.

Signs and Symptoms

- Lack of interest or pleasure in being touched or cuddled
- Violent reactions to attempts of physical closeness
- Blank response and lack of expression to verbal stimulation
- No fear of separation from their parents
- Fascination in strange repetitive behaviors, develops rituals
- Bizarre body movements such as rocking, twirling, flapping arms
- Severe temper tantrums
- Self-destructive acts such as hand-biting and head-banging
- Slow speech development, loses previous ability to say words or sentences
- Echolalia or echoing words
- Lack of the use of pronouns such as "I" or "me"
- Wants to play alone: retreats into own world

Diagnostic Tests

- Complete history, physical, and neurological exam
- Vision and hearing test
- Electroencephalography
- Radiographic studies of the skull
- Urine screening
- Nutritional history
- Developmental tests-speech, intelligence and behavioral

Treatment

- Behavioral modification
- Pharmacotherapeutics
- Individual/family therapy

Therapeutic Nursing Management

- Nurses must recognize that autism places great stress on the entire family.
- Establishing a relationship between the nurse and the child is essential.
- Familiar toys or other valuable objects from home reduce the child's anxiety during doctor's appointments or hospitalization.
- Nurses must provide a safe environment.
- Introduce the child to new situations slowly and gradually.

- Keep communication direct and brief, with only one request given at a time.
- Parents should be provided information about support groups, education, intervention strategies and techniques, facilities such as camps and group homes, and options for respite care.

Critical Thinking Exercise: Nursing Management of the Child with Autism

Situation: A 3-year-old has been recently diagnosed with autism. The parents state that they are overwhelmed with the diagnosis of autism. The nurse is formulating a teaching plan structured by the characteristics related to autism.

1. Utilizing the three defined categories of autism, identify the challenges of parenting and the appropriate nursing interventions.

   Inability to relate to others:

   Inability to communicate with others:

   Limited activities and interests:

2. Link the following long term goals to improve developmental characteristics (create table with option to link or match options).

   Long term goals:

   Promotion of normal development

   Language development

   Social interaction

   Learning

Developmental characteristics:

a. Child is able to complete morning routine (brush teeth and hair, dress self) with minimal supervision.

b. Child is able to communicate needs.

c. Child is able to acknowledge another person (adult or child) present.

d. Child progresses from identified point in learning development.

e. Child will eat a nutritionally-based meal by feeding self.

f. Child is able to participate in a brief conversation.

g. Child is able to participate in an interaction without feeling frustrated or anxious.

h. Child demonstrates activities in which learning is evident.

i. Child will relate to parents and siblings by communication of needs.

j. Child utilizes appropriate words throughout an interaction.

k. Child is accepting of others around.

l. Improvement is noted in completing activities of daily living successfully.

Developmental or Psychosocial Disorders CHAPTER 67

Nursing Management of the Child with Attention Deficit Hyperactivity Disorder

> **Key Points**
>
> - Attention deficit hyperactivity disorder (ADHD) is a condition characterized by inattention, hyperactivity, and impulsivity.
> - Diagnosis is generally made when the child reaches school-age if difficulty with learning, behavioral, and social expectations is observed.
> - Goals of collaborative management:
>   - Provide early recognition, diagnosis, and treatment.
>   - Identify the child's strengths and areas of needed improvement.
>   - Promote self-esteem.
>   - Promote optimal growth, development, and self-image.
> - Important nursing diagnoses (actual and potential) are:
>   - Impaired social interaction
>   - Altered thought processes
>   - Risk for injury
>   - Self-concept disturbance
>   - Knowledge deficit
>   - Ineffective family and individual coping
>   - Altered family processes
>   - Risk for violence
>   - Risk for self harm
> - **Key Terms/Concepts:** Inattention, hyperactivity, impulsivity, dopamine, reticular activating system of the brain, and stimulant medications

Overview

Attention deficit hyperactivity disorder (ADHD) refers to a developmentally inappropriate pattern of behavior including hyperactivity, impulsivity, and inattention. The symptoms of ADHD must be present before the age of seven and are not accounted for by other learning or mental disorders. Children with ADHD are usually average to above average intelligence. The condition occurs more often in boys. Boys exhibit more behavioral problems and girls demonstrate poor academic performance. With ADHD, every aspect of the child's life is affected. Socially, children with ADHD have difficulty forming and maintaining relationships. There is repeated maladaptive behavior causing negative reactions from others that may lead to the formation of a low self-image in the child.

The family, care providers, day care staff, and teachers should be aware of the need to set and reinforce boundaries for those with ADHD. Instructions to the

> client should be consistent when a behavior or violation occurs. Consistency is also important in enforcing limits.

Risk Factors

- Children with a decreased amount of dopamine
- Norepinephrine or serotonin
- Family history of ADHD
- Alteration of the reticular activating system of the mid-brain
- Boys affected 6:1
- Environmental factors: chaotic or abusive home (family history of substance abuse, learning disabilities, conduct or antisocial disorders, depression)

Diagnostic Tests

- History– self report, parental anecdotes, teacher evaluations
- ADHD checklists and assessment tools

Signs and Symptoms

- Inattention to details
- Careless work habits
- Often loses things necessary for tasks, activities or school
- Poor organizational skills
- Poor attention span for developmental age
- Poor listening skills
- Inability to follow directions, wait turns in games or group situations
- Inability to complete tasks
- Easily distracted by internal or external stimulus
- Increased motor function
- Difficulty sitting, fidgety
- Difficulty playing quietly
- Impulsivity
- Often talks excessively or inappropriately
- Often engages in dangerous activities without considering the possible consequences, but not for the purpose of thrill seeking
- Decreased appetite
- Insomnia

Therapeutic Nursing Management

- Assist with screenings and psychological testing.
- Assess and document behaviors carefully and objectively.
- Provide education regarding parenting skills and techniques for behavior modification.

- Provide medications as ordered. Educate child and family regarding dosage and side effects.
- Monitor growth regularly
- Praise appropriate behavior. Encourage family to use behavior charts and other techniques to reinforce positive behavior.
- Emphasize promoting the child's self-esteem.
- Support the child using biofeedback technique for treatment.
- When working directly with, counseling or educating the child with ADHD it is imperative to do so in a quiet environment with few distractions.

Pharmacology

- Stimulant medications:
    - Methylphenidate (Ritalin)
    - Dextroamphetamine (Dexedrine)
    - Pemoline (Cylert) used less frequently
    - Adderall (Amphetamine mixture)

Complications

- Learning difficulty
- Academic underachievement, academic failure
- Social isolation
- Emotional problems, depression, anxiety
- Injuries related to high risk behaviors
- Self-inflicted injury
- Child abuse

Critical Thinking Exercise: Nursing Management of the Child with Attention Deficit Hyperactivity Disorder

Identify 10 behaviors that may be associated with **inattention** in an 8-year-old boy.

1.
2.
3.
4.
5.
6.
7.
8.
9.
10.

Identify 10 behaviors that may be associated with **hyperactivity/impulsivity** in a 14-year-old boy.

1.
2.
3.
4.
5.
6.
7.
8.
9.
10.

Developmental or Psychosocial Disorders   CHAPTER 68

Nursing Management of the Child with Failure to Thrive

Key Points

- Failure to thrive (FTT) is a disorder that manifests as a failure to achieve adequate growth and development.
- Failure to thrive (FTT) causes and influences are complex and vary according to individual circumstances.
- Goals of collaborative management:
  - Correct the underlying problem/disease if possible.
  - Correct nutritional deficiencies and establish a pattern of weight gain.
  - Restore optimal body weight and composition.
  - Educate family about nutritional needs and feeding techniques.
  - Prevent complications (vitamin deficiency, anemia, stress ulceration, infection, and developmental delays).
- Important nursing diagnoses (actual or potential) are:
  - Altered nutrition: Less than body requirements
  - Altered growth and development
  - Activity intolerance
  - Fluid volume deficit
  - Risk for injury
  - Ineffective breastfeeding
  - Knowledge deficit
  - Altered family processes
  - Altered parenting
  - Risk of infection
- **Key Terms/Terms/Concepts**: Organic failure to thrive, nonorganic failure to thrive, idiopathic failure to thrive, feeding resistance, ineffective breastfeeding

Overview

Infants and children who fail to obtain and/or use calories effectively for appropriate weight gain are classified as **failure to thrive** (FTT). By definition, the weight of children with FTT is consistently below the fifth percentile on the growth chart. The disorder is categorized by the etiologic factor: organic failure to thrive (e.g., heart disease or AIDS) and nonorganic causes (e.g., disturbances in mother-child relationship).

Nurses play a vital role in the identification of the child with FTT through the physical assessment and observation of family interaction. Accurate assessment of the child's height, weight, health history, nutritional history, and feeding practices is needed for diagnosis of the condition.

Risk Factors for Nonorganic FTT

- Disturbance in mother-child relationship
- Marital discord
- Economic pressure
- Parental immaturity
- Low tolerance for stress
- Single parenthood
- Alcohol and drug abuse
- Infant drug withdrawal
- Oral aversion or protection (related to past unpleasant experiences such as force feeding or suctioning)
- Gastroesophageal reflux disease (GERD)

Causes for Organic FTT

- Congenital heart defects
- Neurologic lesions
- Gastroesophageal reflux
- Cystic fibrosis
- Microcephaly
- Chronic renal failure
- Malabsorption syndrome
- AIDS
- Cleft lip/palate

Signs and Symptoms

- Weight loss or failure to gain
- Irritability
- Disturbance of food intake (anorexia, pica, abnormal consumption of food)
- Vomiting and diarrhea
- General neuromuscular spasticity
- Most commonly a weight (and sometimes height) below the 5th percentile (some recognized authorities use the 3rd percentile)
- Developmental delays
- Hypotonia
- Unresponsive to cuddling
- Distrust of caretakers

Diagnostic Tests and Lab

- History and physical
- CBC and electrolytes: Acidosis from starvation is common.

Nursing Management of the Child with Failure to Thrive

Therapeutic Nursing Management

- Assess for risk factors and symptoms.
- Collaborate with the multidisciplinary team regarding physiological and psychosocial issues impacting the child's growth and development.
- Provide developmental screening.
- Collaborate with dietitian for nutritional screening and support.
- Assess home feeding practices:
    - Feeding location, routines, and potential distractions
    - If breastfeeding, ask mother about latching on, suck/swallow coordination, and breast emptying.
    - If bottle-feeding, ask type of formula and how it is mixed (correct concentration).
    - Feeding schedule (how often and how long)
    - Supplements and snacks given on a regular basis
    - Child's usual behavior patterns during feeding
- Provide increased-calorie formula and supplements as ordered.
- Provide frequent nutritious snacks and small meals.
- Use supportive feeding techniques.
- Educate family regarding supportive feeding techniques.
- Provide consistent caregiver who knows the child's routine and feeding style.
    - Develop feeding routines and rituals (favorite utensils/dishes, high chair, etc.).
    - Feed in a quiet room with minimal distractions.
    - Maintain a calm, unhurried approach during feeding.
    - Smile and give frequent child eye contact.
    - Use simple directions, encouragement, and praise.
    - Assess and work with the infant's sucking and swallowing rhythm.
    - Introduce new foods and textures gradually.
    - Do not force feed, scold or punish the child for not eating.
    - Limit feeding to 30 minutes or less.
- Monitor intake, output and weight.
- Administer nasogastric, nasojejunal, or gastrostomy feedings as needed.

Pharmacology

- Multivitamin
- Iron supplement
- Caloric supplements (Polycose, medium chain triglycerides [MCT], avocado, margarine)

Complications

- Malnutrition
- Dehydration

- Fluid and electrolyte imbalances
- Developmental delays
- Language delays
- Learning disabilities
- Social behavioral problems
- Vitamin deficiencies
- Anemia

Critical Thinking Exercise: Nursing Management of the Child with Failure to Thrive

Situation: The nurse is caring for the four children described below. Which child CURRENTLY has failure to thrive? Identify the characteristics in each child are associated with failure to thrive.

1. A 6-week-old with a 4-day history of watery diarrhea and vomiting associated with acute gastroenteritis. The infant's admission weight was 5 kg. This was 0.5 kg less than what he weighed in the pediatrician's office 3 days prior. On admission, the infant had a weak cry, dry lips, sunken fontanel, and an increased heart rate. After fluid replacement, the infant's weight increased to 5.4 kg.

    Current failure to thrive? _____ Yes _____ No

    Characteristics associated with failure to thrive:

2. A 3-month-old with gastroesophageal reflux. The child's mother tells the nurse that the amount of "spit-ups" after feeding has decreased since she began giving antireflux medicine (metoclopramide) before the feeds. The infant's pattern of weight gain has improved since the medication was initiated. The infant's growth chart measurements are within normal limits.

    Current failure to thrive? _____ Yes _____ No

    Characteristics associated with failure to thrive:

3. A 9-month-old infant with a congenital heart defect who has been hospitalized several times since birth. Her height and weight are below normal for her age. She is admitted with respiratory difficulty and upper airway congestion. The nurse assesses the following: thin extremities, sparse hair, poor head control, upper airway congestion, dry cough, pale skin, and irritability. The mother asks for a bottle to feed the baby. During feeding, the nurse notes that the baby initially sucks eagerly but

quickly becomes tachypneic, sweaty, and irritable during the feeding. The mother tells the nurse that this is how the baby usually acts during feeding.

Current failure to thrive? _____ Yes _____ No

Characteristics associated with failure to thrive:

4. A 15-month-old with a history of prematurity. He was hospitalized for one month after birth for respiratory distress and feeding intolerance. He is currently seen in the clinic for a well baby exam and immunization. His mother reports that her son is a "picky eater" like his other siblings. She tells the nurse that he eats best when he is in his high chair and he can eat using his fingers. The child is alert, active and appears well nourished with fat folds noted on arms and legs.

Current failure to thrive? _____ Yes _____ No

Characteristics associated with failure to thrive:

Developmental or Psychosocial Disorders CHAPTER 69

Nursing Management of the Child with Anorexia Nervosa

> **Key Points**
>
> - The incidence of anorexia nervosa (AN) and other eating disorders are increasing in the United States, particularly among adolescent females.
> - Anorexia nervosa (AN) is characterized by altered body image, behaviors aimed at causing significant weight loss (extreme dietary restriction, obsessive exercise, and/or purging), morbid fear of being fat and amenorrhea in post-menarchal females.
> - The precise causes of anorexia nervosa (AN) are unknown. It is commonly believed that it is a psychological disorder leading to altered perception of body image, extreme fear of being fat and/or desire to delay puberty.
> - Anorexia nervosa (AN) can lead to a wide range of physiological consequences (cardiovascular, neurological).
> - Goals of collaborative management:
>   - Identify disorder and initiating treatment.
>   - Correct the fluid and electrolyte imbalances.
>   - Correct nutritional deficiencies and establish a pattern of weight gain.
>   - Restore optimal body weight and composition.
>   - Educate the child and family regarding proper nutrition and exercise moderation.
>   - Provide ongoing support.
>   - Prevent complications (vitamin deficiency, anemia, stress ulceration, cardiovascular complication, and developmental delay).
> - Important nursing diagnoses (actual or potential) are:
>   - Altered nutrition: Less than body requirements
>   - Altered growth and development
>   - Fluid volume deficit
>   - Risk for injury
>   - Impaired social interaction
>   - Altered family processes
>   - Noncompliance with treatment plan
>   - Risk for self-harm
>   - Altered sexuality pattern
> - **Key Terms/Concepts:** Self-esteem, body image disturbance, malnutrition, caloric requirements, failure to thrive, purging behavior

Nursing Management of the Child with Anorexia Nervosa

Overview

Anorexia nervosa (AN) is an eating disorder primarily occurring in adolescent and young adult females. There is a major body image disturbance, which is manifested by starvation. These clients also have an intense fear of obesity. The weight loss is brought about by: less-than-body requirement of food intake, intense and excessive exercise, and purging through use of laxatives or induced vomiting. The result is weight loss or failure to gain expected weight for growth (<85%). This illness can be, and too often is, life-threatening. AN has been linked with altered family processes, a desire to delay puberty, and other psychological disorders in some individuals. The onset of AN generally occurs around the time of menarche and may be triggered by an adolescent crisis (for example: sexual abuse, parental divorce, and onset of menstruation). The exact etiology of eating disorders remains unclear.

Anorexia nervosa is closely related to bulimia nervosa (an eating disorder characterized by binge eating followed by purging [self-induced vomiting]). Lack of dietary intake can result in severe changes in the body's nutritional status and fluid/electrolyte balance. AN can lead to delayed puberty, impaired growth, hematological, cardiovascular, neurological and renal complications and death.

Bulimia nervosa is also an eating disorder thought to have psychological roots. Bulimia is characterized by binge eating (up to 5000 calories at a sitting) followed by guilt and fear of weight gain, which is alleviated by purging. Purging may be through self-induced vomiting, use of laxatives, and sometimes through intense, excessive exercise and/or use of diuretics. These clients likely have trouble expressing feelings and tend to be impulsive. Although weight fluctuations can be great in a very short period of time these clients generally remain at a near-normal weight. Therefore the disease of bulimia is often unknown to those close to the client. Complications of the disease may include: hypochloremic alkalosis, dizziness, syncope, dehydration, electrolyte imbalances, dental caries and discoloration of the teeth, hemorrhoids and rectal bleeding.

Risk Factors

- Adolescent female, middle-to-upper class family
- Chronic depression
- Body image disturbance
- Genetic or physiological predisposition
- Sociocultural influences
- Impaired physiological development
- Dysfunctional family
- Sexual abuse

Signs and Symptoms

Physical

- Gradual or sudden weight loss
- Emaciated appearance, weight less than 85% for height/age
- Amenorrhea

- Dry skin with a yellowish discoloration
- Brittle nails
- Dental caries (from acid in emesis)
- Lanugo over back and extremities
- Cold intolerance
- Abdominal pain
- Constipation
- Low blood pressure, pulse, and temperature
- Frequent trips to the bathroom (purging, laxatives, etc.)
- Wearing baggy, layered clothes to hide weight loss

Emotional/Behavioral
- Low self-esteem
- Obsessive behaviors
- Chronic depression
- Emotionally distant or restrained
- Decreased socialization with peers
- Low frustration tolerance
- Poor impulse control
- Repetitive, strenuous exercise
- Preoccupation with food and/or eating
- Change in eating behaviors
- Use of laxatives and/or emetic agents
- Ritualistic behaviors, particularly around issues of food

Diagnostic Tests and Labs

- History and physical
- Height and weight
- Electrolytes (electrolyte imbalances, hypoglycemia)
- CBC (anemia)
- Growth hormone levels: increased
- Plasma cortisol levels: increased
- Thyroid hormones: T3 low, T4 low normal, TSH normal

Therapeutic Nursing Management

- Correct fluid and electrolyte imbalances. Administer intravenous fluids as needed.
- Collaborate with psychology, psychiatry, and social services to address emotional and social issues.
- Collaborate with nutritional services to determine nutrient needs.
- Administer nasogastric (NG) and/or total parenteral nutrition (TPN) feedings as indicated.

- Observe eating patterns and monitor caloric intake.
- Monitor weight at regular intervals. Stabilize weight.
- Assess self-esteem.

Pharmacology

- Multivitamins
- Antianxiety medications and/or antidepressants
- Prokinetic agents during early refeeding

Complications

- Bone: Osteoporosis, fractures
- Cardiovascular: Bradycardia, hypotension, dysrhythmias, mitral valve prolapse, cardiac structure changes, congestive heart failure (during refeeding)
- Central nervous system: Nonspecific EEG changes, cerebral structural changes
- Renal: Hypokalemia, hyponatremia, hypochloremia, alkalosis edema, renal calculi
- Gastrointestinal: Constipation, abdominal distention, dental caries
- GU: Amenorrhea, delayed puberty
- Endocrine: Low T4 and T3 levels
- Hematological: Anemia, bleeding
- Death

Critical Thinking Exercise: Nursing Management of the Child with Anorexia Nervosa

Complete the following statements related to anorexia nervosa:

Altered nutritional status is related to

Fluid volume deficit is related to

Decreased cardiac output is related to

Decreased activity tolerance and fatigue is related to

Bowel incontinence and diarrhea is related to

Constipation is related to

Risk for infection is related to

Skin breakdown and poor healing is related to

Confusion and memory loss is related to

Loneliness is related to

Altered growth and development is related to

Noncompliance with the treatment plan is related to

Powerlessness and hopelessness are related to

Risk for self-harm is related to

Knowledge deficit is related to

Developmental or Psychosocial Disorders CHAPTER 70

Nursing Management of the Child with Adolescent Pregnancy

> **Key Points**
>
> - The incidence of adolescent pregnancy has increased dramatically in the past several decades.
> - Prevention of adolescent pregnancy is best accomplished by providing accurate and realistic information about pregnancy and parenthood, access to birth control and a safe environment for questions and discussion.
> - Education, guidance, and instructions should be appropriate to the age, maturity level, and knowledge base of the client.
> - Goals of collaborative management:
>   - Prevent the unplanned pregnancy.
>   - Provide prenatal care and education to pregnant females.
>   - Support infants born to adolescent parents.
> - Important nursing diagnoses (actual or potential) are:
>   - Self-concept disturbance
>   - Self esteem disturbance
>   - Body image disturbance
>   - Anxiety and fear
>   - Altered health maintenance
>   - Impaired social interaction
>   - Caregiver role strain
>   - Ineffective family coping
>   - Altered family processes
>   - Knowledge deficit
> - **Key Terms/Concepts**: Pregnancy, prevention, contraception, prematurity, and parenting skills

Overview

Many adolescents are socially, educationally, emotionally, and economically unprepared for the realities of pregnancy and parenthood. The normal developmental progression of the adolescent is abruptly changed. For most adolescents, pregnancy marks the end of their own childhood. The risk of complications of pregnancy (pregnancy-induced hypertension, infection, and gestational diabetes) and neonatal problems (prematurity, sepsis, low birth weight, and intrauterine drug exposure) are increased due to lack of sporadic prenatal care, poor nutrition, and lifestyle choices.

Risk Factors

- Adolescent sexual activity
- High risk behavior (alcohol and drug use)
- Lack of contraceptives
- Lack of knowledge regarding contraception
- Dysfunctional home life

Signs and Symptoms

- Refer to OB review module or OB textbook for signs and symptoms.

Nutrition

Nutritional needs in adolescent pregnancy are often different from adult women. Many adolescents are experiencing rapid growth and the pregnancy increases the nutritional needs. The needs depend on the gynecological age of the adolescent (the number of years between the age in years and the age at menarche). If the gynecological age is less than 2 years the pregnant teen will compete with the requirements of the fetus to meet her own nutritional needs. Because the adolescent diet is often high in salt, sugar, and fatty foods while low in protein, vitamins, and minerals, the nurse must make dietary counseling a priority with pregnant teens to ensure the health of both the teen and the fetus. The nurse should set weight gain goals with the pregnant adolescent at the first prenatal visit, if possible. It is imperative to explain why gaining weight is important during pregnancy. Nutritional counseling should continue into the postpartum period to ensure good nutrition of the parent(s) and child.

Therapeutic Nursing Management

- Extensive teaching should include:
    - Diet: good nutrition is a major concern
    - Prenatal iron and folic acid especially important
    - Physiological and psychological changes of pregnancy
    - Parenting skills
    - Preparation for labor and delivery
    - Newborn care
- Discuss plans for birth decisions and plans for the baby.
- Assess the amount of the father's participation.
- Assess for complications during pregnancy.

Complications

- Pregnancy-induced hypertension, diabetes, anemia, hemorrhoids
- Preterm labor
- Low birth weight infant
- Postpartum hemorrhage
- Altered parent-infant bonding and attachment

- Interruption of normal adolescent development
- Ineffective coping
- Altered family processes
- Altered parenting, child neglect and/or abuse
- Poverty

Critical Thinking Exercise: Nursing Management of the Child with Adolescent Pregnancy

Fill in the blank

1. Adolescents experience the feelings of sexual desire due to _____ development and _____ changes.

2. Adolescents often engage in risk taking behaviors due to a belief that "it _____ happen to _____."

3. Adolescents have a tendency to experiment with new experiences without considering the _____ .

4. Many adolescents engage in sexual activity due to _____ _____ and/or a desire to be _____ .

5. The use of _____ and _____ by teens increases the likelihood of pregnancy and sexually transmitted disease due to suppressed inhibition.

6. Some adolescent females chose to get pregnant because they want to have someone to _____ .

Identify which of the following intervention strategies are recommended to help prevent adolescent pregnancy:

a. Provide accurate and realistic information about sexual activity and birth control.
b. Dispel myths related to contraceptive methods and getting pregnant.
c. Discuss the physiological changes associated with pregnancy.
d. Forbid the adolescent from spending time alone with his or her peers.
e. Discuss the realities of parenthood in terms that are meaningful to adolescents. Describe how caring for a newborn infant will affect their social activities, educational goals and economic situation.
f. Have young teens continuously care for an egg or other fragile object to simulate the constant commitment needed to care for an infant.

g. Have teens attend a support group for young parents or invite a teen parent to come to school to discuss their situation with their peers.
h. Do not allow the adolescent to leave the house at night or on weekends.
i. Provide a safe, open environment for teens to ask questions and discuss their thoughts.
j. Reinforce the adolescent's personal, family, and/or spiritual values related to the value of abstinence.
k. Tell the adolescent that they will be severely punished if they have sex before marriage.

Critical Thinking Exercise Answer Keys

Critical Thinking Exercise: CHAPTER 1
Child's Vital Signs Answer Key

Based on the following information received during report, identify which of the vital signs for each child are abnormal (increased, decreased) or normal. This should be based on the normal vital signs for the child's age and the child's illness.

1. 4-year-old with asthma. The vital signs are: HR 128-135, RR 30-35, BP 93/48, and axillary temperature 98° Fahrenheit (F).

    - Slightly increased heart rate
    - Normal blood pressure and temperature

    These vital signs in an acutely ill child could become worse in a child with asthma. The nurse should pay particular attention to the respiratory rate and heart rate in this client.

2. 7-year-old with gastroesophageal reflux who is bundled with 2 thick blankets. The vital signs are: HR 100-110, RR 20-30, BP 96/54, axillary temperature 99.8° F.

    - Normal respiratory rate, heart rate and blood pressure
    - Slightly increased temperature

    The child's increased temperature may be due to overbundling of covers or from an infection. The nurse should remove excess bedding and reassess the temperature to determine if the temperature is increasing or decreasing.

3. 8-month-old with pneumonia. The vital signs are: HR 160-180 dropping to 60's occasionally during the previous shift, RR 76, BP 112/72, axillary temperature 99.5° F.

    - Increased respiratory rate
    - Increased heart rate with periods of bradycardia
    - Increased blood pressure
    - Slightly increased temperature

The child's tachycardia with periods of bradycardia (heart rate dropping into the 60's) is a dangerous sign that the child is unstable. The child's increased respiratory rate is also concerning, particularly because she has pneumonia. The increased blood pressure is another possible sign that she is in distress. The increased temperature is also of concern, but is a lesser priority to the other abnormal vital signs. This child requires immediate attention and intervention to prevent a possible cardiopulmonary arrest.

4. 2-month-old with fever and otitis media. The vital signs are: HR 165-175, RR 32-40, BP 108/64, rectal temperature 102.5° F. (Taken immediately prior to report, no intervention initiated.)

- Increased temperature
- Increased heart rate
- Increased blood pressure

A young infant with a fever and high heart rate could rapidly deteriorate. The high heart rate is most likely related to the fever. Cooling measures and administration of antipyretics are the usual interventions for increased temperature.

Critical Thinking Exercise: CHAPTER 2
Child with Pain Answer Key

Describe the "Reality" and why the "Myth" is false in each of the following statements:

"Myth"	"Reality"
Infants don't feel pain because they have immature neurologic systems.	Infants and children have demonstrated physiological, behavioral, and hormonal responses to pain. The effects of pain experienced by infants and young children may last into adulthood.
A child who is sleeping or lying quietly is not in pain.	Children who are in pain may deny that they are feeling pain. Sleep and/or lack of movement do not mean the child is not in pain. Children may avoid movement because they are afraid that movement will hurt.
Nurses and doctors are the best people to judge how much pain a child is feeling.	The child is the best authority on pain level. The parents of infants and young children are the experts about their child's normal reactions. They can often detect subtle signs of pain.
Children lack the ability to talk about their pain.	Children as young as 3 years old can rank their pain level using an age appropriate rating scale. Older children can point to the place on their body or a diagram where they feel pain. Children may use other words to indicate pain such as "boo-boo," "owe," or "hurt."
Infants and young children shouldn't be given narcotics because of the side effects.	Infants with moderate and severe pain may need narcotics for pain control. Respiratory depression and hypotension can be prevented with proper dosing and monitoring.
Children who receive narcotics for pain are at risk for addiction.	Addiction to pain medication in children is extremely rare.

Nursing Care of Children

Critical Thinking Exercise: CHAPTER 3
Child's Hospitalization and Illness Answer Key

Identify interventions and rationales for each of the following children.

Child	Interventions	Rationale For Intervention
A 7-month-old female with a congenital heart defect is hospitalized for congestive heart failure. She has been irritable and difficult to console.	• Assess if irritability is related to disease process. • Facilitate family presence at bedside whenever possible. • Provide consistent nursing staff. • Arrange to have a volunteer hold and rock the baby. • Place the baby in a room near the central station.	The irritability may be related to hypoxia or other problems related to the CHF. Once this is ruled out, address the infant's basic needs (trust vs. mistrust). Crying without comforting and/or lack of stimulation may lead to distress. Providing caregivers who address the comfort and care needs is important for infants. Room placement near the central station may help reduce response time to crying.
A 14-month-old male who is hospitalized with acute gastroenteritis and dehydration has not slept more than one hour without awakening.	• Address pain management needs. • Promote home routine related to bedtime (brushing teeth, book, etc.). • Provide a quiet, darkened room. • Allow parent to lie in bed or crib next to the toddler. • Post "do not disturb" sign outside the room during designated nap/ sleep times.	This toddler's difficulty may be related to the change in routine caused by the hospitalization. Distress can be heightened when a child has no prior experience with hospitalization. Maintaining home rituals can help normalize the bedtime routine. Providing parental comfort can help minimize the toddler's distress. Protecting the toddler's sleep during nap times and recognizing signs of discomfort can also help promote adequate

Child's Hospitalization and Illness Answer Key

Child	Interventions	Rationale For Intervention
A 4-year-old hospitalized male with acute appendicitis repeatedly wakes up crying after having nightmares.	• Address pain management needs. • Explain procedures honestly using concrete terms. • Promote expression of feelings using medical play (collaborate with Child Life as available). • Encourage family member to spend the night at the bedside. • Leave a small light on at night.	Explaining procedures in terms the child can understand can help allay fears. A preschool-age child's tendency for fantasy and magical thinking may be heightened when the pain and trauma of appendicitis and surgical intervention is experienced. Medical play can help the child express and work through fears. A light in the room can help prevent fantasies and fears related to darkness.
An 8-year-old hospitalized female with asthma has eaten very little from her meal trays in the last few days.	• Talk to the child about the reason for her lack of eating. • Provide the child's favorite foods (allow food from home as possible). • Create a game in which the child can earn a reward or points for eating. Involves eating food the toddler normally eats at home.	The refusal to eat may be related to a lack of appetite due to the medical condition. It may also be a reaction to hospitalization or dislike of the foods provided. Offering favorite foods and asking the child about why she is not eating may help determine the cause of the anorexia. A game that rewards eating can help serve as a motivation, help achieve a sense of accomplishment and control (developmental tasks for this age).
A 15-year-old female with leukemia expresses a desire to be left alone in a darkened room.	• Establish a rapport with the teen. • Ask her to discuss her feelings. • Provide a phone at the bedside. • Encourage her friends to visit. • Encourage use of a journal. • Collaborate with Psychology.	Adolescents with chronic illness may become depressed due to their separation from peers, altered body image, lack of self-esteem, and feeling "different." Connecting adolescents with peers and encouraging expression of feelings may assist them with coping.

Critical Thinking Exercise: CHAPTER 4

Death and Dying Involving a Child Answer Key

Situation: The parents of a 15-year-old boy who has died suddenly from an injury sustained in a motor vehicle accident asks the nurse how to best explain what happened to his 6-year-old brother. The father told the nurse that his 6-year-old son believes that he caused his brother's death because they had a fight that morning.

1. What is the best way to explain the death to the 6-year-old?

    Help the child to understand that the death is not his fault. Feeling guilty or responsible for the accident and death is a common reaction of children of this age group. Explain the events in concrete terms. Reinforce his understanding that death is permanent. Give permission for the child to grieve in his own way.

2. What grief reactions should the nurse anticipate when caring for this family? What interventions are most appropriate when caring for a family after the death of their child?

    Each family member will have his or her own way of dealing with the tragedy. Immediately after a sudden death, families express shock and disbelief. Some may want to talk, while some may want to be left alone. The family members may express a range of emotions from hostility and anger to depression and sadness. It is important that the nurse maintain a nonjudgmental and supportive approach while helping each member express their grief in their own way. Nurses should make every effort to provide a private environment with flexible visitation to accommodate the family's needs. It is also important to allow the family members time hold or sit next to their child's body if they want to do this. The nurse should collect all belongings for the family. Offering spiritual care and other resources to assist the family with their grief is also important.

Situation: The parents of a 3-year-old with cancer have just been informed that their child's condition is terminal due to extensive metastasis.

3. The parents ask the nurse what a child of this age understands about death. What is the nurse's best response?

   Most preschool-age children believe death happens to other people. They often are very curious about death and may ask many questions about the subject. Their tendency for magical thinking and imagination may lead to misconceptions and fears related to pain and mutilation. Children of this age do not understand that death is permanent. For example, the child may ask if a grandparent who has died will be coming to visit on their birthday.

4. What are the appropriate interventions for this child?

   Address comfort needs of the child. Provide pain relief measures as indicated. Encourage the parents to maintain as normal an environment as possible. Provide play activities that are best suited for the child's interests and physical abilities. Allow flexible visitation for parents, siblings and other family members whenever possible. Encourage a family member to spend the night with the child. Support family members with their grief with therapeutic communication. Provide information to family members regarding available resources to help deal with the loss of their child.

Critical Thinking Exercise: CHAPTER 5

Child's Nutrition Answer Key

Select the appropriate response for the following case study. Explain the rationale for your response.

1. The mother of a 2-year-old is concerned because her son has not been eating well during mealtimes at home. What is the nurse's best response?
   a. "You need to give him a daily multivitamin to help increase his appetite."
   b. "It is common for toddlers to eat less. Try giving him small meals and snacks."
   c. "It is best for children to eat three meals a day. Limit snacks to increase his appetite."
   d. "If you give him more milk and juice, it will make up for his lack of eating at meals."

   Correct answer: **b**

   Rationale: It is common for toddlers to develop picky eating habits. "Food jags" are common with this age group. Giving the toddler manageable portions at mealtimes and nutritious snacks throughout the day helps meet the child's nutrition needs while avoiding mealtime battles. Giving a toddler more milk and juice can lead to nutritional deficits related to an unbalanced diet. Giving a multivitamin will not increase a child's appetite but may help meet the nutritional needs. Families should discuss the need for supplemental vitamins with their healthcare provider.

2. The mother of a 13-month-old asks the nurse what finger foods are best. Which of the following is the best answer?
   a. A celery stick
   b. A hot dog
   c. Grapes
   d. Dry cereal

   Correct answer: **d**

   Rationale: Older infants and toddlers enjoy self-feeding using their hands. At 13 months of age, a toddler is able to pick up small pieces of cereal without assistance. This is the best choice for a toddler. Carrot sticks, hot dog slices, and large fruit pieces could cause choking because of their size and hardness. It is important to chop fruit and pieces of meat into very small pieces to prevent a choking hazard. Many parents find it convenient to keep a small bag of cereal in the diaper bag when away from home.

3. Matching: Match the age normally associated with development of each eating behavior listed.

i	6-year-old	a. Eats larger pieces of table food
a	3-year-old	b. Uses strong sucking reflex
f	7-month-old	c. Controls diet to lose weight
h	5-month-old	d. Enjoys cooking simple recipes
e	13-month-old	e. Eats chopped table food
j	6-month-old	f. Begins self-feeding
c	15-year-old	g. Uses a fork and spoon with ease
g	4-year-old	h. Begins taste preferences
d	9-year-old	i. Eats breakfast to help with attention at school
b	3-week-old	j. Begins eating rice cereal

Critical Thinking Exercise: CHAPTER 6
Child's Medications Answer Key

Situation: Identify the correct order for each of the steps for administering a PRN dose of oral acetaminophen to a 9-month-old child. Explain the rationale for each step.

Step	Order	Rationale for Step
Invite the father to assist and/or give suggestions for techniques.	9	Families who are accustomed to administering medication at home often have good suggestions for how their child best takes medications. Involving the father in administration validates his role as caretaker, supports the infant's emotional needs, and may increase the likelihood of successful medication administration.
Wash hands.	5	This step is needed to prevent inadvertent infection.
Educate the infant's father at the bedside regarding the need for the medication.	8	Family teaching is an important part of medication administration.
Calculate correct dosage.	3	This step ensures that the amount of medication is appropriate for the child based on weight.
Prepare a bottle of juice.	7	It is recommended to having a "chaser" ready for the infant to drink immediately after the medication.
Calculate amount to be drawn up from the bottle of acetaminophen.	4	This step is needed to ensure the appropriate amount of medication is given based on the available medication concentration. This step should be done after the appropriate dosage has been verified. The liquid format was selected based on the infant's age.
Draw up the acetaminophen from the bottle using a syringe.	6	A syringe is the best way to accurately measure the medication. It is also the easiest way to administer a liquid medication to a 9-month-old infant.
Offer the infant a sip of juice from a bottle.	11	The juice helps rinse the medication taste from the mouth. Sucking on a bottle often acts as a way to soothe and calm the infant.
Verify medication order.	2	This step is needed to ensure the appropriate medication will be administered.
Document the medication administration and response on the medical record.	12	Documentation should be done after the medication is administered. If a medication is given PRN, the child's response based on premedication assessment should be noted.

Child's Medications Answer Key

Step	Order	Rationale for Step
Identify the need for the PRN medication based on the order.	1	Identification of the child's condition that warrants the medication is the first step in administering a PRN medication. Acetaminophen is frequently ordered PRN for fever or comfort.
Squirt the medication into the back of the infant's mouth between the teeth and gums.	10	This allows the infant to swallow the medication and decreases the likelihood of spitting or coughing up the medication.

Critical Thinking Exercise: CHAPTER 7

Child's Growth and Development Answer Key

Situation: A 16-month-old is admitted to a pediatric unit for observation after removal of a small toy that she aspirated earlier that day. Select the appropriate response and explain why this is the best answer.

1. When assessing the child for the first time, what is the best approach to initiate contact?
    a. Call the child by name before picking her up.
    b. Reassure the child that you are not going to hurt her.
    c. Smile and get the child to talk by asking her to tell you her name.
    d. Talk softly to the child at her eye level while she is in her mother's arms.

   Correct answer: **d**

   Rationale: **The best way to approach a frightened toddler is to allow her to remain in a parent's arms while gently and slowly approaching her at eye level. Verbal reassurance and conversation is less effective in this age group.**

2. Which of the following is a priority teaching need for a family with a 16-month-old child?
    a. Toilet training guidelines
    b. Instructions for preschool readiness
    c. Information on home safety assessment
    d. Guidelines for weaning toddlers from bottles

   Correct answer: **c**

   Rationale: **The teaching priority for any child admitted for accidental injury is safety and injury prevention. Home safety assessment is one of the most important safety teaching topics for active toddlers. The other topics listed above are more appropriate for a slightly older child.**

Child's Growth and Development Answer Key

3. Matching: Match the age normally associated with the developmental task listed.

d	3-year-old	a. Fears body mutilation
a	4-year-old	b. Develops social smile
i	11-year-old	c. Anterior fontanel closes
b	5-month-old	d. Vocabulary of 850 words
h	9-year-old	e. Reads and writes
g	13-year-old	f. Begins picking up objects with fingers
f	8-month-old	g. Menarche begins
e	7-year-old	h. Begins to excel in sports
j	20-month-old	i. Pubic hair develops
c	13-month-old	j. Scribbles drawings

Critical Thinking Exercise: CHAPTER 8

Child with Oxygen Therapy Answer Key

Situation: A 13-month-old with bronchiolitis is receiving 1 L of oxygen via a nasal cannula. The nurse responds to an alarm of the pulse oximeter. Upon arrival at the room, the nurse notes that the pulse oximeter is reading 75%. The nurse also notes that the child is crying and kicking his legs. The pulse oximeter probe on the right foot has loosened. The oxygen cannula is lying beside the child in the bed.

1. What should the nurse do first? Why?

    The nurse should immediately assess the child for signs of respiratory distress, level of consciousness and color. The child's kicking could indicate that he is agitated due to hypoxia.

    The nurse should promptly replace the nasal cannula and secure it with tape. Once it is determined that the respiratory status is stable, the pulse oximeter probe should be moved to another extremity and taped securely.

2. After the initial interventions, the child has the following signs: cyanosis, oxygen saturation level of 86%, moderate retractions, and cough. What actions should be taken next?

    The amount of oxygen should be immediately increased. The nurse should determine possible causes of respiratory distress and take the appropriate measures to address them. The child should be positioned with the head of bed upright in the "sniffing position." Suctioning should be initiated if the child is struggling with his secretions. The nurse should closely monitor for signs of improvement. If the respiratory distress continues, the nurse should request additional assistance because this child is at a high risk for rapid deterioration.

3. If this child does not improve, what alternative oxygen delivery devices may be needed? What are the challenges of using these devices with toddlers?

    If the child's clinical condition does not improve with airway management techniques and increasing oxygen level via nasal cannula, alternatives should be considered. This is a challenge with toddlers because they are too big for oxygen delivery in an incubator or oxygen hoods. As a general rule, toddlers do not tolerate oxygen masks. An agitated toddler may also actively resist being put into a mist tent. Having a parent hold his/her child and provide "blow-by oxygen" may be the least threatening way to administer oxygen to a frightened and agitated toddler. Once the child calms, his respiratory status may improve because his oxygen needs have decreased. If the child's condition continues to deteriorate, especially if he has a decreased level of consciousness, he will need immediate intervention to prevent a respiratory arrest. At this time, the child may need to be intubated and mechanically ventilated to support his breathing.

Critical Thinking Exercise: CHAPTER 9
Child with Cystic Fibrosis Answer Key

Situation: A 10-month-old male infant with a neonatal history including meconium plug is admitted with respiratory difficulty, recurrent bronchitis, and poor weight gain. The health care provider suggests a potential diagnosis of cystic fibrosis.

1. What additional history questions should the nurse ask the family?

   Does anyone in your family have CF?
   > CF is an inherited autosomal recessive disorder that is genetically transmitted. Assess for potential CF carriers in the family.

   Does the baby taste salty when you kiss him?
   > Increased sodium and chloride in the sweat may result in a salty taste when parents kiss their baby.

   Will you describe the baby's typical stools?
   > Assess for the characteristic stool pattern for children with CF (large, fatty, foul-smelling; steatorrhea)

   Does the baby have a persistent cough or thick mucous?
   > Thick, tan or yellowish secretions with cough are commonly associated with CF.

   When did you notice that your baby was not gaining weight as expected?
   > CF frequently leads to persistent weight loss or lack of weight gain (failure to thrive) due to malabsorption of nutrients.

2. What are the most important interventions for the infant and family at this time?

   - Address acute respiratory difficulty with oxygen administration, percussion, postural drainage, oxygen, suction, positioning, and antibiotics
   - Address fluid, electrolyte with IV fluids and electrolyte replacement as needed
   - Support family and provide ongoing information
   - Address nutritional needs with enteral nutrition when respiratory status has stabilized
   - Facilitate diagnostic testing for CF
   - Initiate treatment protocol for CF (vitamins, pancreatic enzymes, etc.)

Critical Thinking Exercise: CHAPTER 10

Child with Asthma Answer Key

Situation: A 6-year-old boy is admitted into the emergency department because of dyspnea, coughing, and wheezing. The boy states that he feels tightness in his chest. Physical findings include pallor with tachypnea and tachycardia.

1. Which health information is most important for the nurse to collect from the parents?

   Have these symptoms occurred previously?
   When did these symptoms develop?
   Which symptoms developed first?
   Are there any factors that could have precipitated the attack?
   Describe the home environment including pets, smokers, types of pillows/linen used.
   Describe the type of heating used in the house.
   Does the child have any food, medication, or dust allergies?
   Is the child taking any medications?

Situation: The child is given a bronchodilator and a metered dose inhaler.

2. Assuming that this is the child's first episode of asthma, prioritize the discharge instructions. (1 is most important).

Instruction	Priority
Avoid milk/milk products.	7
Drink large amounts of water.	6
The child should trigger the inhaler as he breathes in.	4
Bronchodilators can cause tachycardia and restlessness.	5
Asthma decreases the size of the airway causing distress.	1
If an attack occurs at home, the child should sit or stand.	3
Attacks of asthma can be prevented by avoiding environmental and emotional triggers.	2

3. Which of the following needs of the child in the case study should be addressed first? Which need should be addressed next?

   a. Difficulty breathing

   Bronchospasm and bronchoconstriction increased mucous secretion and airway edema contribute to the narrowing of air passages and interfere with airflow during an acute asthma attack. This becomes a priority-nursing problem. Unresolved respiratory distress can lead to respiratory failure.

   b. Anxiety

   Respiratory distress and lack of oxygen can lead to agitation and anxiety as the child struggles to breathe.

   c. Risk for potential adverse reaction to medications

   Medications used for asthma have potential side effects. Albuterol can cause hypertension, tachycardia, palpitations, and CNS stimulation. Steroids can cause hypertension, gastrointestinal upset, immunosuppression, and endocrine complications.

Critical Thinking Exercise: CHAPTER 11
Child with Tonsillitis and Tonsillectomy Answer Key

1. Which of the following children is most likely to receive a tonsillectomy?
    a. 4-year-old with viral adenoiditis with nasal speech
    b. 2-year-old with bronchopulmonary dysplasia and gastroesophageal reflux
    c. 5-year-old with obstructive sleep apnea and frequent sore throats
    d. 1-year-old with recurrent otitis media and bronchiolitis
   Correct answer: c **A 5-year-old with obstructive sleep apnea and frequent sore throats**

2. List three indications for tonsillectomy in children.
    Repeated tonsillitis
    Airway obstruction and/or sleep apnea due to enlarged tonsils
    Chronic feeding difficulty due to inability to swallow from enlarged tonsils

3. Identify each of the following nursing intervention as Appropriate or Not Appropriate when caring postoperatively for a child who has just tonsillectomy and explain your responses.

    Appropriate Placing in a side-lying position **assists with keeping the airway patent if the child has difficulty swallowing or if there is bleeding from the incision site.**

    Not Appropriate Suctioning of the oropharynx routinely **is not recommended because it can cause trauma to the incision site.**

    Not Appropriate Providing bright colored red Jell-O **Red-colored fluids and foods are not recommended because it can look like fresh blood.**

    Not Appropriate Providing warm milk and cookies **Milk is not routinely recommended because it may lead to throat clearing and trauma to the incision. Cookies are generally too hard to be considered part of the soft diet recommended**

    Appropriate Administer pain medication **as needed to address the child's postoperative pain**

4. Identify the earliest sign of hemorrhage in a child who has had a tonsillectomy.
    a. Labored breathing and increased respiratory rate
    b. Decreased heart rate

c. Frequent throat clearing with restlessness
d. Dark brown emesis
e. Pallor

Correct answer: c   **Frequent throat clearing with restlessness**

Rationale: **The earliest signs of hemorrhage after tonsillectomy may be subtle. Look for frequent swallowing, throat clearing, and/or restlessness. Increased heart rate and breathing pattern changes would follow the initial signs. Late signs include pallor (due to blood loss) and bradycardia (due to poor airway control). Brown emesis indicates the blood is old. Bright red color with emesis is associated with fresh bleeding.**

Critical Thinking Exercise: CHAPTER 12
Common Respiratory Illnesses in Children Answer Key

Situation: A pediatric nurse is working at a community walk-in clinic. It is one of the most common months for respiratory infections and the nurse assesses a variety of respiratory conditions.

1. Match the symptoms on the left with the illness on the right.

f	Hoarseness of the voice with no associated symptoms	a.	Allergic Rhinitis
g	Exudates in the throat, headache, fever, painful swallowing	b.	Epiglottis
d	Body aches and chills, nasal discharge and inflammation, cough	c.	Anaphylaxis
e	Tonsillar edema and inflammation, difficulty swallowing	d.	Common Cold
b	High fever, protrusive tongue, drooling	e.	Tonsillitis
a	Watery eyes and nose, headache, itching of eyes, nose, and pharynx	f.	Laryngitis
c	Hives, itching, swelling of eyes, lips and tongue, respiratory distress	g.	Strep Throat

2. What is the most common cause of bronchiolitis?

   Respiratory Syncytial Virus

3. Who is at greatest risk of severe illness with respiratory syncytial virus (RSV)?

   Young infant

4. What diagnostic test is definitive for RSV?

   Nasal swab for RSV

Nursing Care of Children

Critical Thinking Exercise: CHAPTER 13

Child with Congenital Heart Disease Answer Key

1. Fill in the blanks:

    a. Four common signs of digoxin toxicity include: **anorexia, nausea, vomiting**, and **irregular cardiac rhythm**.

    b. Infants with complex congenital heart defects may have difficulty gaining weight because of **feeding difficulty**.

    c. **Diuretics** are frequently administered to children with complex cardiac defects to prevent fluid retention.

    d. A child who has a high hematocrit related to a congenital heart defect is vulnerable to **clotting (thrombosis, stroke)**.

    e. Chronic cyanosis leads to **clubbing** of the fingers.

2. Match the heart defect with the symptom or description

h	Ventricular septal defect	a.	Opening between the right and left atrium
a	Atrial septal defect	b.	Increased BP in upper extremities
f	Patent ductus arteriosus	c.	Cyanotic episodes called "Tet spells"
g	Pulmonary stenosis	d.	Aorta and pulmonary artery are reversed
e	Aortic stenosis	e.	Decreased blood flow into the aorta
b	Coarctation of the aorta	f.	Usually closes shortly after birth
c	Tetralogy of Fallot	g.	Decreased blood flow to the lungs
d	Transposition of the great vessels	h.	Opening between the right and left ventricle

Critical Thinking Exercise: CHAPTER 14

Child with Hodgkin's Disease Answer Key

Situation: A slender 14-year-old female is newly diagnosed with Hodgkin's disease. Her primary care provider first suspected the disease during a routine exam. The girl denied having any symptoms at the time of diagnosis except for feeling tired and not eating much.

1. What is Hodgkin's disease?

    Hodgkin's disease is a type of cancer that originates in the lymphoid system. It is most often detected when firm lymph nodes are discovered. Hodgkin's disease occurs most often in adolescents and young adults.

2. What symptoms did the primary care provider most likely find during the routine exam that led to the detection of the Hodgkin's disease?

    Symptoms include painless firm lymph nodes in the neck and axillary areas. Since the nodes are painless, they may go unnoticed unless the girl happened to touch the area containing the firm nodes.

    Anorexia and weight loss are evident because the girl is slender and has a history of "not eating much". Since many teenage girls engage in regular dieting to control their weight, this girl's weight loss and poor appetite may not have been recognized as a sign of illness.

    Fatigue is also associated with Hodgkin's disease. The girl's fatigue may have been mistakenly attributed to her lack of adequate nutritional intake and/or a lack of sleep.

3. What diagnostic tests and assessments should be anticipated to determine if there is spread of the disease to other parts of the body?

    History questions (assess for symptoms related to various body systems)
    Assess the neck (assess for additional nodes)
    Auscultation of the lungs (evaluate lung involvement)

Abdominal assessment and palpation (assess for nodes and distention)
CBC (assess WBC count and differential, assess for anemia)
Lymph node biopsy in various nodes (assess for Reed-Sternberg cells)
Chest x-ray (evaluate mediastinal involvement)
CT scan, MRI (evaluate thoracic and/or abdominal involvement)
Bone marrow aspiration (evaluate bone marrow involvement)
Lymphangiography (evaluate retroperitoneal involvement)

# Critical Thinking Exercise: CHAPTER 15
Child with Leukemia Answer Key

1. Which of the following is most frequently associated with the EARLY stages of acute leukemia?
    a. Fever and pallor
    b. Abdominal pain and swelling
    c. Headache with double vision
    d. Painful and frequent urination

    Correct answer: **a Fever and pallor**

    Rationale: **Leukemia often first presents with fever and pallor. Abdominal pain, swelling, headache, and painful urination are not typical symptoms of leukemia.**

2. What is the most common cause of death in children with leukemia?
    a. Hemorrhage
    b. Infection
    c. Metastasis
    d. Drug toxicity

    Correct answer: **b Infection**

    Rationale: **Although children with leukemia are at risk for injury due to bleeding problems and the toxic effect of chemotherapy, the most common cause of death is infection due to immunosuppression (inability to effectively fight infection). Leukemia diagnosed and treated early usually has a good prognosis.**

3. Why are children with leukemia prone to bleeding episodes?

    Children with leukemia have problems with platelet formation.

Nursing Care of Children

4. Which of the following interventions is most appropriate when caring for a child receiving chemotherapy?
   a. Tell the parents that if their child will not have any long-term effects.
   b. Encourage the child to drink orange juice for breakfast.
   c. Monitor rectal temperature every 4 hours.
   d. Administer medication to prevent nausea.

   Correct answer: **d Administer medication to prevent nausea**

   Rationale: **Nausea is a common side effect of chemotherapy. It is best controlled when antiemetic medications are given before the nausea occurs. It is unrealistic to tell the parents that there will not be any long-term effects. Orange juice is not recommended because the acidity can cause irritation to the mouth and throat. Rectal temperatures should not be done in children with cancer.**

5. Which of the following is most appropriate to help 6-year-old girl adjust to her chemotherapy related hair loss?
   a. Wait to discuss the hair loss with the child until it begins to happen
   b. Encourage the girl's parents to help her select a wig or cap to wear
   c. Remove the mirrors from the child's room to prevent her from seeing bald head
   d. Avoid discussing the topic of hair loss because she is too young to understand

   Correct answer: **b Encourage the girl's parents to help her select a wig or cap to wear**

   Rationale: **Wigs and caps are often used to help improve self-esteem that may be lost because of hair loss from chemotherapy. Children should be given information regarding what to expect in terms that they can understand before chemotherapy is initiated. Trying to shield children from seeing themselves in mirrors is not an effective strategy.**

Critical Thinking Exercise: CHAPTER 16

Child with Iron Deficiency Anemia Answer Key

Situation: At a routine clinic visit, the nurse documents the following assessment data for a 22-month-old child: pallor (especially of the mucous membranes), limp muscle tone, restlessness, low energy levels, and a systolic heart murmur. The nurse reviewing the laboratory report notes the hemoglobin is 9.8 g/100 mL and hematocrit is 32%.

1. Place an **X** by the information that should be included in the child's history to support the diagnosis of iron deficiency anemia.

    Amount of milk the child is drinking per day **X**
    Child's food preferences **X**
    Child's eating patterns **X**
    Mother's feelings about the child ____
    Family's socioeconomic status **X**
    Family's living arrangements **X**
    Number of siblings in the household ____
    Does the child eat dirt or paint? **X**
    Percentile ranking of growth and development on a growth chart **X**
    Is the child is up to date with immunizations? ____
    Has the child has been taking prednisone or salicylates? ____

After the primary care provider's assessment, the child is started on a daily dosage of ferrous sulfate.

2. Place an **X** by the instructional information that should be given to the child's mother regarding the administration of the medication and treatment of anemia.

    X Provide juice enriched with vitamin C, which will aid absorption.
    X Give iron supplement via straw to prevent discoloration of teeth.
    X Include iron-rich food in diet: including eggs, cheese, green vegetables, dried apricots.
    X Children over age 6 months should not receive more than 32 ounces of milk per day.
    X Discuss the side effects of the iron supplement: constipation, dark-colored stools, nausea.
    ____ Cost of medication and foods
    X Keep iron supplement in a safe place to avoid accidental overdose.
    X Provide nutritious snacks and finger foods that reflect the child's developmental stage.

Child with Iron Deficiency Anemia Answer Key

X   Signs and symptoms of anemia
X   Iron stores return to normal after 4-6 weeks of treatment.
X   The importance of returning for follow-up lab work

Critical Thinking Exercise: CHAPTER 17
Child with Hemophilia Answer Key

Situation: A mother brings her 13-month-old son to the emergency department with a small laceration on his forehead from a fall against the edge of a coffee table. The mother sought treatment when she was unable to stop the bleeding. The mother tells the nurse that she noticed that her son seemed to bruise easily and had bleeding with teething. She stated that she didn't think that her son could have hemophilia because no one on his father's side of the family has this disease. She had heard it was a genetic disorder in males.

1. What part of this history is consistent with a diagnosis of hemophilia?
    Bleeding during teething
    Bruising easily
    Uncontrolled bleeding with small laceration

2. What part of the mother's understanding of hemophilia is incorrect?
    It is an inherited disorder from the maternal side (X-linked recessive).
    Females are the carriers.

3. What laboratory studies should the nurse anticipate?
    CBC
    Platelet count
    Prothrombin time (PT)
    Partial thromboplastin time (PTT)
    Bleeding time
    Fibrinogen
    Thrombin clotting time

4. Why do children with hemophilia have problems with bleeding?

> Children with hemophilia have a deficiency of clotting factors (most commonly Factor VIII and/or Factor IX). These are essential components of the clotting cascade. Therapy for children with hemophilia includes factor replacement.

5. What family teaching should be done with this mother?

> Protect the child from harm by removing or padding sharp edges.
>
> Have the child play on grass or other soft surfaces whenever possible.
>
> Use a soft toothbrush to avoid dental caries.
>
> Do not give aspirin or aspirin-containing products.
>
> Use ice packs for painful joints if needed.

Critical Thinking Exercise: CHAPTER 18

Child with Sickle Cell Disease Answer Key

Situation: A 5-year-old African American female is admitted with complaints of pain in her arms and legs. She has a three-day history of upper respiratory infection with fever, vomiting and decreased oral intake. The nurse caring for the child makes the following assessments: heart rate 136 beats/minute, respiratory rate 30 breaths/minute, blood pressure 90/85 mmHg, temperature 101.3° F, dusky mucous membranes, cough, delayed capillary refill and no tears.

1. What are the most important interventions for this child at this time?

    Administer oxygen.

    Provide IV hydration.

    Manage pain.

    The best approach to caring for acutely ill children is to do an ABC (airway, breathing, circulation) prioritization. Oxygen is needed because of the child's tachycardia, tachypnea, cough, and dusky mucous membranes. Circulatory support with IV hydration is needed because of the child's sickle cell disease. It is also needed because of her 3- day history of vomiting with decreased oral intake, tachycardia, decreased urine output, and dry lips. Pain management is also an important aspect of managing sickle cell crisis. This child was admitted with complaints of pain.

2. What laboratory data is important for this child?

    Oxygen saturation: to assess the adequacy of oxygenation

    Complete blood cell count: to assess the RBC, hematocrit, and hemoglobin. To assess the white blood cell count and differential for signs of infection

    Sputum culture: to assess for respiratory infection

    Chest x-ray: to assess for signs of pulmonary infection and acute chest syndrome

    Electrolyte panel: to assess for electrolyte imbalance related to vomiting and dehydration

3. What family teaching is appropriate for this child and family?

    Seek prompt medical attention with the first sign of infection.

    Identify the signs of hypoxia, dehydration, and sickle cell crisis.

    Identify and avoid the potential causes of dehydration: fluid loss, decreased intake, fever, heat exposure, or overexertion.

    Provide adequate hydration and fluids.

    Provide adequate rest.

    Seek routine immunization.

Critical Thinking Exercise: CHAPTER 19

Child with a Blood Transfusion Answer Key

Situation: A previously healthy 8-year-old lost a large amount of blood after being shot in the upper arm in by his mother's boyfriend during a domestic dispute. The boy's vital signs were stabilized after the bleeding was stopped. A 15-cc/kg blood transfusion was ordered.

1. What are key assessments needed prior to initiating the blood transfusion?

    - Baseline vital signs for later comparison (temperature, pulse, respiration, and blood pressure)
    - Spiritual or personal reasons for the child or family to refuse a blood transfusion
    - History of previous blood transfusions (assess for possible hypersensitivity reactions and the need to premedicate with acetaminophen and antihistamines)

2. The boy tells the nurse that he heard that he could get AIDS or other diseases from a transfusion. How should the nurse respond?

    - Tell the child that all blood is tested to make sure that it does not contain the AIDS virus or other diseases.
    - Explain that he needs the blood transfusion because of the amount of blood he lost after the accident.
    - Assess for residual concerns. Ask the child's mother if she has any concerns before initiating the blood transfusion. If the nurse cannot address her questions and/or concerns satisfactorily, the health care provider should be contacted.
    - The nurse should remember that the child's parent(s) has (have) a right to refuse treatment, including blood transfusions. In some areas, informed written consent for transfusion is needed except in an emergency.

3. Ten minutes into the transfusion the child complains of tightness in his chest and difficulty breathing. The nurse notes that he is wheezing and slightly cyanotic. What interventions are needed at this time?

    - The nurse should immediately call for assistance. Wheezing, dyspnea, chest tightness, cyanosis, are signs of transfusion reaction. It should be treated as a medical emergency since it can lead to hypotension, shock, and death.

- The transfusion should be immediately stopped and the IV will need to be flushed.
- Assist the child in maintaining his airway by having him to sit upright (the position of comfort with respiratory distress) and administer 100% oxygen.
- Keep the child calm and reassure him that he will be feeling better soon.
- Vital signs and additional data and should be assessed and recorded.
- Promptly notify the health care provider to obtain additional orders.
- Administration of additional fluids, medications, and/or other treatments may be needed.

Critical Thinking Exercise: CHAPTER 20
Child with Seizures Answer Key

Situation: A 2-year-old male is admitted after a seizure at home. The nurse obtains the following information from the child's mother: the child had generalized jerking of his arms and legs lasting one to two minutes with vomiting and cyanosis. He had been on Phenobarbital since nine months of age when he was diagnosed with a febrile seizure disorder. He has had two prior incidents of seizures since diagnosis.

1. What additional questions should the nurse ask the mother?

    - Has the child been taking his medication on a regular basis?
    - When was the last phenobarbital level drawn?
    - Did the child have a fever at home?
    - Could the child have accidentally ingested a medication or chemical?
    - Did the child have any history of a head injury?
    - Did the child fall or hit his head during the seizure?

2. What child assessment should be made at this time?

    Vital signs including temperature measurement
    Respiratory assessment and oxygen saturation level
    Neurological assessment
    Signs of injury

3. Shortly after admission, the mother calls the nurse to the room because her child is having another seizure. What interventions are needed for this child during and immediately after the seizure? List in order of priority.

    - Turn to child to the side.
    - Remove any sharp or potentially harmful objects.
    - Provide oxygen blow-by.

- Closely observe duration, activity, and child's condition during the seizure.
- Call for help if seizure persists or if child deteriorates.
- Promptly report seizure activity to health care provider.
- Administer anticonvulsants as ordered.
- Accurately record information in chart.
- Provide emotional support and education to family.
- Draw anticonvulsant levels as indicated.

4. The child's mother admits that she had not been giving her son his phenobarbital at home because he hates the taste of the syrup. How should the nurse respond?

Educate the mother about the importance of maintaining a therapeutic medication level and administering all prescribed doses.

Discuss alternative ways to administer phenobarbital (administering crushed tablets instead of the elixir) with the healthcare provider.

Check to see if the mother uses a "chaser" to help rinse the taste from the child's mouth after the medication is given.

Help family identify creative strategies to gain child's cooperation (allowing him to squirt the medication, using a sticker chart, reading a favorite book, etc.).

Critical Thinking Exercise: CHAPTER 21
Child with Bacterial Meningitis Answer Key

Instructions: Place each of the following signs and complications of bacterial meningitis in the correct box(s). Items may be placed in more than one location.

Apnea	Fever or hypothermia	Photophobia
Behavioral changes Blindness	Full or tense fontanel	Poor feeding
Brudzinski sign	Hallucinations	Poor muscle tone
Bulging fontanel	Headache	Septic shock
Cardiovascular collapse	Hearing loss	Seizures
Cold extremities	High-pitched cry	Sensitivity to noise
Cranial nerve damage	Hydrocephalus	Stupor or coma
Cyanosis Chills	Irregular breathing pattern	Vomiting
Diarrhea	Irritability	Weak cry
Extreme irritability	Kernig sign	Weak suck
Facial muscle paralysis	Nuchal rigidity	Weight loss
Fever	Opisthotonos	

	Early	Late/Complications
Neonate	Weak cry Poor muscle tone Vomiting Diarrhea Weak suck Fever or hypothermia Irritability Apnea, irregular breathing pattern Seizures Full or tense fontanel Cyanosis	Bulging fontanel Seizures Apnea Cyanosis Cardiovascular collapse

Nursing Care of Children

Child with Bacterial Meningitis Answer Key

	Early	Late/Complications
Infant/Young Child	High-pitched cry Bulging fontanel Vomiting Poor feeding Fever Extreme irritability Irregular respiratory pattern Seizures	Apnea Cyanosis Cardiovascular collapse Cold extremities Hallucinations Stupor or coma Seizures Hydrocephalus Blindness Hearing loss Shock Facial muscle paralysis Cranial nerve damage
Older Child/Adolescent	Fever Vomiting Headache Chills Extreme irritability Behavioral changes Kernig sign Brudzinski sign Nuchal rigidity Photophobia Sensitivity to noise Seizures	Opisthotonos Cold extremities Hallucinations Stupor or coma Seizures Hydrocephalus Blindness Hearing loss Septic shock Facial muscle paralysis Cranial nerve damage

Critical Thinking Exercise: CHAPTER 22

Child with Reye's Syndrome Answer Key

1. What combination of factors is commonly believed to trigger Reye's syndrome?

    a. Use of salicylates (aspirin or aspirin-containing medications)

    b. Children under 18 years old, particularly between 4 years and 14 years of age

    c. Viral infection (most prevalent in the winter months)

2. The parent of a school-age child asks the nurse how she would know if her child had Reye's syndrome. How should the nurse respond?

    Children in the earliest stage of Reye's syndrome may become more quiet than normal, have a loss of appetite, and begin vomiting.

    This may progress to lethargy with changes in speech and/or coordination.

    You should immediately call your health care provider if you notice any of these symptoms.

    If your child becomes difficult to arouse or has difficulty breathing, you should immediately activate the emergency response system (call 911)

3. What can happen if Reye's syndrome is not identified and treated promptly and/or if the child does not respond to treatment?

    There is a high likelihood that the child will not survive.

    If the child does survive, he could suffer permanent brain damage causing mental retardation, developmental delays, speech difficulties, hearing impairments, and/or a seizure disorder.

    Other body organs such as the kidney, pancreas, and intestines can also be damaged.

Critical Thinking Exercise: CHAPTER 23
Child with a Head Injury Answer Key

Situation: A 14-year-old male is admitted to a pediatric medical/surgical unit after falling off his skateboard three hours prior to admission. Witnesses at the scene reported a brief loss of consciousness. The child does not recall the events. Initial assessment reveals a healthy appearing adolescent who is alert and oriented. He reports having a headache and vomiting once since the fall.

1. What additional assessments are important for this child?

    - Assess vital signs for signs of increased ICP or hypovolemia from bleeding
    - Assess respiratory and circulatory status
    - Assess for signs of external skin injury and bleeding
    - Assess for signs of increased intracranial pressure (continued vomiting, persistent headache, speech changes, visual changes, LOC changes, neurological changes)
    - Assess LOC (confusion, disorientation, irritability, lethargy, stupor, and coma)
    - Assess for other neurological changes (coordination, weakness, muscle tone, reflexes, and pupillary changes)
    - Continually reassess for neurological changes

2. What diagnostics tests should the nurse anticipate for this child?

    - CT or MRI: to visualize cranial structures and assess injury
    - CBC: to assess for bleeding, and possible preoperative preparation
    - X-rays: to visualize C-spine alignment

3. Shortly after admission, the child has a generalized seizure lasting 1-minute followed by a decreased level of consciousness. What are the priority interventions for this child?

    Protect the child during the seizure.
    Call for assistance.
    Turn the child to his side and open the airway during the seizure.

Administer oxygen.

Administer bag-mask ventilation if needed.

Prepare for possible endotracheal intubation.

Suction the airway as needed.

Notify the health care provider and obtain orders.

Administer anticonvulsants.

Continually assess for signs of neurologic deterioration.

Place an intravenous line for fluids, medications and diagnostic procedures.

Prepare for diagnostic testing (CT, MRI) if not already completed.

Provide emotional support to child and family.

Transfer to intensive care unit.

Prepare for possible surgical intervention.

Prepare for possible placement of an intracranial pressure-monitoring device.

Critical Thinking Exercise: CHAPTER 24

Child with a Brain Tumor Answer Key

Situation: A 7-year-old male is admitted after a large brain tumor was discovered during an MRI scan. The boy has a history of recurrent headaches, vomiting, and blurred vision. Upon admission, the child is awake, alert, and oriented with vital signs within the normal range for his age.

1. What changes in vital signs should the nurse anticipate if the brain tumor were large enough to cause increased intracranial pressure (ICP)?

    Increased or decreased heart rate
    Respiratory pattern changes
    Possible temperature instability
    Possible change in blood pressure

2. What should the nurse ask the child and parent about the vomiting?

    - How often does the vomiting occur? (To determine the frequency of the vomiting and if the child is in danger of becoming dehydrated from extensive fluid losses)
    - Does it occur most frequently in the morning? (A characteristic of vomiting related to increased ICP)
    - Is the vomiting projectile? (A characteristic of vomiting related to increased ICP)
    - Has the child also had a fever, diarrhea, or other signs of an infection? (To rule out other reasons for the child's vomiting)

3. What assessments would indicate that the child's neurological functioning and/or level of consciousness are deteriorating?

    Additional changes or worsening of the child's vision
    Increased severity of the headache or vomiting
    Change in gait, coordination, or balance
    Muscle weakness, paralysis, spasticity, or change in muscle tone

Behavioral changes such as irritability, confusion/speech changes, lethargy, or unresponsiveness

Seizure activity

4. What nursing interventions are indicated for this child and family?

Continually assess for signs of neurologic deterioration.

Provide emotional support and education to the child and family.

Provide quiet, darkened room.

Prepare for additional diagnostic testing.

Prepare for surgical intervention as indicated.

Administer medications and treatments as ordered.

Critical Thinking Exercise: CHAPTER 25

Child with Cerebral Palsy Answer Key

Situation: A 2-year-old born at 26 weeks gestational age was recently diagnosed with cerebral palsy (CP). The child's parents have many questions about their daughter's diagnosis.

1. Which of the following statements would most help the parents to have an accurate perception of CP?
    a. The child will probably be very intelligent because most children with CP compensate for their disorder by developing significantly superior cognitive abilities.
    b. The child will eventually outgrow the disorder if she has consistent physical and occupational therapy when she is young.
    c. CP is a progressive condition characterized by increasing neuro-muscular deterioration.
    d. CP was most likely caused by hypoxic damage when she was a critically-ill premature infant.

   Correct answer: **d CP was most likely caused by hypoxic damage when she was a critically-ill premature infant.**

   Rationale: **Birth trauma and prematurity are risk factors for CP. It is impossible to predict intelligence in children. Many children with CP also have some degree of mental retardation. CP is a nonprogressive, chronic disorder that cannot currently be cured.**

2. Which of the following assessments is most characteristic of CP?
    a. Unusual hand and foot creases
    b. Vomiting, diarrhea and high fever
    c. Hypertonicity and developmental delay
    d. Periorbital edema and pulmonary congestion

   Correct answer: **c Hypertonicity and developmental delay**

   Rationale: **CP is often not diagnosed until two years of age or older. Abnormal muscle tone and developmental delay are often the earliest signs of CP. The other symptoms are not typically associated with CP.**

3. What medication should the nurse expect to administer to help decrease muscle tone?
   a. Metoclopramide
   b. Methotrexate
   c. Beclomethasone
   d. Baclofen

Correct answer: **d Baclofen**

Rationale: **Baclofen is a relatively new medication that has been successful in decreasing spasticity. It is usually administered orally.**

4. Which of the following are most important to families with children who have cerebral palsy?
   a. Reversing the degenerative processes that have occurred.
   b. Identifying the underlying defect that is causing the disorder.
   c. Promoting optimal cognitive and physical functioning.
   d. Assisting the family in finding counseling resources.

Correct answer: **c Promoting optimal cognitive and physical functioning.**

Rationale: **The main goal for children with CP is to optimize cognitive and physical functioning. This is accomplished through a multidisciplinary approach to therapy and prevention of secondary complications. CP is not a degenerative disease. It is not possible to pinpoint the exact cause of CP. Internet-based resources may be helpful for some individuals. Families should be cautioned that some Internet-based information might not be accurate. They should be encouraged to verify the accuracy of any information that they find on the Internet.**

Critical Thinking Exercise: CHAPTER 26
Child with Strabismus Answer Key

Identify each of the following statements about strabismus as **TRUE** or **FALSE**.

1. The terms "lazy eye," "cross-eyed," or "squint" are commonly used to describe three different conditions of the eye.

    FALSE

    Rationale: **Strabismus or esotropia is a malalignment of the eyes. It is commonly referred to as "lazy eye," "cross-eyed," or "squint."**

2. Strabismus is caused by deformation of the ocular socket and unequal shape of the eyeballs.

    FALSE

    Rationale: **Strabismus is caused by an imbalance or weakness in the eye muscles.**

3. Assessment of strabismus is done by watching for eye deviation when the child is focusing on an object.

    TRUE

    Rationale: **Strabismus is detected when one eye deviates from the point of fixation. Also assess for squinting or closing one eye to see when focusing on an object.**

4. Strabismus should be treated as soon as possible during the first 3 months of life.

    FALSE

    Rationale: **Strabismus is common and benign until four months of age. This is due to the weakness of young infants' supporting eye muscles.**

5. Visual loss is a common result of untreated strabismus.

    TRUE

    Rationale: **Strabismus should be treated to prevent permanent visual loss.**

6. A child with strabismus would be expected to have difficulty building with blocks and assembling puzzles.

   TRUE

   Rationale: **Strabismus causes inaccurate judgment when picking up objects and difficulty with focusing. These skills are needed for building with blocks and assembling puzzles.**

7. A child with strabismus who has photophobia, dizziness, and headache probably has meningitis.

   FALSE

   Rationale: **Photophobia, dizziness, and headache are probable side effects from the child's strabismus. A thorough assessment should be done to rule out other neurologic disorder with similar symptoms.**

8. Treatment involves covering the affected eye to rest the weak muscles.

   FALSE

   Rationale: **Treatment is done using occlusion therapy. This involves covering the unaffected eye in order to exercise the weak eye muscles of the affected eye.**

9. Both young children and older children are at risk for noncompliance with treatment because they don't like wearing an eye patch.

   TRUE

   Rationale: **Young children may be intolerant of the discomfort of wearing a patch over their eye. Older children may have self-esteem and body image issues because they looking different from their friends. Some children may be teased and called names such as "pirate." Emotional support and a creative approach are needed to address the issues faced by children of various ages.**

10. Surgical removal of the eye may be needed if noninvasive treatment is ineffective.

    TRUE

    Rationale: **Surgical correction of strabismus is done by shortening the eye muscles and realigning them to produce binocular vision (vision using two eyes).**

Critical Thinking Exercise: CHAPTER 27

Child with Type I Insulin-Dependent Diabetes Mellitus Answer Key

1. What factors most commonly lead to hyperglycemia in a client with Type I diabetes mellitus?

    - Disease process: Lack of insulin production due to damaged beta cells in the pancreas
    - Not enough insulin (e.g., insulin dose that is too low for the client's needs)
    - Too much sugar (e.g., over administration of IV fluids with glucose or excessive food consumption)
    - Mismatching sugar intake and insulin administration (e.g., administering insulin between meals instead of immediately prior to meals)

2. What factors most commonly lead to hyperglycemia in a client who is taking insulin?

    - Too much insulin (e.g., dose is too high)
    - Too little sugar (e.g., insulin dose is administered but client refuses to eat)
    - Mismatching sugar intake and insulin administration (e.g., administering insulin between meals instead of immediately prior to meals)
    - Increased use of glucose (e.g., if the client has a fever or acute illness)

3. What are the most common early signs of Type I diabetes mellitus?

    Polyuria, polydipsia, polyphagia, weight loss, and fatigue

4. Identify the key signs and symptoms for hypoglycemia and hyperglycemia:

	Hypoglycemia	**Hyperglycemia**
Onset	Serum glucose < 70 mg/dL	Serum glucose > 160 mg/dL

	Hypoglycemia	Hyperglycemia
Blood Glucose	Rapid	Slow
Urine Dipstick	Urine glucose & ketones negative	Urine glucose positive May have ketonuria
Respiratory System	Shallow breathing No fruity breath odor	Deep rapid breathing Kussmaul respirations Fruity breath odor
Cardiovascular System	Full pulses Tachycardia	Weak pulses Tachycardia
Neurological System	Irritability, anxiety, confusion, Weakness, tremors Progressing to decreased LOC Seizures	Fatigue Visual changes (blurring) Lethargy Progressing to decreased LOC, coma
Skin	Diaphoresis, pallor Cool, clammy	Dry, flushed skin
Gastrointestinal System	May have hunger	Nausea, vomiting Abdominal pain
Fluid status (hydration)	Normal hydration	Thirst, increased urine output, weight loss, signs of dehydration

Critical Thinking Exercise: CHAPTER 28

Child with Diabetic Ketoacidosis Answer Key

Situation: A 17-year-old with a seven-year history of Type I diabetes mellitus is admitted after "passing out" at his senior prom. He is currently conscious with slurred speech. He admits to having "a few beers with his friends" earlier that night. His initial serum glucose is 500 mg/dL.

1. List seven additional history questions that would be helpful for this child.

    - Amount of alcohol consumed
    - Did the child take any drugs that day?
    - Last insulin dose and amount
    - Last glucose level
    - Home glucose monitoring history and routine
    - Usual insulin dose and administration routine
    - Dietary habits
    - Prior history of alcohol ingestion and/or recreational drug use
    - History of depression and/or difficulty coping with his illness
    - Child's understanding of the risk of alcohol ingestion and noncompliance with diabetic regimen

2. List at least five assessments that are most important for this child during initial stabilization.

    - Assess LOC for signs of intoxication vs. signs of decreased LOC from DKA.
    - Assess vital signs for hypertension, tachycardia, and respiratory pattern changes (Kussmaul breathing).
    - Assess for respiratory difficulty related to decreased LOC and/or intoxication.
    - Assess hydration status: skin turgor, urine output, membranes (dry or moist), pulses, and sunken eyes.
    - Assess breath for ketones (fruity odor) vs. alcohol odor.
    - Assess behavioral patterns for signs of depression and/or anger.
    - Assess urine for ketones and glucose.
    - Reassess blood glucose levels at least hourly and after treatment.

3. Identify at least ten interventions appropriate for this child (list in order of priority).

- Place on a cardiorespiratory monitor.
- Place an intravenous line.
- Administer IV bolus insulin dose.
- Administer IV fluids.
- Reassess child's vital signs, neurological status, and glucose level.
- Draw labs to identify serum electrolyte imbalances.
- Draw blood gas to identify acid-base balance and assess respiratory function.
- Measure and record accurate intake and output.
- Monitor for clinical signs of electrolyte imbalance (hyperkalemia, hypokalemia, hypocalcemia, and hyponatremia).
- Monitor for signs for hypoglycemia and hyperglycemia.
- Provide information regarding status and immediate plan to child and family.
- Encourage child to talk with a counselor who can help him with coping strategies.
- Reinforce reasons why it is important to comply with treatment regimen. Give the child an opportunity to ask questions and dispel misconceptions.

Critical Thinking Exercise: CHAPTER 29
Child with a Clubfoot (Talipes Equinovarus) Answer Key

Identify each of the following statements about clubfoot as TRUE or FALSE.

1. Clubfoot is a positional deformity that can be manipulated to a normal position.

    FALSE

    Rationale: **Metatarsus adductus is the positional deformity. Clubfoot is an anatomic deformity.**

2. An infant with clubfoot will need to have foot casts that are replaced every six weeks.

    FALSE

    Rationale: **Casts need to be replaced weekly for the first month and then every two weeks to allow room for the infant's rapid foot growth and to correct the deformity.**

3. A child with clubfoot may need surgery if the casts do not sufficiently correct his feet.

    TRUE

    Rationale: **Surgical intervention is used when casts are unsuccessful.**

4. Most individuals with clubfoot will be severely deformed for the remainder of their life.

    FALSE

    Rationale: **Most cases of clubfoot can be corrected without lasting effects.**

5. Children with clubfoot often do not need treatment because their feet strengthen and straighten as they grow.

   FALSE

   Rationale: **Clubfoot is a congenital malformation of the foot, involving a congenital malformation or the bones, muscles, tendons of foot, ankle, and lower leg, leading to plantar flexion, inverted heel, and an adducted forefoot.**

6. Surgery should be considered if deformity persists despite casting and manipulation.

   TRUE

   Rationale: **Some cases of clubfoot will require surgical intervention. Various techniques may be used; most involve cutting the tendons and pin placement.**

7. Most children who have had their clubfoot corrected successfully will have no signs of the defect.

   FALSE

   Rationale: **Although the correction is achieved, most individuals will have a slightly smaller foot and less developed calf muscle on the affected side.**

Critical Thinking Exercise: CHAPTER 30

Child with Fractures Answer Key

Situation: A 10-year-old female is admitted to the pediatric unit after an open reduction for a fractured femur. While crossing the street, she was struck by a car and injured. She sustained no other injuries except superficial lacerations. Upon arrival the nurse notes that the child is alert and oriented with an intact spica cast.

1. What nursing assessments are important for this child?

    - Assess superficial lacerations.
    - Assess level of consciousness.
    - Monitor vital signs.
    - Assess hydration status.
    - Conduct a neurovascular assessment: color, pulse, temperature, capillary refill, movement, and sensation of the extremity.
    - Assess for edema.
    - Pain assessment; identify position of comfort and assess need for analgesia.
    - Assess for muscle spasm.
    - Assess emotional needs.
    - Assess knowledge base and information.

2. What physical and emotional complications is this child at risk for developing within in the next 3-7 days?

    - Decreased circulation/neurovascular compromise (related to the injury, swelling, and/or compression from the cast)
    - Skin breakdown (related to pressure areas from the cast and immobility)
    - Infection (related to open injuries and/or immobility)
    - Constipation (related to immobility)
    - Pain
    - Sleep disturbance (related to discomfort, positioning, and/or hospitalization)
    - Emotional distress, anxiety, or fear (related to social isolation, boredom, separation from peers, missing school and/or feelings about the accident)

- Respiratory complications/pneumonia (related to immobility)
- Compartment syndrome (related to compression from severe edema)
- Fat embolism/pulmonary embolism (related to broken bone)

3. Identify complications related to skeletal fractures.
   - **Tissue loss from gangrene**
   - **Contracture**
   - **Limb deformity**
   - **Leg length discrepancy**
   - **Nerve damage**
   - **Damage to the joint**
   - **Altered growth (if growth plate is affected)**
   - **Pulmonary embolism**

Critical Thinking Exercise: CHAPTER 31

Child with Traction Answer Key

Identify the correct response for each of the following items. Explain the rationale for each response selected.

1. The nurse caring for a child in skeletal traction should question which of the following orders?
    a. Administer acetaminophen (Tylenol®) every four hours PRN pain.
    b. Release traction for 30 minutes every shift.
    c. Elevate the foot of the bed.
    d. Perform neurovascular checks every eight hours.

    Correct answer: **b Release traction for 30 minutes every shift.**

    Rationale: **Under normal circumstances, skeletal traction should not be released. Appropriate care of a child with a fracture and traction includes routine neurovascular checks, pain assessment and management, and elevation of the foot of the bed as ordered.**

2. Which of the following is most appropriate for assessing circulation and sensation?
    a. Color, temperature, movement, sensation, and capillary refill of the extremity
    b. Degree of motion and ability to position the extremity
    c. Length, diameter, and shape of the extremity
    d. Amount of swelling, intensity of pain, and presence of drainage on the dressing

    Correct answer: **a Color, temperature, movement, sensation, and capillary refill of the extremity**

    Rationale: **Neurovascular assessment should include identification of signs of circulation (color, temperature, and capillary refill), sensation, and movement. The other assessments listed are not generally associated with routine neurovascular assessment.**

3. A 5-year-old Chinese-American client is hospitalized with skeletal traction for a fractured femur. The nursing assistant tells the nurse that the child has shown little interest in eating the food on his meal trays. Which of the following assumptions is most likely to be accurate?
    a. The child is spoiled and angry that he is in the hospital.
    b. The child needs less food since he is on bed rest and not playing as usual.

c. The child is probably eating between meals and is spoiling his appetite.
d. The child may have culturally-related food preferences.

Correct answer: **d The child may have culturally-related food preferences.**

Rationale: **It is important to consider the influence of cultural and individual food preferences when assessing lack of appetite in a hospitalized child. Children on bed rest do not necessarily need less food since other factors may increase metabolic demands (infection, healing, pain, fever, etc.). Lack of eating should not be assumed to be due to behavior problems or snacking without further information.**

Critical Thinking Exercise: CHAPTER 32
Child with Scoliosis Answer Key

Identify five nursing interventions for each of the following problems of a 16-year-old female who has had surgical placement of rods for scoliosis.

Fluid loss
- Assess dressing for signs of bleeding.
- Assess for edema.
- Administer continuous maintenance IV fluids.
- Closely monitor blood pressure and heart rate.
- Administer fluid bolus as needed.

Pain
- Frequently assess pain using a 1-10 pain scale.
- Administer pain medication promptly when needed.
- Encourage the child to listen to her favorite music with headphones.
- Place telephone within reach; allow her to make calls to friends as desired.
- Use assistance to log roll as quickly and effortlessly as possible.

Difficulty sleeping
- Help child find her position of comfort.
- Administer medications as needed for pain.
- Provide quiet, darkened environment at night.
- Make every attempt to minimize number of times the child is awakened at night.
- Encourage the family to bring in favorite pillow or blanket.

Lack of self esteem due to body image changes
- Develop a trusting relationship (provide consistent caregivers).
- Ask open ended, non-threatening questions.
- Use active listening techniques.
- Avoid offering solutions unless requested.
- Assist the child in identifying strategies to improve her self-esteem and body image (make-up, clothing, scarves, etc.).

Critical Thinking Exercise: CHAPTER 33
Child with Juvenile Rheumatoid Arthritis Answer Key

Situation: A 10-year-old female is admitted with a diagnosis of juvenile arthritis (JA).

1. What assessments are important for this child?

    - Assess number of joints affected.
    - Assess joint mobility and range of motion.
    - Assess knees, ankles, elbows, and other joints for swelling.
    - Assess for painless joint swelling.
    - Take temperature: assess for low-grade fever.
    - Assess for fatigue and malaise.
    - Assess for enlarged lymph nodes.
    - Assess for hepatomegaly and splenomegaly.
    - Assess for vision changes.
    - Assess hydration status.
    - Assess nutritional status.
    - Assess emotional state and coping response.
    - Assess knowledge level.

2. List interventions might be helpful in decreasing the pain associated with JA.

    Apply heating pad to affected joints.
    Have the child take a warm bath.
    Administer NSAID medications.
    Position the child to reduce joint strain.
    Use non-pharmacological pain management techniques (distraction, biofeedback, etc.).

3. List interventions that assist with self-care and mobility in children with JA.

>Suggest the parent buy loose-fitting clothing with elastic that is easy to put on and remove.
>Provide a walker or cane for ambulation.
>Encourage regular exercise and mobilization of the joints to prevent contractures.
>Provide adaptive appliances designed to assist the child with eating, drinking, and grooming.
>Teach use of splints to prevent flexion contractures.

4. Matching: Match the symptoms with the type of JA:

b	High fever spikes	
a	Occurs during first 6 months of the disease	a. Pauciarticular
c	Five or more joints affected	b. Systemic
b	Red rash on trunk and extremities	c. Polyarticular
a	Four or fewer joints affected	

Critical Thinking Exercise: CHAPTER 34
Child with Muscular Dystrophies Answer Key

Situation: A 4-year-old male presents with an arm laceration that he received after falling off his tricycle. His mother tells the nurse that he is clumsy and seems to be weaker than her other children especially when he tries to get up from the floor. Diagnostic tests are scheduled to determine if the child has muscular dystrophy (MD).

1. What additional history questions should the nurse ask the child's mother?

   Is there anyone else in your family with MD?
   Can you explain what you are seeing when you notice his muscle weakness?
   When did your child first stand? Walk? Run?
   Does he use his hands to brace himself on his legs when he gets up from the floor (Gowers' sign)?
   Can you describe what his typical walk looks like?
   Have you noticed any other problems with coordination? Does he have any difficulty handling feeding utensils or feeding himself?

2. What assessments are important for this child?

   Assess laceration for bleeding and need for cleaning.
   Ask the child to walk (assess for waddling, wide base stance).
   Assess the child's ability to rise from the floor (Gowers' sign).
   Ask the child to raise his arms above his head to assess for upper body strength.
   Assess muscle strength and tone of each extremity.
   Assess calf muscles for pseudohypertrophy.
   Assess hips and shoulders for tone and stability.
   Assess face for tone and mobility.
   Assess the respiratory status.

3. What type of muscular dystrophy most resembles the child's symptoms?

> **Duchenne (pseudohypertrophy) MD**
>
> This type occurs in males with an average age of onset at 3-5 years old. The child is within this age range and has some of the classic symptoms (waddling gait, clumsiness, and Gowers' sign).

4. Matching:

b	Gowers' sign	a.	Tracheostomy and mechanical ventilation by late adolescence
e	Delayed motor development	b.	Uses hands on legs to brace the legs when rising from the floor
d	Duchenne muscular dystrophy	c.	Muscle replaced with fatty and connective tissue
a	Progressive respiratory weakness	d.	Manifests in boys
c	Pseudohypertrophy of the calf	e.	Infants and toddlers

Critical Thinking Exercise: CHAPTER 35

Child with Burns Answer Key

Situation: A nurse is working in the Emergency Department at a community hospital when the staff is notified of a day care center fire with explosion, probably in the kitchen. Several children are being transported to the Emergency Department with varying degrees of burns.

1. Matching:

b	Reddened, discolored area with a moist weeping surface	a.	Superficial (first degree)
a	Sunburn	b.	Partial thickness (second degree)
d	Deep burn to the muscle, bone and fascia	c.	Full thickness (third degree)
a	Tender, slightly swollen, and red skin	d.	Full thickness (fourth degree)
c	Leathery brown with little surface moisture		
b	Open blisters and reddened burns		

2. Identify each of the following burns as minor, moderate, or major (severe).

Major	Partial and full thickness burns on face, neck, torso, arms and hands
Major	First- and second-degree burns on legs covering 5% of the body surface
Moderate	Full thickness burn on calf involving 3% of the body surface
Major	Full thickness burns (third-and-fourth degree) on 50% of the body surface
Moderate	Partial thickness burn on the back covering 25% of the body surface
Minor	Small, red, tender area on the forearm after being burned by the tip of an iron

Critical Thinking Exercise: CHAPTER 36

Child with Eczema Answer Key

Situation: A mother has brought her 9-month-old daughter to a rural clinic. The daughter is diagnosed with eczema of the cheeks, knees, and elbows. The mother and nurse discuss strategies for care and troubleshoot any potential problem situations.

1. From the list below, select correct interventions. Identify the rationale for all interventions.
    a. Use a mild detergent in the laundry.
    b. Stay in a warm environment.
    c. Utilize latex gloves during care.
    d. Utilize a room humidifier.
    e. Apply topical steroids.
    f. Administer lotions with pleasing scents.
    g. Obtain adequate rest/naps.
    h. Bathe 3 -4 times a day.
    i. Allow child to play in bubble bath.
    j. Assess for secondary skin infections.
    k. Administer an antihistamine.
    l. Bathe in a tepid bath with mild soap.
    m. Clip nails to prevent scratching.
    n. Place a thick layer of ointment on skin.
    o. Modify diet.
    p. Cover with a wool blanket.
    q. Soak in cornstarch and water.
    r. Wear cotton clothes.
    s. Utilize cool, wet compresses.
    t. Apply emollient following bath.

Rationale for selections:
1. To hydrate the skin: **d, l, q, s, t**
2. To relieve pruritus: **e, k, q, s**
3. Reduce inflammation: **e, r, m**
4. Prevent and control secondary skin infections: **j, m**

Critical Thinking Exercise: CHAPTER 37
Child with Impetigo Answer Key

Identify each of the following statements regarding impetigo as **TRUE** or **FALSE**. Explain the rationale for each response.

1. Impetigo is a noncontagious autoimmune disease causing skin irritation when exposed to the sun.

    FALSE

    Rationale: **Impetigo is a superficial bacterial infection of the skin. It is highly contagious.**

2. Impetigo can be spread from one child to another by sharing the same brush.

    FALSE

    Rationale: **Impetigo is highly contagious. Contact with an infected object such as a brush can result in cross contamination and spread of infection.**

3. Reddened macular lesions develop into small vesicles that become pustules and rupture leaving moist erosions. The dried exudate forms honey-colored lesions.

    TRUE

    Rationale: **This is the typical pattern of lesion development and healing.**

4. Rubbing alcohol solution in a tepid bath is used to dry and heal the lesions.

    FALSE

    Rationale: **Rubbing alcohol will dry the skin and may lead to further cracking. Crusted lesions are softened with 1:20 Burrow's solution compresses.**

5. Topical antibiotic ointment may be used to treat infected skin lesions.

> **TRUE**
>
> Rationale: **Impetigo is a bacterial infection that is best treated with antibiotic therapy. Topical antibiotic ointments such as Bacitracin, Polysporin, Neosporin, or Bactroban are most frequently used to treat the infection.**

6. Providing interventions for pruritus will help the child with impetigo feel more comfortable.

> **TRUE**
>
> Rationale: **Pruritus and scratching is associated with the spread of infection. Pruritus is experienced due to drying and crusted lesions.**

Critical Thinking Exercise: CHAPTER 38

Child with Diaper Rash Answer Key

Situation: A 9-month-old is brought to the clinic for a regular check up. Upon physical examination, redness and excoriation of the diaper area is noted. The mother states that the child has had reddened areas for approximately two weeks.

1. The nurse recognizes that this is the first child of a young mother, and infant care instruction is necessary. Regarding general skin care, as well as specific care of diaper rash, what instruction would be essential?

    General skin care includes keeping the body bathed and dressed appropriate to the climate. Infants should be bathed regularly especially in the summer. The skin should be assessed for any redness, abrasion or excoriation. Lotions may be utilized but should not include perfumes as this could cause irritation. Powder helps keep the skin dry, but talc is very dangerous if breathed into the lungs. Plain cornstarch or cornstarch based powder is safer.

    If diaper rash should occur, it is important to keep the skin dry. Allow air to circulate; thus avoid rubber pants. Change diaper as soon as it is soiled to decrease skin wetness, alter diaper/skin pH, and eliminate fecal enzymes. Apply ointment to protect the skin.

2. Create and evaluate a care plan selecting nursing diagnoses, interventions, goals and outcomes to evaluate the effectiveness of care.

    Nursing diagnosis: **Impaired skin integrity related to redness in the diaper and skin excoriation**

    Nursing interventions:
    - Assess diaper area at each visit.
    - Instruct mother on utilizing absorbent diapers.
    - Instruct on proper ointment administration.
    - Watch mother care for diaper area.
    - Verbally assess mother's understanding of care.

Outcome: **Mother will verbalize three factors that will improve the integrity of the skin in the diaper area.**

Goal: **Skin integrity will be intact without signs of redness.**

Evaluation: **Mother will verbalize completing frequent diapering, applying a skin protecting ointment, and allowing air to circulate around the diaper area.**

Critical Thinking Exercise: CHAPTER 39
Child with Head Lice (Pediculosis Capitis) Answer Key

1. Fill in the blank:

    Head lice occur in children in **all** socioeconomic groups.

    Head lice are spread through **direct** contact with infected objects.

    The feeling of the lice crawling and the saliva on the skin causes **itching**.

2. Matching:

e	Permethrin	a.	One month
i	Pyrethrin shampoo	b.	Eggs
c	Lindane	c.	Kwell
b	Nits	d.	Treats Itching
g	Louse	e.	Treatment of choice for infants and young children
f	Incubation period of eggs	f.	7-10 days
d	Diphenhydramine (Benadryl)	g.	Adult organism
a	Female adult life span	h.	48 hours
h	Lifespan if away from host	i.	RID

3. Answer the following questions:

    a. How should families be instructed to look for signs of the organisms?

    Separate the hair with a tongue blade.
    Inspect the child's head closely for whitish-gray nits attached to the hair shaft.

Nursing Care of Children

Child with Head Lice (Pediculosis Capitis) Answer Key

b. How should families be instructed to treat head lice?

Remove nits by combing with fine-toothed comb dipped in hot vinegar.
Treat with the prescribed medicated shampoo, creme rinse, or lotion (Permethrin, Pyrethrin, or Lindane).
Wash bedding and clothing with hot water, then use a hot dryer.
Spray mattresses with disinfectant.
Dry clean wool clothing or place it in hot clothes dryer for 20 minutes.
For itching: Keep the child's nails trimmed and clean, administer Benadryl if needed.

c. What should the nurse teach the family to prevent the spread or reinfection of head lice?

Notify close contacts of infection (family, friends, school, daycare, etc.).
Discourage children from sharing hats, scarves, coats, hair ornaments, combs, and brushes.
During slumber parties, clean bedding should be used for each child.

Critical Thinking Exercise: CHAPTER 40

Child with Dermatophytosis (Ringworm) Answer Key

Situation: A student nurse is teaching a junior high health class about ringworm. To illustrate the point, the student nurses made a drawing on poster board and utilized a mapping perspective concept. Placing the tinea in the center of the poster board, what other information is a priority to be included regarding each of the areas of infection? Specifically and creatively relate the information to the junior high class.

Place tinea in the center. In the four corners include the following: Tinea Capitis, Tinea Corporis, Tinea Pedis and Tinea Cruris

1. Creatively depict information of each of the fungal infections:

    The poster board could reflect an age appropriate interest, such as, sports and peer relationships and how ringworm can impact these activities.

    a. Tinea Capitis **Ringworm of the scalp**

    Tinea Capitis is transmitted through combs, towels, hats or direct contact. It begins with a small papule on the scalp and spreads, leaving patches of baldness.

    Age appropriate information: Do not share objects that come in contact with head such as, hats, combs, brushes, etc.

    b. Tinea Corporis **Ringworm of the body**

    Tinea Corporis is frequently contracted by contact with an infected cat or dog. Topical antifungal agents are used in treatment.

    Age appropriate information: Wash following contact with pets

    c. Tinea Pedis **Athletes foot**

    Transmission is by direct or indirect contact with skin lesions of infected people. Contaminated sidewalks, floors, pool decks and shower stalls can spread the condition.

    Age appropriate information: Wash the feet following use of public showers, wear sandals if in contact with public surfaces such as pool decks.

d. Tinea Cruris **Jock itch**

   Tinea Cruris is frequently transmitted by fungal infection in warm moist areas of groin. Athletes commonly have in the groin area and inner thighs.

   Age appropriate information: Wash the groin area and keep the area clean and dry. Sitz baths may be soothing.

Critical Thinking Exercise: CHAPTER 41
Child's Immunizations Answer Key

1. Match the immunizations that are on the schedule for a child of each the following ages:

c	Birth	a.	DPT, HIB, polio & Pneumococcal vaccine & Hepatitis B #2
a	4 months old	b.	DPT, Polio, & MMR
d	6 months old	c.	Hepatitis B #1
f	2 months old	d.	DPT, HIB, Polio, Pneumococcal vaccine & Hepatitis B #3
b	5 years old	e.	Make up vaccinations
e	11 years old	f.	HIB, Polio, Pneumococcal vaccine, Varicella, MMR, & Hepatitis B #3 (if not already administered)

2. The mother of a 3-week-old infant is concerned because her baby has only had one immunization since birth. Has the infant missed any scheduled immunizations?

   Instruct the parent that this is appropriate. Review the current immunization schedule: Hepatitis B vaccine is given at birth and the next scheduled immunizations are routinely given at two months of age (Hepatitis B #2, DPT, Hib, polio, and pneumococcal vaccine).

3. The father of a 15-month-old asks the nurse to give the IM vaccination in his daughter's buttocks so she does not have to see the needle. What should the nurse tell the father?

   Inform the parent that the preferred IM injection site for children under the age of two is the vastus lateralis. The gluteal muscle in this age group should be avoided due to potential problems with the sciatic nerve and interference with walking. Avoid showing the toddler the syringe or needle prior to injection. Encourage the child's father to provide comfort and support to his daughter before, during, and/or after the injection.

4. A 4-month-old child presents for routine immunization with lethargy, tachycardia, fever of 104° F, and decreased urine output over the past 24 hours. Should the nurse give the immunization? Why or why not?

   This infant has a moderate-to-severe illness as evidenced by the tachycardia, decreased LOC, high fever and decreased urine output. This condition should be stabilized prior to vaccination. If this infant had only had a mild illness, immunizations would have been given as scheduled.

Critical Thinking Exercise: CHAPTER 42

Child with Oral Candidiasis (Thrush) Answer Key

Situation: A 12-week-old is brought to the pediatricians' office for a follow-up visit. The nurse brings the infant into the room and questions the mother about the recent upper respiratory infection and antibiotic completion. The mother states that the infant's symptoms have improved; he is sleeping better, but is not eating well.

The physician examines the oral cavity and discovers white patches on the tongue, palate and inner aspect of the cheek.

1. Correlate the past history of the infant with the symptoms described. How is it best to explain the occurrence to the mother?

    When assessing a normally healthy infant, the white patches on the tongue, palate and inner aspect of the cheeks are most likely linked to the treatment of the infection. The infant completed an antibiotic for an upper respiratory infection. Antibiotics often change the normal flora of the mouth causing the symptoms. The white patches can be uncomfortable thus potentially causing the infant to have poor oral intake.

2. In what other instances would it be a priority to complete teaching related to thrush?

    It is priority to complete teaching related to thrush in the following circumstances:

    An asthmatic child who is utilizing an inhaler. The mouth should be rinsed following the use of an inhaler.

    An immunosuppressed child such as cancer patients or patients with AIDS. Opportunistic infections grow in individuals with low defenses.

3. What instruction is most effective in providing treatment for thrush?

    Thrush is treated by using topical nystatin (Mycostatin) over the surfaces of the oral cavity four times daily. Nursing care is directed toward preventing the spread of infection down the gastrointestinal tract and correctly applying the topical medication.

To correctly administer the medication: cleanse the infant's mouth with water following a feeding then distribute the nystatin (Mycostatin) suspension over the affected oral surfaces. The remainder of the dose is deposited into the mouth and swallowed to treat any gastrointestinal lesions. To prevent relapse, therapy should continue for at least three days after symptoms disappear.

Critical Thinking Exercise: CHAPTER 43

Child with Human Immunodeficiency Virus (HIV) and Acquired Immunodeficiency Syndrome (AIDS) Answer Key

Situation: A 17-year-old client presents with a recurrent upper respiratory tract infection, cough, fever, enlarged lymph nodes, and weight loss. She tells the nurse that she has been sleeping more than usual and has been sweaty at night. She admits to participating in sexual partner trading games at 2-3 parties during the past year. She did not remember using a condom during intercourse.

1. How is HIV most commonly spread?

    - Unprotected sexual contact
    - Sharing contaminated needles during IV drug use
    - Direct contact with infected blood and body fluids
    - Spread from infected mother to infant (least common of the methods listed above)

2. What typical adolescent beliefs and behaviors increase their risk of becoming infected with the HIV virus?

    - Developmental belief common among adolescents that they are invincible– "it won't happen to me."
    - Developmental task of forming identity, which may lead to using sex to help achieve a feeling of being desirable and loved
    - Multiple sexual partners
    - Unprotected sexual contact
    - Use of alcohol and recreational drugs

3. Identify the factors in the 17-year-old female's history and presentation that are associated with HIV infection.

    - History of multiple sexual partners without use of protection
    - Enlarged lymph nodes
    - Weight loss
    - Night sweats

Child with Human Immunodeficiency Virus (HIV) and Acquired Immunodeficiency Syndrome (AIDS) Answer Key

- Sleeping more than usual (may indicate malaise or fatigue)
- Recurrent upper respiratory tract infection (possibly an opportunistic infection related to decreased immunity)

4. Tests reveal that the adolescent does have an HIV infection. What nursing interventions are needed at this time?

   - Treat current respiratory symptoms (oxygen, antibiotics, airway support).
   - Provide emotional support and information to the adolescent and family about the disease, precautions, and treatment plan.
   - Support the teen in informing all sexual contacts of the need to be tested for HIV.
   - Prevent transmission of the disease by using appropriate precautions.
   - Protect the client from additional infections.

Critical Thinking Exercise: CHAPTER 44
Child with Otitis Media Answer Key

Situation: A 7-month-old infant is brought to the clinic with a fever of 102° F. The infant's mother reports that her baby has had a "runny nose" and cough for the last three days. The infant is crying and is irritable. The primary care provider assesses red, bulging tympanic membranes and diagnoses bilateral otitis media. Amoxicillin is to be given at home every six hours for ten days.

1. The child's mother asks the nurse what she can do to prevent additional ear infections. What should the nurse tell the parent about risk factors associated with otitis media?

    - Explain that infants who are bottle fed in supine position are more prone to ear infections because their ear passages (eustachian tubes) are relatively short and flat as compared to older children. If the infant is bottle fed, elevate the head during feeding. Tell the mother not to prop the bottle in the baby's mouth or put the infant to bed with a bottle.

    - Inform the mother that parental smoking has also been linked with an increased incidence of ear infections.

    - Explain that infants who are exposed to other sick children and/or have a respiratory illness may have a greater chance of getting infected. Explain that there are more ear infections in the winter months because infants and children tend to get more infections in the winter.

    - Discuss the peak age range of three months to three years.

2. The child's mother then asks the nurse if her baby will suffer any damage from the infection. What should the nurse tell her?

    - In general, ear infections that are identified and treated early will leave no lasting effects.

    - It is important for her to administer all of the medication to prevent complications and/or reinfection.

    - Untreated ear infections can lead to hearing loss and/or more serious infections, such as meningitis.

3. What instructions should the nurse give the mother regarding the antibiotics?

- Give all doses of medication until it is gone (the full ten days).
- Give at approximately the same time each day.
- Store the medication in a safe place to avoid accidental overdose.
- Shake the bottle before drawing up the amount needed. Use the dropper or a syringe to squirt the medicine to the side of the mouth and wait for the child to swallow it.
- Do not repeat the dose if the child spits, drools or vomits the medicine. Do not mix the medicine in the child's bottle.
- Call your doctor if your child develops diarrhea, rash, or other symptoms.

Critical Thinking Exercise: CHAPTER 45
Child's Varicella-Zoster Infection (Chickenpox and Shingles)
Answer Key

1. Matching:

B	Contagious period begins	a.	Provides passive immunity 92 hours after exposure
E	Most commonly infected	b.	1-2 days after the rash develops
C	Time for vesicles to crust	c.	One week
I	Crusting usually begins	d.	10-21 days
G	Shingles infection	e.	5-9 year olds
H	Contagious period ends	f.	Infants and immunocompromised children
D	Incubation period	g.	Elderly adults
A	VZIG	h.	When lesions have dried
F	Increased risk for complications	i.	24-48 hours after the fever

2. Fill in the blank:
   a. The typical chickenpox rash lesions progress from a **macular** to **popular** rash, then forms **vesicles** before erupting into **open** lesions.

   b. Children with varicella may have a slight fever and malaise **24** to **48** hours before the rash appears.

   c. A nurse should wear a **gown**, **gloves**, and a **mask** when bathing a child with draining varicella lesions.

   d. **Shingles (zoster)** is a secondary varicella-zoster infection caused by activation of the latent infection in the dorsal root ganglion.

Critical Thinking Exercise: CHAPTER 46
Child with Rubeola (Measles) Answer Key

1. List the following rubeola symptoms in the order in which they occur.

    2 Fever, Koplik spots, photophobia, no rash

    4 Red rash on the face, trunk, and legs

    6 Positive convalescent serum measles titers

    5 Brown rash over entire body

    3 Maculopapular rash along on the head and neck

    1 Fever, cough, and a runny nose without a rash or Koplik spots

2. A 5-year-old with rubeola is admitted to the hospital. What should the nurse do for the following symptoms?

    a. Cough and upper respiratory congestion
       Assess adequacy of breathing (oxygen saturation, respiratory effort, respiratory rate).
       Elevate the head of the bed.
       Provide cough suppressants as needed.
       Administer oxygen and suction needed.

    b. Fever
       Administer antipyretics as ordered.
       Provide cooling measures.

    c. Photophobia and headache
       Maintain a quiet, darkened room.
       Provide analgesics as needed.

d. Eye irritation from conjunctivitis

   Administer saline drops for moisture.

   Instruct child not to rub eyes.

e. Rash

   Apply a topical lotion.

   Bathe in a colloid solution.

   Administer medications for itching as ordered.

f. Emotional distress

   Encourage family members to stay with the child.

   Provide activities that the child can do while on bedrest (VCR with the child's favorite videos, drawing, coloring pictures, action figures, etc.).

   Maintain the child's bed as a "safe zone" by avoiding painful procedures in bed.

Critical Thinking Exercise: CHAPTER 47
Child with Rubella (German Measles) Answer Key

1. Explain why each of the children listed below is at risk for acquiring rubella.

    All of these children are at risk because they have not been immunized.

    a. A 7-year-old child attending home school:

    Vaccinations are required for all children entering school. Children who attend school at home may not be fully immunized.

    b. A 10-year-old child from a family visiting from a foreign country:

    Routine vaccination does not occur in all countries as it does in the United States. This child is at risk because of the unknown vaccination status.

    c. A 1-year-old healthy infant:

    Routine MMR vaccination is scheduled for 15 months. This child is younger than the typical vaccination time therefore does not have the immunity protection.

    d. A 2-year-old with chronic respiratory illness and frequent hospitalizations:

    Young children with chronic illness may not have received their routine vaccinations. The child's chronic illness and lack of immunity put him at increased risk.

    e. A 3-year-old child from a family without medical care who is sharing a small one bedroom apartment with 2 other families:

    The lack of medical care puts this child at risk for missing routine well childcare and immunizations. The close living quarters puts this child at risk for infectious disease exposure.

2. Identify which of the following children with rubella is at greatest risk for serious complication associated with the disease. Explain your rationale. Discuss the risk of complications associated with rubella for the remaining children.

    a. A 7-year-old male with fever, nasal drainage, enlarged lymph nodes, and a rash on his face

Child with Rubella (German Measles) Answer Key

b. A 16-year-old female with diarrhea, nausea, and positive Forchheimer's sign
c. A 1-year-old female with a rash on her head and neck, irritability, decreased appetite, and sleep disturbance
d. A 3-year-old male with chills, joint pain, vomiting, diarrhea, anorexia, and a rash over entire body

Answer: **The 16-year-old girl is at greatest risk for being pregnant because of her age and gender.** Congenital rubella is associated with the most serious complications of maternal rubella exposure (growth retardation, deafness, cardiac defects, retinopathy, cataracts, mental retardation, encephalitis, diabetes, and thyroid disorders). Young children with diarrhea, vomiting, poor feeding, anorexia, and fever are at risk for fluid loss and dehydration. Presence of the rash on the head and neck only is an indicator that the disease is in an earlier stage. These children should be closely monitored for complications during the acute phase of their illness.

Critical Thinking Exercise: CHAPTER 48
Child with Epstein-Barr Viral Infection (Mononucleosis)
Answer Key

1. Discuss why each of the following children may be at risk for acquiring EBV. Identify which of the following children is at greatest risk for acquiring this disease. Explain your rationale.

   a. 4-year old twins imitating kissing seen on television:

   EBV is spread through oral-salivary route. Imitating kissing may cause exposure to the virus. This exposure would most likely not be as long or as frequent as adolescent kissing. Four-year old twins are at lower risk for having the infection to transmit.

   b. A 16-year old male who tells the nurse he enjoys "making out" with his 16-year-old girlfriend:

   These teens are at greatest risk for obtaining the disease because of their age and behavior patterns that are commonly associated with disease transmission.

   c. A 1-year-old infant who puts a pacifier in his mouth after picking it up off the carpet:

   The usual route of transmission is through saliva or blood. The risk of acquiring EBV from a pacifier would probably be less than other scenarios described.

   d. A 7-year-old who shares a bedroom with his parents and two younger siblings:

   Close contact is likely in crowded living conditions. There may be some risk of acquiring the disease due to exposure if any of the adults had the disease. This risk is less than the direct contact of the 16-year-olds.

2. A 15-year-old with EBV tells her nurse that her disease is really upsetting her. Describe five or more reasons why an adolescent with EBV might be distressed.

   - Decreased ability to cope with distress related to fatigue and discomfort
   - Physical discomfort from the sore throat, headache, abdominal pain, fever and/or bed rest
   - Hunger and/or thirst related to not being able to swallow without pain
   - Lack of sleep related to illness
   - Boredom related to bed rest and activity intolerance

- Anxiety and/or anger related to missing schoolwork, friends, and social activities
- Depression or frustration related to duration of illness
- Fear of losing boyfriend/friends related to having an infectious disease and need for bed rest
- Low self esteem related to change in activity level and social isolation

Critical Thinking Exercise: CHAPTER 49
Child with Rheumatic Fever Answer Key

Fill in the blank:
1. Rheumatic fever is a complication of **group A beta-hemolytic streptococci** pharyngitis and is self-limiting.

2. The dangerous complication associated with rheumatic fever is **rheumatic heart disease**.

3. The inflammatory, hemorrhagic, bullous lesions that result from rheumatic fever are known as **Aschoff bodies or nodules**.

4. Rheumatic heart disease may require **valve replacement** surgery due to the thickening and deformity of the **heart valves**.

5. Minor manifestations of rheumatic fever noted on the Jones Criteria from 1992 include **arthralgia** and **fever**.

6. The gold standard in treating rheumatic fever is **penicillin**.

7. The best way to prevent rheumatic fever is to ensure **adequate antibiotic treatment of** streptococcal pharyngitis.

Identify 5 teaching points for the family of a child with rheumatic fever.
1. **The importance of bedrest during the acute febrile phase of the disease**

2. **The need for follow-up care for 5 years due to the susceptibility of recurrence of the disease**

3. **The need for antibiotic prophylaxis prior to dental work or some invasive procedures**

4. **The importance of taking the prescribed antibiotic until it is all gone**

5. **The need to restrict activity until the fever resolves**

Critical Thinking Exercise: CHAPTER 50
Child with Gastroenteritis/Diarrhea Answer Key

Situation: A 6-month-old male is admitted to the hospital with diagnosis of gastroenteritis/diarrhea. He is alert but listless. The child is pale with sunken eyes. VS-101.6 - 146 - 42. The child is refusing all oral food and fluids. The parent reports that the child has vomited 6 times and has had numerous diarrhea stools. Currently watery diarrhea is noted. Abdomen is soft with hyperactive bowel sounds. The nurse notes that the child cries and pulls his legs to the abdomen.

Following a detailed health history and physical assessment, the nurse begins to formulate a plan of care with nursing diagnosis. The nurse has started with the following NANDA approved nursing diagnosis. Enter the symptoms, both from the scenario above and your knowledge of the disease process that could complete the nursing diagnosis statement. Explain rationale for the choices.

Risk for Impaired Parent/Infant Attachment related to: **infant fussiness, infant not being content with being comforted secondary to abdominal cramping, parental frustration secondary to infant behavior.**

> Rationale: **The infant with gastroenteritis and abdominal cramping as evidenced by pulling up the legs and fussiness is difficult to soothe. During the acute phase of the disease process, the infant and the family is unable to rest properly leading to frustration of both the infant and parents. Parents may question their parenting ability and ability to comfort their infant.**

Risk for caregiver role strain related to: **being the primary caretaker of an ill child, child fussiness, demands of caring for the infant and other children in the home, trying to care for infant and work**

> Rationale: **Caring for the infant is demanding. The infant needs comforting, frequent diapering, and frequent offering of rehydrating fluids. Satisfying all of the needs is difficult enough without also adding the demands of additional children, work responsibilities and duties in the home. The caretaker must understand the need to rest when the child rests to preserve energy for care.**

Impaired comfort related to: **abdominal pain, nausea, reddened diaper area**

> Rationale: **Gastroenteritis produces nausea, vomiting, and diarrhea. The child exhibits signs of pain by crying and pulling up his legs. Comfort needs to be given to the child and attention to meticulous diapering so as not to avoid skin breakdown. The child is fussy**

and uncomfortable throughout this disease process. This child has had recurrent vomiting and diarrhea to the extent of watery stools. Due to the frequent stools, diaper changes are important so not to have skin breakdown. Frequently the anal area will be reddened from irritation.

Interrupted family processes related to: **the demand of parenting an ill child, restructuring family obligations secondary to the child's illness.**

> Rationale: **When the family has an ill child, that child impacts the family process within the home. Many times, roles will be altered so that one parent is committed to caring for the child while the other continues with the family's schedule.**

Fluid volume: Deficient related to: **decreased desire to ingest fluids/solids, inability to tolerate fluid/ nutrition, leading to poor intake along with vomiting and/or diarrhea.**

> Rationale: **Signs of dehydration are noted in this child as the child is listless, pale with sunken eyes. The child has vomited several times and had many stools. Other factors to consider may be skin turgor, mucous membranes and last urination.**

Hyperthermia related to: **progression of the disease process, elevated temperature readings**

> Rationale: **The child's temperature is currently elevated. Consideration should be made to dress the child lightly to not further elevate the temperature. Children often have poor temperature regulation and may consequently have a febrile seizure.**

Ineffective infant feeding pattern related to: **inability to tolerate foods/fluids**

> Rationale: **Feeding patterns will be disrupted during the disease process due to the vomiting, diarrhea and cramping. Even when the child is vomiting, consideration should be made to offer rehydrating fluids. If the child continues to be unable to tolerate fluids, an intravenous solution should be started until the child is able to tolerate fluids.**

Knowledge: Deficient related to: **disease process, progression of the disease, comforting measures, oral rehydration, and skin care.**

> Rationale: **Having an ill child is very stressful. Being unsure of the nature of the disease and measures to care for a sick child makes the disease process more stressful. Specific guidelines and instruction with follow up can assist the parent in making the correct decisions to combat the disease process. Assessing the child's symptoms can also provide needed knowledge during the treatment phase.**

Nausea related to: **inability to tolerate solids/liquids, progression of the disease process**

> Rationale: Nausea/vomiting is classic sign of gastroenteritis. This child has had frequent episodes. Nausea/vomiting is uncomfortable for the child and leads to a fluid deficit.

Nutrition: Less than body requirements: **inability to tolerate diet**

> Rationale: Even though the child is listless, the body is working to eliminate the infective agent. Without being able to tolerate nutrition, the body has less than is needed and many times will draw on bodily resources of vitamins, minerals and fat during this time period. It is not uncommon for a weight loss to be noted during the disease process.

Risk for impaired skin integrity related to: **reddened diaper area, excoriation/bleeding around the anus**

> Rationale: Due to the change in content, consistency and frequency of bowel movements, the diaper area is frequently red and sore. Excoriation and bleeding may also be noted. A soothing protective agent to the skin area is commonly necessary couples with frequent diaper change to protect the skin integrity.

Identify the 3 nursing diagnosis (2 physical and 1 psychosocial) that are priorities. Justify your answer.

1. Fluid volume: Deficient

    It is extremely important to preserve the fluid balance in an infant. Oral rehydration fluid may be utilized in the early stages of the disease process; however, if the disease process continues, hospitalization, laboratory monitoring of electrolytes and an intravenous solution may be needed.

2. Impaired skin integrity

    It is also important to maintain diaper area with meticulous care. Skin breakdown can easily occur due to the status of the stools. The skin often times is unable to tolerate the nature and frequency of the stools

3. Caregiver role strain

    Regardless of the circumstances of the lives of the parents, caring for an ill infant places stress on the caregiver and family. During the acute phase of the disease process, the caregiver is frequently attending to the infant. Sleep is often compromised during the process.

Critical Thinking Exercise: CHAPTER 51
Child with Cleft Lip and Palate Answer Key

Identify each of the following statements regarding **preoperative care** of an infant with cleft lip and palate as **TRUE** or **FALSE**.

1. Family members should be encouraged to participate in cares as soon as possible after birth.

    TRUE

    Rationale: **Parents may need encouragement to hold, feed, and provide care for their baby due to fear of making a mistake or difficulties with attachment. Family members may need time to work through emotional issues and grieving the loss of their "perfect baby."**

2. Keep the infant flat and in the prone position to prevent aspiration.

    FALSE

    Rationale: **The infant is best-positioned upright and side lying to protect the airway.**

3. Feeding best done by nurses who can ensure the child's safety.

    FALSE

    Rationale: **Caregivers need practice to enable them to use correct feeding techniques at home. Nurses should encourage caregivers to feed while providing instruction, feedback, and suggestions regarding their technique. Most parents caring for an infant with a cleft palate develop expertise regarding the best feeding techniques for their baby.**

4. Feed by holding the infant parallel to arm. Direct nipple towards the gums. Allow the child to suck until the seal is broken.

    FALSE

    Rationale: **The infant should be held upright for feeds. Fluids need to be directed towards the back of the mouth. The infant should be burped frequently. Infants with cleft lip and palate are generally unable to develop a seal when sucking due to their defect.**

5. Use an orthodontic appliance to promote alignment of the maxilla.

> **TRUE**
>
> Rationale: **These devices assist in the proper development of the teeth and shaping of the mouth. Parents should be instructed how to clean and properly place the device.**

Identify each of the following statements regarding **postoperative care** of a child with cleft lip and palate as **TRUE** or **FALSE**.

---

6. The child will have a smooth, straight incision to prevent the lip from notching.

> **FALSE**
>
> Rationale: **A staggered suture line (Z-plasty method) is used to prevent scar tissue contraction and lip elevation.**

7. The child will need to wear elbow restraints after surgery to prevent injury to the surgical site.

> **TRUE**
>
> Rationale: **Elbow restraints prevent the child from being able to touch the incisional area.**

8. The child will be encouraged to sip water slowly through a straw.

> **FALSE**
>
> Rationale: **Sucking and placing devices in the mouth is discouraged. Sipping from a cup is the preferred method of fluid administration.**

9. A medicated pacifier will be used to decrease postoperative pain.

> **FALSE**
>
> Rationale: **Postoperative pain medication is generally administered via the oral, rectal or IV routes. Sucking on pacifiers is discouraged in the postoperative period due to the potential trauma to the surgical site.**

Critical Thinking Exercise: CHAPTER 52
Child with Pinworm Infection (Enterobiasis) Answer Key

Situation: A 5-year-old male presents to the health care provider's office with a one-week history of rectal itching, restlessness, and perianal irritation. Pinworms are suspected.

1. What causes the rectal itching and perianal irritation in children with pinworm infections?

    The female pinworms living in the lower intestine come out of the anus at night to lay eggs in the perianal region. The sensation causes the child to scratch.

    Perianal irritation occurs from repetitive scratching.

2. What factors are associated with the spread of pinworms?

    Contact with infected fecal material such as other children's diapers in preschool or daycare

    Sleeping in the same bed as another child infected with pinworms

    Nail biting and/or thumb sucking (spreads from oral-fecal route)

3. How should the nurse instruct the family to obtain a pinworm specimen?

    Touch tongue blade wrapped with cellophane tape to child's perianal area upon awakening in the morning. This should be done before he uses the bathroom or bathes

4. What instructions should the nurse give the family regarding treatment of a pinworm infection?

    Wash the bedding and garments with hot water.

    Scrub and trim the child's fingernails.

Give the prescribed anthelmintic medications to the child and family members.

Do not allow the child to share a bed while infected.

Notify the child's daycare or preschool as needed.

Give a second dose of the medication after 2 weeks as indicated.

5. What instructions should the nurse give the family regarding prevention of recurrent pinworm infections?

Seek prompt medical attention with continued scratching.

Keep the child's nails clean and trimmed short.

Discourage nail biting and thumb sucking.

Continue to wash the bedding in hot water.

Practice good hygiene: change underwear and pajamas frequently.

Critical Thinking Exercise: CHAPTER 53
Child with Hypospadias Answer Key

Situation: A nursery room nurse is completing an admission assessment on a newborn. Upon review of systems, it is noted that the child has hypospadias.

1. What anatomical changes would the nurse document in the admission assessment and identify the nursing responsibilities.

    Documentation would include: the position of the urethra on the penis, any presence of chordee, any discharge from the penis, any discoloration of the skin

    Nursing responsibilities: Documentation of voiding (character, color, amount), notification of pediatrician, education of family, delay of circumcision

2. If the family declines surgical repair of the hypospadias, what difficulties could be anticipated in the future?

    Voiding pattern: Although there are no problems with voiding, the boy can not stand and void in the normal position due to the location of the urethra.

    Psychological consequences of being different and bullied may lead to a poor self concept and embarrassment around the peers.

    Waiting for surgical repair could be additionally painful for the boy due to physical maturation.

3. What post operative education following repair is necessary for the parents?

    Hypospadias repair may require diversion of urine with a silicone stent or feeding tube to promote optimal healing and to maintain the position and potency of the newly formed urethra. Parents are taught to care for the indwelling catheter with an irrigation technique, when indicated. Parents need to be instructed on emptying the urinary bag, measuring the output, preventing kinking of the tubing, preventing infection and frequent diaper changes. A tub bath should be avoided until healing is complete. An increased fluid intake is encouraged. Limited sedentary activities are suggested until the client is seen for post surgical follow-up by the surgeon.

Critical Thinking Exercise: CHAPTER 54
Child with Wilms' Tumor Answer Key

Situation: A 4-year-old female is admitted with a Wilms' tumor. The child's mother tells the nurse that her daughter has been fussy and her clothing seems too tight around her enlarged abdomen. The nurse's initial assessment reveals the following: pronounced abdominal distention and low-grade fever with an increased respiratory rate, heart rate, and blood pressure. The child cries and pulls away when her abdomen is approached.

1. Which of the child's symptoms are characteristic of Wilms' tumors?

   Age 4 (peak age)

   Fussiness (sign of not feeling well)

   Clothing too tight and enlarged abdomen (from the tumor)

   Hematuria (renal involvement)

   Fever (inflammatory response)

   Tachypnea (from the enlarged abdomen)

   Increased blood pressure (from possible kidney involvement)

   Pulling away when her abdomen is approached (guarding response)

2. What preoperative interventions are indicated for a child with a Wilms' tumor?

   Protect the abdomen from palpation and excess manipulation (prevent capsule rupture and spread of the cancer cells).

   Provide teaching to the child using simple explanations of what will occur and medical play (teach at child's developmental level).

   Provide education and emotional support to the child and family.

3. What are the priority postoperative interventions for a child who has had a Wilms' tumor removed?

    Monitor and support respiratory status.
    Assess and manage pain.
    Maintain NG tube patency.
    Monitor bowel sounds.
    Maintain NPO status and IV fluids until bowel function returns.
    Assess wound for bleeding and signs of infection.
    Change wound dressing as indicated.
    Provide emotional support to the child and family.

Critical Thinking Exercise: CHAPTER 55
Child with Nephrotic Syndrome Answer Key

Identify the reason each of the following interventions is important when caring for the child described in the case study.

Situation: A 2-year-old boy has been admitted to the pediatric unit with a diagnosis of nephrotic syndrome. His mother states that he has had a five-day history of irritability, poor appetite, and vomiting and woke up today with swelling around the eyes. She also says his urine output has decreased significantly in the past 24 hours, even though he has gained 4 pounds.

Intervention	Rationale
Elevate head of bed to semi-Fowler position.	Provides baseline for further care helps detect hypovolemia from excessive fluid shifts.
Obtain urine for urinalysis.	Proteinuria is characteristic of this condition. Need a baseline for the evaluation of the effectiveness of treatment. Urine specimen may be difficult to obtain if future output is low.
Assess for signs of infection.	Provides a baseline to evaluate treatment weight is expected to decrease after diuresis begins.
Measure abdominal girth.	Ascites is common and measurement provides documentation that treatment is effective.
Administer prednisone per order.	Prednisone rapidly reduces proteinuria and edema.
Assess for skin breakdown	After administering prednisone, the urine output should increase the goal is for diuresis without protein loss.
Daily weights	Steroids mask the signs of infection. They suppress the immune system.
Take the vital signs q 4 h.	Elevation of the head of the bed reduces periorbital edema and facilitates breathing.
Provide high-protein, low-salt, high- potassium diet.	Due to nausea and vomiting, providing solid food is not a priority.
Monitor I and O.	Edematous skin breaks down easily.

Critical Thinking Exercise: CHAPTER 56
Child with Acute Glomerulonephritis Answer Key

1. Describe how the following symptoms manifest in acute glomerulonephritis and nephrotic syndrome.

Symptom	Acute Glomerulonephritis	Nephrotic Syndrome
Edema	Present	Markedly present
Hematuria	Significant	Mild or none
Proteinuria	Mild to moderate	Severe
Blood pressure	Hypertensive	Normal or hypotensive
Anorexia	Present	Present
Pain, discomfort	Headache, abdominal, edema, activity intolerance	Related to massive edema, activity intolerance
Fatigue, activity intolerance	Present	Present
Serum albumin/protein levels	Minimally decreased	Markedly decreased
Serum lipid levels	Normal	Increased
Serum electrolyte levels	Normal or altered	Normal
Hemoglobin and hematocrit	Normal or decreased	Increased
Serum creatinine and BUN	Normal or increased	Normal
Serum streptococcal antibody titers	Increased	Normal
Age at onset	Preschool, young school-age (5-7 years)	Toddler, preschool (2-6 years)

2. Compare and contrast nursing interventions appropriate when caring children with acute glomerulonephritis and nephrotic syndrome.

Nursing Intervention	Acute Glomerulonephritis	Nephrotic Syndrome
Intake and Output	Strict	Strict
Weight Measurement	Daily	Daily
Diet	Low salt	Low salt, high protein
Fluids	Fluid restriction	No fluid restriction, administer fluids for hypotension
Positioning	• Reposition every 2 hours (prevent skin breakdown and pulmonary complications) • Activity as tolerated	• Reposition every 2 hours (prevent skin and pulmonary complications) • Pillows on bony prominences • Activity as tolerated
Skin care	• Clean skin well • Assess for breakdown	• Clean skin well, assess for breakdown • Pressure reduction mattress
Medications	• Antihypertensives • Diuretics • Antibiotics (prevent or treat infection)	• Corticosteroids • Immunosuppressive agents (disease resistant to steroids) • Diuretics (possible) • Albumin (possible) • Antibiotics (prevent infection)

Critical Thinking Exercise: CHAPTER 57
Child with Urinary Tract Infections Answer Key

1. Matching:

e	Intravenous pyelogram	a.	Invasion of a bacterial pathogen
a	Bacterial infection	b.	Blood in the urine
g	Urinalysis	c.	White blood cells in the urine
k	Neurogenic bladder	d.	Stopping and starting of the urinary stream
d	Stranguria	e.	Radiocontrast is used to assess the kidney, ureters and bladder
i	Vesicoureteral reflux	f.	Bedside urine test for blood, protein, glucose and pH
h	Suprapubic aspiration	g.	Urine test for white blood cells, hematuria, and organisms
b	Hematuria	h.	Urine sample obtained directly from the bladder using a needle
j	Urine culture	i.	Back flow of urine into the ureter and kidney.
f	Hematuria	j.	Urine test for bacterial infection
l	Clean catch	k.	Incomplete bladder emptying due to inadequate innervation
c	Pyuria	l.	Non-invasive method of collecting a urine sample

2. Answer the following questions:

   a. Why are uncircumcised males more prone to urinary tract infections than circumcised males?

   Circumcision is the removal of foreskin from the prepuce of the penis. Fecal bacteria may colonize in the foreskin of the uncircumcised penis, thus increasing the incidence of UTI in these children. Proper cleaning of the foreskin during bathing is recommended for all uncircumcised males.

   b. Why are children with spina bifida and spinal cord injury prone to urinary tract infections?

   Children with spina bifida and spinal cord injuries have decreased innervation to their bladders. This causes incomplete bladder emptying (neurogenic bladder). The urine that remains in the bladder (urinary stasis) provides a medium for bacterial growth causing a UTI.

   c. Why should children be taught go to the bathroom and not to ignore the urge to urinate?

   Ignoring the urge to urinate can lead to retention of urine in the bladder. The resulting urinary stasis is a medium for bacterial growth that leads to UTI.

Critical Thinking Exercise: CHAPTER 58
Child with Sexually Transmitted Disease Answer Key

Situation: A 16-year-old female is admitted with abdominal pain and purulent vaginal discharge. After conversing privately with the nurse, the child revealed that she participated in a sexual activity with several different partners in the past two months. She told the nurse that she did not use condoms during sexual intercourse. The child also hinted that she had been sexually abused as a child but refused to divulge any additional information on this subject.

1. What aspects of the child's history put her at risk for contracting a sexually transmitted disease (STD)?

   Teenage
   Lack of education
   Unprotected intercourse
   Multiple partners
   Sexual abuse history

2. How is this disease diagnosed?

   History
   Symptoms
   Culture of the vaginal discharge

3. What are the appropriate interventions for this child?

   Administer antibiotics.
   Manage pain.
   Educate regarding how to avoid risk of reoccurrence of infection and unwanted pregnancy.
   Referral for counseling related to possible history of sexual abuse

4. The child asks the nurse if there will be any long-term problems because of this disease. How should the nurse respond?

> **Untreated infections can lead to pelvic infection and abscesses.**
>
> **Tissue damage from the infections can also lead to fertility problems. The risk of infertility increases with each incidence of infection therefore, prevention of reoccurrence is very important.**

Critical Thinking Exercise: CHAPTER 59
Child with Sudden Infant Death Syndrome Answer Key

1. Identify which of the following sleeping conditions follows the current SIDS prevention recommendations.
    a. Infant in a home where both parents are smokers
    b. Prone positioning on a quilted blanket
    c. Infant sleeping in hot room and covered with a heavy blanket
    d. Supine positioning on a sheepskin with small stuffed animals at the foot of the bed
    e. Side-lying on a firm mattress and covered with a thick blanket
    f. Use of a small pillow under an infant's head during sleep
    g. None of the above responses are correct.

2. What things should the nurse tell the family to DO to prevent SIDS?

    Get prenatal care.
    Seek medical care when the infant is ill.
    Position on back for sleep.
    Use a firm mattress with a fitted crib sheet.
    Breast-feed to help the immune system.
    Keep the room and infant's temperature comfortable.

3. What things should the nurse instruct the family to AVOID to prevent SIDS?

    Positioning prone during sleep
    Placing sheepskins, comforters, fluffy blankets, or pillows under the baby
    Using thick, fluffy blankets or comforters to cover the baby
    Placing stuffed animals in the crib
    Overbundling the baby during sleep
    Smoking during pregnancy
    Allowing people to smoke near the infant

Critical Thinking Exercise: CHAPTER 60
Abused Child Answer Key

Situation: A 9-year-old female presents in the emergency department with a spiral fracture of her left arm, dislocated right shoulder, and several small circular burns on her arms. The child's mother tells the nurse that the child was hurt when she fell out off her bed two days ago. When the nurse asks the child's mother about the presence of several old bruises and scars on the back of the child's arms and legs, the mother claims that the child is very clumsy. The mother also told the nurse that she had no idea how her daughter received the burns.

1. What parts of the child's presentation and history are suspicious for child maltreatment? Why?

    Spiral fracture of her left arm and a dislocated right shoulder (possibly related to forceful arm twisting)

    Small circular burns are not typical of accidental burns. They are characteristic for intentional burns made from cigarettes. There does not appear to be an explanation for how the burns occurred.

    The child's injuries do not appear to match the explanation. The average bed is only a few feet off the floor. It is unusual for this to lead to a dislocated shoulder and spiral fracture.

    The presence of several old bruises and scars on the back of the child's arms and legs. Most children who fall while playing sustain cuts and bruises to their hands, front of the legs and knees. Bruises and scars on the back of the child's arms and legs are more likely to be inflicted from being hit by another person.

    The two-day delay in seeking medical care. Families who have caused an injury may be reluctant to seek medical care for fear of others discovering their secret.

2. What additional questions should the nurse ask the mother and the child?

    Ask the mother describe the events and details about how the child got hurt.
    Ask the mother for details regarding how the child received the old injuries and the burns.
    Ask the child to describe what happened that day (away from her mother).
    Ask the child if she knows how she got the burn marks on her arms.
    Ask the child to tell you how she got her bruises and scars on her arms and legs.

3. What else should the nurse assess?

- Assess for additional cuts, bruises, burns or fractures in various stages of healing.
- Assess for signs of sexual abuse (urinary frequency, urinary burning, pain, and rectal or vaginal trauma).
- Assess the child's and mother's affect, behavior patterns and mood.
- Assess the parent-child relationship and interaction pattern.

4. Identify nursing interventions that are appropriate for this child and family.

- Address the child's physical and pain management needs.
- Collaborate with social services in reporting the suspected abuse to the appropriate authorities.
- Maintain a safe environment for the child to discuss her feelings, thoughts, and/or events.
- Provide dolls, crayons, modeling clay or other types of play to help the child relax and begin to working through her feelings.
- Maintain a nonjudgmental and supportive attitude when interacting with the child and family.
- Monitor for inconsistencies in the child and/or caregiver's account of how the injury occurred.

Critical Thinking Exercise: CHAPTER 61
Child with Lead Poisoning (Plumbism) Answer Key

Identify if each of following clients has a **high** or **low** likelihood of having lead poisoning or an increased lead level.

1. A 2-year-old female is seen in a clinic with a history of irritability, decreased appetite, vomiting, and weight loss over the past month. Her father tells the nurse she has not been as active as usual over the last several months. The child cries and guards when her abdomen is approached. The father works in a foundry where lead is used.

    High. This child has some of the symptoms associated with moderate lead poisoning: irritability, vomiting, guarding the abdomen (probable abdominal pain). This is further confirmed because her symptoms have been present for one month. The child's exposure was most likely related to her father's job in a foundry where lead is used.

2. An 8-year-old male is brought to the health care provider's office with a two-week history of constipation. The boy's mother also reports that her child has been complaining about difficulty seeing the blackboard and often has a headache at school. The mother reports that the only possibility of lead exposure was a stained glass-making workshop she attended 2 days ago. The child did not attend the workshop with his mother.

    Low. Although this boy has some symptoms that may be associated with lead poisoning (constipation and headache), there could be many reasons for the symptoms. His headache and difficulty seeing the blackboard is probably related to a need for glasses, a common problem among school-age children. His constipation could be related to a diet low in fiber or other gastrointestinal illness. The mother's participation in a stained glass workshop without her son only 2 days prior makes this a very low likelihood of the boy's exposure.

3. A 4-year-old boy presents in a clinic with vomiting, muscle tremors, and lethargy. He has a history of attention deficit disorder and experienced unexplained weight loss and loss of developmental milestones over the past 6 months. When asked, his mother tells the nurse that she owns orange earthenware dishes she bought while traveling outside the United States one year ago. She also tells the nurse that these are her favorite dishes and has been routinely using them to prepare the family meals.

    High. This boy's symptoms of muscle tremors, lethargy, and vomiting are suggestive of advanced lead poisoning and central nervous system toxicity. His history of attention deficit disorder, weight loss, and loss of developmental milestones over the past 6 months

Child with Lead Poisoning (Plumbism) Answer Key

are suspicious for chronic lead ingestion. The family's bright orange earthenware dishes have a high likelihood of containing lead-based glazes. The child's exposure is most likely due to eating the food contaminated by the lead in these dishes.

1. A 5-year-old girl presents with a 3-day history of fever, vomiting, nausea, diarrhea, and abdominal pain. Her brother and sister both had acute gastroenteritis the week prior. She lives in a house built in 1982.

    Low. Although this girl has some of the symptoms associated with lead poisoning (vomiting, abdominal pain, and diarrhea), her fever and three-day history of nausea, vomiting, and diarrhea are most likely due to the same acute gastroenteritis illness that her brother and sister experienced. She has no identified risk factors for lead poisoning. Her home was built after 1970 when lead-based paint was outlawed.

Critical Thinking Exercise: CHAPTER 62
Child with Acetaminophen Poisoning Answer Key

Situation: A 2-year-old presents in the emergency department at 4 p.m. after ingesting 40–50 children's chewable acetaminophen tablets at approximately 3:15 p.m.

1. What initial symptoms should the nurse anticipate?

   Since the ingestion was less than one hour ago, the onset of symptoms may not have occurred. At 2-4 hours after ingestion, the nurse should anticipate nausea, vomiting, pallor, malaise, and diaphoresis

2. Rank the following interventions in order of priority. Explain the rationale for the rank order.

Intervention	Rank order	Rationale for rank order
Administer syrup of ipecac.	1	Ipecac should be administered as soon as possible after ingestion.
Gastric lavage	2	Lavage is used to further empty the stomach of gastric content.
Administer activated charcoal.	3	This binding agent acts to absorb the toxic agent. It should be given in lieu of or after gastric lavage and the induction of vomiting.
Obtain a serum acetaminophen level.	4	This level is needed to determine the need for the N-acetylcysteine administration.
Administer N-acetylcysteine.	5	N-acetylcysteine is the antidote for acetaminophen overdose. An initial dose is given, followed by 17 additional doses every 4 hours.
Monitor liver function tests.	6	Liver function test abnormalities will begin after ingestion and peak at 72-96 hours.
Educate family regarding home safety needs.	7	Home safety is an important topic. This teaching is likely to be most effective after the child's status has been stabilized.

3. The child's mother asks the nurse to explain the signs of liver damage. What should the nurse tell her?

   Liver damage is assessed by taking blood and monitoring liver enzymes (ALT, AST), blood clotting (PT) and bilirubin levels. The child will also be assessed for abdominal pain, jaundice and decreased level of consciousness.

Critical Thinking Exercise: CHAPTER 63
Child with Substance Abuse Answer Key

1. Match the level of risk for substance abuse for each of the following adolescents.

b	13-year-old male caught experimenting with inhalant drugs in his friend's garage. He claims he only occasionally uses inhalants. He begs the neighbor not to tell his parents because of fear of severe punishment.	a. Low risk of substance abuse
b	14-year-old girl who is described as "popular" at school. She was sexually abused when she was ten years old. She gives a vague answer when asked if she uses drugs or drinks alcohol. She does admit to smoking cigarettes.	b. Moderate-to-high risk of substance abuse
a	15-year-old female who reports having many friends and a good relationship with her parents. She admits to having tried alcohol once but denies current use because she doesn't like the way it made her feel.	
b	16-year-old male with a blood alcohol level above the legal limit after a recent auto accident. He recently received his driver's license and his own car. He reports that his parents don't care when he comes home at night.	

2. What are the risk factors for substance abuse in the adolescents described above?

    Adolescent age group (prone to experimentation, feeling invincible, and peer pressure)
    History of sexual abuse
    Lack of parental supervision
    Prior experience with drugs and alcohol
    Inflexible parenting style with severe punishment

3. Identify interventions to assist families with members who are at risk for substance abuse.

    Offer substance abuse education for the adolescent (formatted for this audience).

    Teach the adolescent and family strategies for preventing substance abuse.

    Teach the family how to identify the signs of substance abuse.

    Support communication and positive family relationships.

    Promote counseling for prior emotional trauma (such as physical or sexual abuse).

    Encourage family counseling to address parenting styles and family relationships when indicated.

    Help families dealing with substance abuse issues identify community support resources.

Critical Thinking Exercise: CHAPTER 64
Child in a Suicidal Crisis Answer Key

1. Identify each of the following statements about suicide as a myth or reality.

Statement	Myth or Reality
Suicide is a disease that affects only adults and adolescents.	Myth (suicide affects children of all ages most common in adults and adolescents)
Parental expectations that are high but realistic can serve as is associated with a low risk of suicide.	Reality
An apparently happy teen involved in school activities that earns A's in school will not commit suicide.	Myth (all children should be evaluated for risk, outward appearances may mask inner feelings)
Past suicide attempts puts a teen at risk for future suicide attempts.	Reality
It is best to ignore a child who has a tendency for fighting and truancy.	Myth (this is a possible sign of suicide risk)
A joke about suicide is not a serious threat.	Myth (treat all talking about suicide as a possible threat)
A person who describes specifics regarding how and where he would commit suicide is at high risk.	Reality
If an adolescent is serious enough to make a suicide attempt, there is not much that can be done to prevent them from succeeding.	Myth (suicide attempts are often a cry for help, prompt intervention is key to "successful" attempts)
Breaking up with a serious boyfriend can lead to a suicide attempt.	Reality

2. Identify which of the following behaviors is associated with children who are at risk for suicide:

   a. Abuses alcohol
   b. Feels sad most of the time
   c. Popular among peers
   d. Gets in fights frequently
   e. From a large family
   f. Involved in sports
   g. Sleeps most of the time
   h. Feels that life is meaningless
   i. Has a low self esteem
   j. Inflexible parents with poor communication skills
   k. Doesn't have an interest in spending time with others
   l. Skips school and gets in trouble frequently
   m. Suddenly starts giving away prized possessions to friends
   n. Parents who are supportive and provide structure
   o. Chronically teased at school for a physical deformity

Key: a, b, d, g, h, i, j, k, l, m, o. The other behaviors (c, e, f, and n) may also be found in children who commit suicide, but are not considered risk factors or signs of possible suicidal behavior.

Critical Thinking Exercise: CHAPTER 65
Child with Down Syndrome Answer Key

Situation: The parents of a child diagnosed with Down syndrome are attending the first meeting of Parents of a Down Syndrome Child Support Group. The new parents are obviously overwhelmed with the diagnosis and seeking information regarding care.

1. Identify the myths associated with the diagnosis of Down syndrome.

    Children with Down syndrome will need to be institutionalized at some point during their life.
    Children will require personal care throughout the lifespan.
    The individual with Down syndrome will always be a burden to society.
    An adult with Down syndrome will always have to live with the parent or be institutionalized.
    Individuals with Down syndrome are always lazy and overweight.
    Communication is difficult for those with Down syndrome.
    Individuals with Down syndrome can not work.
    Individuals with Down syndrome can be violent if they do not get their way.
    The child with Down syndrome learns little over the lifespan.
    Individuals with Down syndrome are unlovable and unloved.
    Family members should try to remain unattached to the child.

2. Define the nurse's role in promoting the true character and abilities of those with Down syndrome.

    The nurse has the role of supporting the child and family. Parental education is essential in providing specialized care correlated with the abilities of the child. Because there are many variations in abilities, a specific plan of care is needed to have the family/child reach full potential. Developing a relationship with the family allows the family to express issues in a safe environment.

    The nurse also has the role of educating the public on the abilities and talents of the individual with Down syndrome. Many individuals work within the community and their talents go far beyond their duties. The nurse can define appropriate roles and work responsibilities.

Child with Down Syndrome Answer Key

2. How does a karyotype determine a person's genetic make-up? What differences in karyotype are seen in the Down syndrome client that are not present in the general population?

A karyotype is a photomicrograph of the chromosomes of a single cell, taken during metaphase, when each chromosome is still a pair of chromatids. The chromosomes are then arranged in numerical order.

The individual with Down syndrome has trisomy 21. This means that there are three chromosomes in the 21st position on the chromosome. A few individuals also have partial dislocation of chromosomes 15 and 21. Down syndrome is the most common chromosomal abnormality.

Critical Thinking Exercise: CHAPTER 66
Child with Autism Answer Key

Situation: A 3-year-old has been recently diagnosed with autism. The parents state that they are overwhelmed with the diagnosis of autism. The nurse is formulating a teaching plan structured by the characteristics related to autism.

1. Utilizing the three defined categories of autism, identify the challenges of parenting and the appropriate nursing interventions.

    Inability to relate to others: **Children with autism do not develop a positive response to social interaction, cuddling, touching or smiling. The child often pulls away and is fretful as a result of the interaction. There is a lack of response to separation from parents. Ritualistic behaviors may occur such as rocking, pulling hair, or banging head. Parents often grieve the loss of closeness with their child. Parenting challenges include finding ways to show attention and love toward the child.**

    Nursing interventions include:
    - Develop techniques to gain the child's cooperation with activities of daily living. The nurse must assist the parent in identifying ways to relate to the child.
    - Encourage the parents to begin a journal of the child's daily behavior and response to stimulation.
    - Identify satisfying ways of promoting relationships between the parent and child.
    - Educate the parents about the importance of maintaining consistency in the home with caregivers and home routines.

    Inability to communicate with others: **Children with autism are slow to develop speech and have difficulty communicating their needs. This is difficult for the parent caring for the child and others in the extended family and/or friends who also care for or want to interact with the child. Social situations for the family are difficult. Echolalia and repetitive behaviors may be uncomfortable for the parents in social situations.**

    Nursing interventions include:
    - Define patterns of behavior that communicate the needs of the child.
    - Develop a list/chart of actions that communicate desires/needs.
    - Advise the parent(s) to arrange time for the baby sitter to get to know the child and

family prior to being left alone with the child.

Limited activities and interests: **Children with autism are self-centered and have little interest in participating in activities. Normal interactions with friends are impaired. It is difficult for parents to encourage the children to participate in structured activities. Social isolation can occur for the parents since the child can not relate in normal age-specific activities.**

Nursing interventions:
- Conduct an activity assessment to identify the sources of pleasure in the child's life.
- Expand the child's activities and experiences slowly, introducing new interactions a little at a time.
- Note changes in behavior that may indicate the child is not coping with the exposure to the activities.

2. Link the following long term goals to improve developmental characteristics (create table with option to link or match options).

Long term goals: **Answer Key**

Promotion of normal development: **a, e, i**

Language development: **b, f, j, i**

Social interaction: **c, g, k**

Learning: **d, h, l**

Developmental characteristics:

a. Child is able to complete morning routine (brush teeth and hair, dress self) with minimal supervision.

b. Child is able to communicate needs.

c. Child is able to acknowledge another person (adult or child) present.

d. Child progresses from identified point in learning development.

e. Child will eat a nutritionally-based meal by feeding self.

f. Child is able to participate in a brief conversation.

g. Child is able to participate in an interaction without feeling frustrated or anxious.

h. Child demonstrates activities in which learning is evident.

i. Child will relate to parents and siblings by communication of needs.

j. Child utilizes appropriate words throughout an interaction.

k. Child is accepting of others around.

l. Improvement is noted in completing activities of daily living successfully.

Critical Thinking Exercise: CHAPTER 67
Child with Attention Deficit Hyperactivity Disorder Answer Key

Identify 10 behaviors that may be associated with inattention in an 8-year-old boy.

1. Frequently makes careless mistakes with schoolwork
2. Has difficulty following directions
3. Requires frequent reminders to follow through with chores
4. Avoids tasks that require concentration
5. Has difficulty completing homework assignments
6. Dislikes reading
7. Loses things needed to complete required activities (pencils, books, papers)
8. Forgets instructions
9. Begins one task and abandons it to begin another
10. Does not appear to listen when spoken to directly

Identify 10 behaviors that may be associated with hyperactivity/impulsivity in a 14-year-old boy.

1. Experiments with drugs and alcohol
2. Fidgets and squirms in seat
3. Expresses a feeling of restlessness when seated or standing in place
4. Stands up and walks around during class
5. Frequently fights with friends
6. Talks excessively
7. Blurts out answers in class
8. Frequently shouts and curses at parents when angry or frustrated
9. Has difficulty waiting for his turn, "takes cuts" in line
10. Engages in constant activity—constantly "on the go"

Critical Thinking Exercise: CHAPTER 68
Child with Failure to Thrive Answer Key

Situation: The nurse is caring for the four children described below. Which child CURRENTLY has failure to thrive? Identify the characteristics in each child are associated with failure to thrive.

1. A 6-week-old with a 4-day history of watery diarrhea and vomiting associated with acute gastroenteritis. The infant's admission weight was 5 kg. This was 0.5 kg less than what he weighed in the pediatrician's office 3 days prior. On admission, the infant had a weak cry, dry lips, sunken fontanel, and an increased heart rate. After fluid replacement, the infant's weight increased to 5.4 kg.

    Current failure to thrive? _____ Yes __X__ No

    Characteristics associated with failure to thrive: **Weight loss, vomiting, and diarrhea. This infant's weight loss was due to his acute illness (gastroenteritis, and dehydration). If his weight loss, vomiting, and diarrhea become chronic, he would most likely develop failure to thrive.**

2. A 3-month-old with gastroesophageal reflux. The child's mother tells the nurse that the amount of "spit-ups" after feeding has decreased since she began giving antireflux medicine (metoclopramide) before the feeds. The infant's pattern of weight gain has improved since the medication was initiated. The infant's growth chart measurements are within normal limits.

    Current failure to thrive? _____ Yes __X__ No

    Characteristics associated with failure to thrive: **Gastroesophageal reflux, vomiting, and poor weight. The gastroesophageal reflux could have led to failure to thrive. However, this infant has improved with weight gain and decreased vomiting since the antireflux medication was initiated. This is confirmed by his growth chart measurements that are within normal limits.**

3. A 9-month-old infant with a congenital heart defect who has been hospitalized several times since birth. Her height and weight are below normal for her age. She is admitted with respiratory difficulty

and upper airway congestion. The nurse assesses the following: thin extremities, sparse hair, poor head control, upper airway congestion, dry cough, pale skin, and irritability. The mother asks for a bottle to feed the baby. During feeding, the nurse notes that the baby initially sucks eagerly but quickly becomes tachypneic, sweaty, and irritable during the feeding. The mother tells the nurse that this is how the baby usually acts during feeding.

Current failure to thrive? __X__ Yes _____ No

Characteristics associated with failure to thrive: **Her multiple hospitalizations and congenital heart defect increase her risk. Her thin extremities, irritability, and poor head control (developmental delay) are all characteristics associated with this disorder. This is further confirmed with the infant's poor feeding behaviors (tachypnea, diaphoresis, and irritability) and her height/weight below normal for age.**

4. A 15-month-old with a history of prematurity. He was hospitalized for one month after birth for respiratory distress and feeding intolerance. He is currently seen in the clinic for a well baby exam and immunization. His mother reports that her son is a "picky eater" like his other siblings. She tells the nurse that he eats best when he is in his high chair and he can eat using his fingers. The child is alert, active and appears well nourished with fat folds noted on arms and legs.

Current failure to thrive? __X__ Yes _____ No

Characteristics associated with failure to thrive: **Prematurity and feeding intolerance, poor eating habits. This toddler is currently active, alert, and well nourished with fat folds on his extremities. At birth (more than one year ago) he was at risk for failure to thrive because of his prematurity and feeding problems. His picky eating and preference for finger foods are normal developmental behaviors for toddlers. If the child's weight loss is associated with "picky eating"; the child may be at risk for failure to thrive.**

Critical Thinking Exercise: CHAPTER 69
Child with Anorexia Nervosa Answer Key

Complete the following statements related to anorexia nervosa:

Altered nutritional status is related to **caloric intake less than body requirements**.

Fluid volume deficit is related to **lack of fluid intake, vomiting, and diarrhea**.

Decreased cardiac output is related to **cardiac dysfunction and hypovolemia**.

Decreased activity tolerance and fatigue is related to **decreased energy stores from lack of adequate caloric intake**.

Bowel incontinence and diarrhea is related to **excess laxative use**.

Constipation is related to **insufficient fiber and fluid intake**.

Risk for infection is related to **suppressed immune system from poor nutrition**.

Skin breakdown and poor healing is related to **lack of subcutaneous fat and malnutrition**.

Confusion and memory loss is related to **malnutrition**.

Loneliness is related to **social isolation and avoiding criticism of others**.

Altered growth and development is related to **the effect of malnutrition on the reproductive system and bones**.

Noncompliance with the treatment plan is related to **the psychological processes causing the illness, the inability to seek assistance and/or comply with the treatment plan**.

Powerlessness and hopelessness are related to **the perceived lack of control over disease and/or symptoms**.

Risk for self-harm is related to **the physiological effects of the disorder, risk for self-injury from excessive exercise laxative use and purging, and the risk of suicide.**

Knowledge deficit is related to **lack of information regarding the risks, complications, and treatment.**

Critical Thinking Exercise: CHAPTER 70
Child with Adolescent Pregnancy Answer Key

Fill in the blank

1. Adolescents experience the feelings of sexual desire due to **sexual** development and **hormonal** changes.

2. Adolescents often engage in risk taking behaviors due to a belief that "it **won't** happen to **me**."

3. Adolescents have a tendency to experiment with new experiences without considering the **consequences**.

4. Many adolescents engage in sexual activity due to **peer pressure** and/or a desire to be **loved**.

5. The use of **drugs** and **alcohol** by teens increases the likelihood of pregnancy and sexually transmitted disease due to suppressed inhibition.

6. Some adolescent females chose to get pregnant because they want to have someone to **love**.

Identify which of the following intervention strategies are recommended to help prevent adolescent pregnancy:

a. Provide accurate and realistic information about sexual activity and birth control.
b. Dispel myths related to contraceptive methods and getting pregnant.
c. Discuss the physiological changes associated with pregnancy.
d. Forbid the adolescent from spending time alone with his or her peers.
e. Discuss the realities of parenthood in terms that are meaningful to adolescents. Describe how caring for a newborn infant will affect their social activities, educational goals and economic situation.
f. Have young teens continuously care for an egg or other fragile object to simulate the constant commitment needed to care for an infant.

g. Have teens attend a support group for young parents or invite a teen parent to come to school to discuss their situation with their peers.
h. Do not allow the adolescent to leave the house at night or on weekends.
i. Provide a safe, open environment for teens to ask questions and discuss their thoughts.
j. Reinforce the adolescent's personal, family, and/or spiritual values related to the value of abstinence.
k. Tell the adolescent that they will be severely punished if they have sex before marriage.

All except d, h, and k.

Bibliography

Ackley, B. & Ladwig, G (2002). *Nursing diagnosis handbook* (5th ed.). St. Louis, MO: Mosby.

Ball, J.W. & Bindler, R.C. (2003). *Pediatric nursing care for children* (3rd ed.). Upper Saddle River NJ: Prentice Hall.

Behrman, RE., Kliegman, R.M., & Jenson, H.B. (2004). *Nelson textbook of pediatrics* (17th ed.). St. Louis: Saunders.

Bond, G.R. (2003). Home syrup of ipecac use does not reduce emergency department use or improve outcome. *Pediatrics*, 112(5), 1061-1064.

Feldman, R. (2002). *Development across the life span* (3rd ed.). Upper Saddle River, NJ: Prentice-Hall, Inc.

Gunn, V. L., Nechyba, C. & Barone, M.A. (Eds.) (2002). *The Harriet Lane handbook* (16th ed.). Philadelphia: Mosby.

Hockenberry, M. J., Wilson, D., & Winkelstein, M. L. (2005). *Wong's essentials of pediatric nursing* (7th ed.). St. Louis, MO: Elsevier Mosby.

Holmes, H. N. (Ed.). (2001). *Professional guide to diseases* (7th ed.). Springhouse, PA: Springhouse Corporation.

Ignatavicius, D., & Workman, M. L. (2002). *Medical surgical nursing* (4th ed.). Philadelphia: W. B. Saunders Company.

James, S. R., Price, D. L., & Schulte, E. B. (2004). *Thompson's pediatric nursing: An introductory text* (9th ed.). Philadelphia: W. B. Saunders.

Jarvis, C. (2004). *Physical examination & health assessment* (4th ed.). St. Louis: Saunders.

McCance, K.L. & Huether, S.E. (2002). *Pathophysiology the biologic basis for disease in adults & children* (4th ed.). St. Louis MO: Mosby, p

Middleton, D. B., Zimmerman, R.K., & Mitchell, K.B. (2005). Childhood vaccine schedule and procedures, 2005. *The Journal of Family Practice*, March 2005 special edition, S16-S25.

Nettina, S. M. (2001). *The Lippincott manual of nursing practice* (7th ed.). Philadelphia: Lippincott Williams & Wilkins.

Pillitteri, A. (2003). *Maternal & child health nursing* (4th ed.). Philadelphia: Lippincott.

Porth, C. M. (2002). *Pathophysiology: Concepts of altered health states*. Philadelphia: Lippincott Williams & Wilkins.

Potter, P.A. & Perry, A.G. (2005). *Fundamentals of nursing* (7th ed.). St. Louis: Elsevier Mosby.

Potts, H. L., & Mandleco, B. L. (2002). *Pediatric nursing: Caring for children and their families*. Clifton Park, NY: Delmar.

Sawyer-Sommers, M. & Johnson, S. (2002). *Diseases and disorders* (2nd ed.). Philadelphia: F.A. Davis Company.

Stapleton, E., Aufderheide, T., Hazinski, M., & Cummins, R. (2001). *Fundamentals of BLS for healthcare providers*. Dallas: American Heart Association.

Tierney, L. M., McPhee, S. J., & Papadakis, M. A. (Eds.). (2002). *Current medical diagnosis & treatment* (41st ed.). New York: Lange Medical Books/McGraw-Hill.

Wong, D. L., & Hockenberry, M. J., Wilson, D., Winkelstein, M.L., & Kline, N.E. (2003). *Wong's nursing care of infants and children* (7th ed.). St. Louis, MO: Mosby, Inc.

Wong, D., Hockenberry-Eaton, M., Wilson, D., Winkelstein, M.L., & Schwartz, P. (2004). *Wong's essentials of pediatric nursing* (6th ed.). St. Louis, MO: Mosby-Yearbook.